Sexual Health

SEXUAL HEALTH

Volume 4

State-of-the-Art Treatments and Research

Edited by Annette Fuglsang Owens
and Mitchell S. Tepper

Introduction by Dr. David Satcher

Praeger Perspectives

Sex, Love, and Psychology
Judy Kuriansky, Series Editor

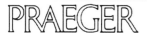

Westport, Connecticut
London

Library of Congress Cataloging-in-Publication Data

Sexual health / edited by Mitchell S. Tepper and Annette Fuglsang Owens ;
introduction by David Satcher.
    p. cm. — (Sex, love, and psychology, ISSN 1554–222X)
  Includes index.
  ISBN 0–275–98775–2 (v.1) — ISBN 0–275–98776–0 (v.2) — ISBN 0–275–
98777–9 (v.3) — ISBN 0–275–98778–7 (v.4) — ISBN 0–275–98774–4 (set)
1. Sex. 2. Sex (Psychology) 3. Sex (Biology) 4. Sexual ethics. 5.
Sex customs. 6. Hygiene, Sexual. I. Tepper, Mitchell. II. Owens,
Annette Fuglsang.
  HQ21.S47364   2007
  306.7—dc22   2006031706

British Library Cataloguing in Publication Data is available.

Library of Congress Catalog Card Number: 2006031706
ISBN-10: 0–275–98774–4 (set)   ISBN-13: 978–0–275–98774–9 (set)
           0–275–98775–2 (vol. 1)   978–0–275–98775–6 (vol 1)
           0–275–98776–0 (vol. 2)   978–0–275–98776–3 (vol 2)
           0–275–98777–9 (vol. 3)   978–0–275–98777–0 (vol 3)
           0–275–98778–7 (vol. 4)   978–0–275–98778–7 (vol 4)
ISSN: 1554–222X

First published in 2007

Praeger Publishers, 88 Post Road West, Westport, CT 06881
An imprint of Greenwood Publishing Group, Inc.
www.praeger.com

Printed in the United States of America

The paper used in this book complies with the
Permanent Paper Standard issued by the National
Information Standards Organization (Z39.48–1984).

10 9 8 7 6 5 4 3 2 1

To my friend, colleague, and coeditor Dr. Annette F. Owens for her selfless dedication and infectious enthusiasm. Annette, this one is for you!
Mitch Tepper

To my husband Wyn and our children Xenia, Saskia, and Evan—wishing them a lifetime of sexual health.
Annette Owens

CONTENTS

FOREWORD

Do people who enjoy sex live longer? At what age does sexual attraction start? Can a tree bark extract help erectile dysfunction?

These are just a few of the issues of interest in the field of sexuality today, and they are among the many issues presented in this impressive four-volume set about sexual health. Noted experts in the field of sexology give the latest up-to-date information about compelling aspects of sexuality. Professionals as well as members of the public will be interested to learn about the role of the chemical oxytocin in love, research findings that sexual enjoyment is indeed related to longevity, proof that the G-spot relieves pain as well as increasing pleasure, and findings that attraction starts as early as age ten.

Statistics about the numbers of men and women of all ages suffering from sexual problems are staggering—up to 8 out of 10 people are dissatisfied with their sex life, and up to half complain of sexual problems that could benefit from professional attention. The need for sexual information—and help—is undeniable.

Readers of these volumes will be engaged by the breadth and depth of the information, from case histories—like those of couples experiencing loving after giving life (i.e. having a baby)—to new biological approaches to treating sexual disorders. There are new developments to keep up with, such as new models of the sexual response cycle that are cyclical rather than linear, and that include precursors like sexual interest and desire that lead to arousal.

These volumes are intelligently divided into major topics of interest from psychological issues (like attraction and communication) to physiological aspects (like the role of hormones and the impact of drug use and medical problems) to cultural considerations (affecting Middle Eastern, Latino, African American and Chinese sexuality) to state of the art treatments and research. Each volume contains valuable resources for further information.

Having been in the field of sexology since its beginnings decades ago—as the protégé of the first group of psychiatrists, psychologists, and health professionals working with the grandfather and grandmother of sex therapy, William H. Masters and Virginia E. Johnson—I have seen the world of sexology grow. Questions about sex—as well as the number of qualified experts—have multiplied. Throughout these years, it has become increasingly evident that healthy sexuality is an essential part of good health in general, and that knowledge about all aspects of sexual functioning is essential to good health. This is exactly what these chapters are about.

I remember all too well when, just a few decades ago, the field of sexology was just developing. A small group of health experts met in a medical school in New York to form a professional organization to study sexuality and to formalize treatments for sexual problems. We called the organization SSTAR—the Society for Sexual Therapy and Research. The acronym provided a metaphoric guiding star for helping people understand themselves as sexual beings and to begin to build a respectable field of study about sexuality. The group grew over the years, and more professionals developed an interest in the growing field of sexology. Other organizations already existed, such as the American Association of Sexuality Educators, Counselors and Therapists, the Society for the Scientific Study of Sexuality, and the World Association for Sexual Health. I, and many of the authors in these volumes, have served on the boards of some of these groups and take an active part in professional activities and public information about healthy sexuality. Indeed, the study of sex has become a legitimate field, so that now students call me and say that they want to study about sex and become sex therapists.

The quest for healthy sexuality has spread around the world. Even "closed" countries like China are developing an open-door policy about sexuality, knowing that healthy sexuality makes for a healthy society. I know this first hand in that country, having taught doctors and public groups there for the past seven years about healthy relationships.

For years, I have been a media sexologist—answering thousands of people's questions about sex on radio, TV, and in newspapers and magazines—recommending books for people to read. Here is a set that can be on everyone's bookshelf as a reference to many issues of interest about sexuality—from fertility to spirituality and cultural mores. This four-volume set is the most up-to-date and comprehensive collection for such valuable information. With its vast diversity of subject matter and chapters written by an impressive group of professionals—including some of the most well-known and respected sexologists, sex researchers and therapists in this country and abroad—it is an essential reading and resource for everyone interested in sexual health, from students to professionals and the public. Readers can find a particular subject, or turn to a new area of interest, and always be engaged in learning about sexual health, which is a fundamental aspect of a healthy life.

Dr. Judy Kuriansky

ACKNOWLEDGMENTS

Acknowledgments are always difficult in that no one person deserves to be first, last, or forgotten, and yet someone will ultimately fall into each of these categories. As we do our best to thank everyone using a combination of chronology, reverse alphabetical order, and spontaneity, we recognize wholeheartedly that it is the contribution of the collective group that makes the publication of four simultaneous volumes possible.

We thank Judy Kuriansky, Series Editor, for inviting us, and then encouraging us, to take on this important work.

We thank our advisors, who committed themselves early on in one way or another and gave of their time in helping to shape the outline of the initial proposal, recruit authors, review chapters in their areas of expertise, and contribute chapters themselves. We acknowledge our advisors here by name only; their academic credentials and affiliations can be found in the back of this book: Beverly Whipple, William Stayton, June Machover Reinisch, Jean Koehler, Gilbert Herdt, Annamaria Giraldi, Eli Coleman, and Alan Altman.

We thank Kelly Ace, who has worked with us in various capacities on a number of critical projects outside of these four volumes and who served as administrative assistant and contributor of two chapters to these works.

We thank our more than 70 contributing authors, who are all listed in the back of this book. It is important to recognize that there is no financial payment to them for their contributions. They have given of themselves and their time because they share in a vision of a world where we can all enjoy sexual health to its fullest.

One other contributor whose biography is not listed in the back of this book will be named here. Thanks to Dr. David Ferguson who encouraged us to include a chapter on iatrogenic causes of women's sexual health problems and managed to find alternative authors when multiple surgeries prevented him from writing.

In a content area as vast as sexual health, not even our internationally renowned and highly sought-after advisors can be experts in every aspect. We are thankful to the following list of ad hoc reviewers and editors, some of whom are also contributing authors to these volumes, for coming through when called upon; their help was greatly appreciated: Sarah Beshers, Robert Birch, Peggy Cohen-Kettenis, Sandra Cole, Judith Cook, Joy Davidson, Dallas Denny, William Finger, Bob Francouer, Yvonne Fulbright, Woet Gianotten, Georgan Gregg, Pat Huston, Shimon Kapnick, Wendy Maltz, Konnie McCaffree, Herbert Samuels, Christian Thrasher, and Heather Turgeon. Beverly Whipple, Sandra Cole, and Woet Gianotten not only answered our questions, but also went above and beyond their roles.

We thank Dr. David Satcher, Director of the Center of Excellence in Sexual Health at the Morehouse School of Medicine and former Surgeon General of the United States, for writing the introduction to these volumes. Dr. Satcher is to be commended for increasing the dialogue on sexual health through the release of the 2001 *Surgeon General's Call to Action to Promote Sexual Health and Responsible Sexual Behavior* and for his continued leadership through the Center of Excellence in Sexual Health.

We thank Debora Carvalko, Senior Acquisitions Editor, Psychology and Health, for guiding us through this project and Shana Jones, Developmental Editor, for helping us to follow up on the final details.

Last, but not least, we thank our families for their patience with us and for graciously giving up shared time together so that we could share our passion with you.

INTRODUCTION

When I was Surgeon General, I worked through a collaborative process with over 100 thought leaders from academic, medical, and religious communities to develop the 2001 *Surgeon General's Call to Action to Promote Sexual Health and Responsible Sexual Behavior*. Policy makers, advocates, teachers, parents, and youth in the area of sexual health were all engaged in the process. The process sought the broadest possible input and brought together a wide range of experience, expertise, and perspective, with an emphasis on using the best available scientific evidence and best practice models in order to improve the health of our nation. At the same time, everyone involved recognized that there were still many different views and beliefs as to the best approach to public health interventions and much research still to be done in the area of sexual health. Diversity in opinions was encouraged because the primary purpose of the *Surgeon General's Call to Action* was to initiate an honest, mature, and respectful national dialogue on issues of sexuality, sexual health, and responsible sexual behavior.

The *Call to Action* focused on the need to promote sexual health and responsible sexual behavior throughout the lifespan. Among many other things, the *Call to Action* was the first step toward the development of guidelines to assist parents, clergy, teachers, and others in their work of improving sexual health and responsible sexual behavior. The *Call to Action* specifically called for providing adequate training in sexual health to all professionals who deal with sexual issues in their work, encouraging them to use this training, and ensuring that they are reflective of the populations they serve.

After issuing the *Call to Action* and finishing my tenure as Surgeon General, I moved on to the Morehouse School of Medicine, where the Ford Foundation funded the Sexual Health Program, an initiative to keep the *Surgeon General's Call to Action to Promote Sexual Health and Responsible Sexual Behavior* alive and to begin to work on the recommendations made within the report. Our overarching goal continues to be to increase the national dialogue around sexual health and responsible sexual behavior.

In my capacity as U.S. Surgeon General and now as Director of the Center of Excellence on Health Disparities at the Morehouse School of Medicine, I have had the opportunity to work with and develop relationships with many of the fine contributors to these four volumes of *Sexual Health*.

Consistent with the fundamental strategies of the *Call to Action* and the Ford-funded Sexual Health Program and new Center of Excellence for Sexual Health at Morehouse School of Medicine, *Sexual Health* contributes significantly to the goal of providing access to thorough, wide-ranging information on sexual health and responsible sexual behavior in a manner that is evidence-based, honest, mature, and respectful. *Sexual Health* is unique in its focused attention both on the positive aspects of sexual health and sexual development through the lifespan, including the importance of pleasurable touch and positive communication, and on moral and cultural issues that are both the roots of responsible sexual behavior and the fuel that drives the debates as to the appropriate public health policies and interventions. In addition to embracing the positive aspects of sex and providing a comprehensive coverage of biological and psychological foundations of sexual health, this work also addresses the difficult issues of sexually transmitted diseases (STDs), sexual violence, sexual dysfunction, and compulsive or addictive sexual behavior, and it considers the interactions and effects of mental illness, developmental disabilities, chronic conditions and acquired disabilities, gender, and minority status on sexual health. *Sexual Health* furthers the work of the *Call to Action* and the Ford-funded Sexual Health Program and Center of Excellence for Sexual Health at the Morehouse School of Medicine in providing a valuable resource for education in sexual health for future and current health care and other helping professionals.

David Satcher, MD, PhD

Chapter One

SEXUAL PROBLEMS AND DYSFUNCTIONS IN MEN

Julian Slowinski

PLACING MALE SEXUAL DYSFUNCTION IN PERSPECTIVE

Male sexual dysfunction is no longer a hushed topic. Thanks to the publicity about the development of recent medical treatment for erection difficulties and other male sexual disorders, the general public is now aware of common male sexual problems. The availability of the drugs Viagra (sildenafil), Cialis (tadalafil), and Levitra (vardenafil) has advanced the ability to treat common male erectile difficulties. The public discussion has also served as a reminder about how much ignorance and myth still limits our general knowledge about sexual functioning. Our attention in the following pages will be on the types of sexual problems men may encounter over their life span. This chapter is closely tied to the following one, "Psychological and Relationship Aspects of Male Sexuality," also by this author. The focus there is on effects of sexual dysfunction on the man and his relationships with his sexual partners. Treatment of sexual dysfunction is briefly mentioned in chapter 2 but is more thoroughly discussed in chapters 3 and 4 of this volume.

What is the incidence of sexual dysfunction among American males? A number of studies have been conducted over the years, some good, and some leaving much to be desired in terms of scientific rigor. Among the most recent studies, The Massachusetts Male Aging Study (Feldman, Goldstein, Hatzichristou, Krane, & McKinlay, 1994) of men in the 40- to 70-year-old age group found that nearly 35 percent of the men interviewed experienced some form of erectile dysfunction that ranged from mild to severe. The results were strongly related to age, health status, and emotional function (Laumann Paik, & Rosen, 1999).

The National Health and Social Life Survey was an extensive study of sexual behavior in the United States. In the male sample, 1,410 men between 18 and 59 years of age were studied. Differences in the areas of sexual dysfunction in the male population ranged slightly by age, marital status, education, and race/ ethnicity. This study found the following prevalence of sexual problems in men: lacking interest in sex (13%–17%), being unable to achieve orgasm (7%–9%), climaxing too early (28%–31%), finding sex not pleasurable (6%–10%), being anxious about performance (14%–19%), and having trouble getting or maintaining an erection (7%–18%) (Laumann et al., 1999).

While the effectiveness of modern medication in reducing symptoms and promoting sexual health has been dramatic, medical interventions cannot address the complexity of all sexual and relationship problems. For treatment to be thorough and for relapse to be avoided, additional factors need to be addressed. Male sexual functioning occurs within a biopsychosocial environment, which includes the physical, emotional, social, and relational aspects of sexual life. A man's sexual functioning is determined and affected by the health of his body and lifestyle, his personal emotional state, the quality of his relationship, and the influence of life and environmental stress.

The study and understanding of human sexual functioning has come a long way from viewing sexual difficulties as being based in either physical or psychological causes. Sexual dysfunctions must be evaluated by exploring the possibility of a combination of factors, which may both contribute to, as well as potentially serve to maintain the problem. Obtaining and maintaining sexual health is the goal.

THE SEXUAL RESPONSE CYCLE: WHAT IS INVOLVED?

We tend to think of sexual response as an automatic biological thing that just happens. Sexual feeling and changes in the body are usually pleasurable and are accompanied by emotional feelings that can move a person to initiate or participate in sexual behavior. Human sexual response was described in detail by research pioneers William Masters and Virginia Johnson (1966). While Masters and Johnson's work focused on sexual arousal leading to orgasm, their efforts contributed to the basis for understanding the biological process of sexual response. Masters and Johnson's model was expanded by Harold Lief (1981) and Helen Singer Kaplan to include the person's inner sexual experience. Lief and Kaplan used the term *DAVOS* to describe the sexual response cycle (*DAVOS* meaning "desire, arousal, vasocongestion, orgasm, and satisfaction"). Difficulties in any of the components of the DAVOS model can either represent problem areas in themselves or can negatively influence other areas of sexual functioning in both men and women. Since this chapter focuses on men's sexual response, the original DAVOS model will be applied here. (The reader interested in women's sexual response is referred to in the appendix of this volume). Case examples, all of which are fictional, have been incorporated in this discussion of the DAVOS model.

Desire is where sexual response begins for most men. Desire can be experienced as being spontaneous or as a growing awareness of sexual interest or tension (some would say "feeling horny"). Desire is a very important component of sexual response. We can't pretend to have desire, but if desire is perceived as a threat instead of as pleasure, it can be denied or inhibited. Many people in today's busy world complain of lack of desire. This lack of desire can be a result of lifestyle habits and stress; hormonal influences; disease; and even medication side effects, any of which can inhibit sexual response. Whatever the cause, lack of desire can affect the rest of the DAVOS cycle. Many sexual problems are caused by people trying to feel or behave sexual when they actually lack the desire to be sexual.

Case Example: Fred visited his doctor complaining of loss of interest in sex. His male hormone levels were within normal limits. He was not taking any medications, which might have caused a problem, and he had no other health problems. His relationship was a good one, and he still was attracted to his wife. Fred just wasn't interested in sex. He didn't fantasize about women like he used to, but really didn't care.

Fred was referred to a therapist where he talked about the many stresses and concerns in his life. He was depressed. In fact, there was a family history of depression. While he did not label his complaints as being related to depression, the warning sign was his loss of sexual desire.

Arousal can feel like desire, but it is both a psychological perception and a biological response of the body. In other words, arousal is feeling "turned on." Masters and Johnson (1966) called this "excitement." Arousal can be both objectively and subjectively experienced. This means both the conscious mind and the body are aware of becoming aroused. Arousal is accompanied by many physical changes, such as increased breathing and heart rate and increased muscular tension. People usually know when they are becoming aroused. However, like desire, arousal can be interfered with by anxiety. Many male sexual dysfunctions are heavily influenced by the presence of anxiety, especially performance anxiety, which will be discussed later in this chapter.

> **Case Example:** Vic complained to his therapist that he was having a sexual problem with a new woman he met at a staff meeting. He had tremendous desire for her but could not become aroused when with her. He could not get an erection in intimate situations with her. It was as if someone had "pulled the plug" from his "turn on" machine. Detailed questioning by the therapist revealed that his new partner was a married woman. Vic was not only consumed with desire for her but also with a healthy dose of anxiety about his boss or her husband finding out about the affair.

Vasocongestion is a genital response to psychological and/or physical sexual stimulation. The mechanism of erection continues to be the focus of much research, but essentially, penile swelling is the result of a combination of chemical, neurological, and blood flow factors that result in increased blood flow to the penis, which causes an erection. Erectile dysfunction (ED) is the manifestation of a problem in vasocongestion.

> **Case Example:** One night, while at a wedding, Pete and his wife, Carol, had too much to drink. When they were home, she admitted to him that she had a fling with the groom when they were in college. Pete considered himself to be open-minded. However, he was upset about the thought of Carol with the other man, even though it happened before he met her. It got to the point were this preoccupation interfered with getting an erection with Carol. He had to seek help.

Orgasm, or "climax," involves the sometimes overwhelming total body feeling of letting go. It is accompanied by increased heart rate and blood pressure as well as brief loss of voluntary muscle control. The French call orgasm "the little death." There are many myths about orgasm, which can interfere with sexual functioning and relationships. Men associate orgasm with ejaculation, but the two events are really separate, although they are often experienced as being simultaneous. Some men complain of ejaculation difficulties such as ejaculating too soon, too late, or even not at all. It is natural for a man to experience a loss of erection following ejaculation and orgasm. This is part of what is called the resolution or refractory phase. Resolution reflects the body returning to its presexually excited state. The refractory phase represents the period of time until a man is again able to get another erection. This time period varies with the individual man, his age, or even the newness of or attraction to his partner. While a young man usually can get a second erection shortly after he has ejaculated, it is considered not unusual for a man in his seventies to take up to two days before he can get another erection.

Case Example: It is important to note that same-sex couples can experience sexual difficulties just as heterosexual couples do. Therapists who deal with same-sex partners know that relationship dynamics between partners are similar whether the couples are straight or gay. This similarity should be kept in mind as the reader progresses through this chapter. What is said for straight couples can apply to gay couples as well. While there are some different expectations about the way men and women are raised in a given society, people are still people, and relationships are still relationships. For example, what is said about Al, a gay young man described in the following example, can be applied to the same situation for a heterosexual couple.

Al was a gay graduate student who enjoyed dating while in college. When he met Dan he was surprised that he was having difficulty controlling his ejaculation whenever he and Dan had sex. He had never had trouble pacing himself and controlling his ejaculation either with previous partners or during masturbation. Something was going on now that began to worry him. Even Dan complained. Al was experiencing premature or rapid ejaculation and didn't know what to do about it. Al did not realize that his worry was only making matters worse. Men with rapid ejaculation complaints need to relax and reduce their anxiety. Typically, a sex therapist may recommend gaining better ejaculation control through stop-start masturbation exercises, which a man can do either by himself or with the assistance of his partner (see the section below).

Al visited a campus counselor who specialized in sexual difficulties. Al and Dan attended therapy sessions as a couple, and the techniques recommended by the therapist helped Al to gain ejaculatory control in his new and exciting relationship.

Satisfaction in sexual activity is a subjective experience. Satisfaction is a very important ingredient in sexual relationships. People tend to evaluate the sexual experience as being good or not, and satisfaction is a key component in the motivation toward further sexual activity with the partner. Dissatisfaction with the sexual relationship can affect the person's response across the sexual response cycle (DAVOS), and sexual dissatisfaction can even result in the development of a sexual dysfunction.

Case Example: Pete and Mary were married for two years before Pete began to complain that Mary never had orgasms during intercourse. As he became increasingly more frustrated, he began to lose interest in having sex with her. She was upset, too. His desire for her was waning. Pete discussed his dissatisfaction with his doctor. It seemed that Pete believed the myth that a so-called real man gives his partner an orgasm during sex. His doctor explained that there was a wide range among women with regard to their orgasmic response during intercourse. Some women reach orgasm easily and consistently, while others take much longer and need intense stimulation (manually, orally, or with a vibrator). Even though there was nothing wrong with trying to pursue Mary's ability to experience coital orgasm, the doctor emphasized that Mary's current level of response was not a reflection on Pete's manhood. Pete was among the many men living out their sex lives hindered by the influence of misinformation and myth.

ERECTILE DYSFUNCTION: WHEN SOMETHING GOES WRONG

Erectile dysfunction, commonly referred to by the abbreviation ED, describes a consistent inability to obtain or maintain an ejection sufficient for satisfactory sexual activity. *Impotence* and *erectile insufficiency* are other terms used to describe erectile dysfunction. Medical terminology, like any other usage, evolves. Just as the term *frigid* is no longer commonly used to describe inadequate female sexual response, the term *impotence* is used less today because of the surplus meaning that the word implies. Perhaps the term *erectile insufficiency* may eventually replace the term *ED* and begin to take on a more common usage.

The criteria for professional diagnosis found in the *Diagnostic and Statistical Manual of Mental Disorders* (American Psychiatric Association, 1994), or *DSM-IV*, state that ED, as well as other sexual difficulties, also causes personal and interpersonal distress. Relationship distress is not to be overlooked when examining sexual difficulties. It cannot be overstated that sexuality resides in the relationship. It is also important to note that ED is not the same problem as sterility or ejaculation problems. Both men with low sperm counts (sterility) and ejaculation problems can be perfectly capable of having good erections.

Neither is erectile dysfunction a recent problem. Historical writings, from Greek mythology to the Bible to the Middles Ages, as well as contemporary literature contain themes and reports of ED and its consequences.

Superstition about the causes of ED were abundant throughout the centuries, as were the various, and usually unsuccessful, treatments. Only recently has medical and psychological knowledge allowed rapid advances toward an accurate assessment and improved treatment of ED and other male sexual dysfunctions.

Erectile dysfunction can occur suddenly or with a gradual onset. It can be a primary problem, in that the man was never able to complete sexual activity with a partner, or present as a recent difficulty following a period of normal functioning. ED can be unpredictable and episodic or ongoing and chronic. It can occur with one type of sexual activity (e.g., intercourse) but not with another (oral sex or masturbation). It can even be related to a particular partner or circumstance. The degree of erectile failure can range from mild to severe. It is important to be aware that occasional erectile problems can be considered within normal limits, often depending on circumstances.

ED can have multiple causes. It can result from a single source, such as physical trauma, or originate in a number of the body systems (neurological, circulatory, as well as hormonal factors). Medication side effects, certain lifestyles, psychological issues, and stress all have the potential to cause ED. Erection problems can affect men of all ages. While older men are more likely to experience erectile difficulties, ED frequently is not the direct result of age but rather of problems in other body systems that affect potency by interfering directly with the mechanism of erections. Finally, decreased orgasmic intensity can also accompany ED.

Estimates of the incidence of ED have varied greatly. Studies have differed in both the criteria used to measure the problem as well as in the quality of the research design. Alfred Kinsey found ED to be rare in men under 35 years of age, but the incidence increased as men aged (Kinsey, Pomeroy, & Martin, 1948). It wasn't until recently that more comprehensive surveys were available to update the early Kinsey findings about the incidence of erectile problems. We have already mentioned that data from the Massachusetts Male Aging Study (Feldman et al., 1994) found that 34.8 percent of men between 40 and 70 years of age had moderate to complete ED. The figures climbed to 52 percent when mild ED was included. The more recent National Health and Social Life Survey found that American men in the 50–59 age group were three times more likely to complain of ED than the younger 18–29 age group. Lack of sexual desire was associated with ED. Nonmarried and postmarried men (divorced, widowed, or separated) were at higher risk for symptoms of ED (Laumann et al., 1999).

Estimates of men experiencing ED range from 20 million to 30 million in the United States. This is a very significant number and suggests that ED, as well as other male sexual dysfunctions, is both a public health concern and a quality of life matter. If one considers that these millions of men have sexual partners, the effects of ED on the general population are quite high.

The medical community today is much more aware of risk factors for ED and is making an effort to educate patients about risks for developing ED. Sexual health requires a generally healthy lifestyle. Environmental and life-style factors such as stress; chronic fatigue; excessive use of alcohol, tobacco or street drugs; being overweight; and lack of exercise are potentially con-tributing factors to ED. Depression is seen both as a contributing cause of ED and also as an effect of loss of adequate sexual functioning. Certain health problems (e.g., diabetes, hypercholesterolemia, or high blood pres-sure) can contribute to ED, as can the side effects of many medications. As a rule of thumb, any medical or health condition that affects the blood vessels or the nervous system can potentially inhibit the erectile process. A functioning penis requires healthy blood circulation and intact nerves to the area. Concerns about medications and medical conditions, which might contribute to sexual dysfunction, should be discussed with a health practitioner.

Despite the high incidence of male sexual problems, it has been estimated that few men actually seek assistance with their problems. This is due in part to men's embarrassment and reluctance to share the problem and the reluc-tance of many health practitioners to inquire about sexual functioning. In addition, until recently, there was little to offer in terms of effective treat-ment. Hopefully, today's media coverage of new treatment options of ED is encouraging men and their partners to seek assistance. Significant help is now available.

EJACULATION DIFFICULTIES

Difficulty controlling ejaculation is a common complaint, which, until recently, has received little attention from the professional community in terms of developing new approaches to treatment. Since there is no average time to reach ejaculation, many complaints about ejaculatory control are sub-jective. What is perceived as a difficulty for one man may not be for another. The medical diagnostic nomenclature places ejaculatory problems within the category of male orgasmic disorders. It defines these disorders as a "persistent or recurrent delay in, or absence of, orgasm following a normal sexual excite-ment phase during which . . . sexual activity is judged to be adequate in focus, intensity, and duration" (DSM-IV, p. 509).

One of the most common ejaculatory problems is premature or rapid ejaculation (PE). Sex therapists Michael Metz and Barry McCarthy (2004) define PE as being the inadvertent and unsatisfying rapid speed of male ejaculation. They describe PE as an inability to decide or choose approximately when he wants to ejaculate in more cases than not, and it is distressing to a man and his partner. The 1994 National Health and Social Life Survey found that nearly 30 percent of the men interviewed felt they climaxed too early during at least one month during the previous year. Less than 10 percent complained of having difficulty ejaculating (Michael, Gagnon, Laumann & Kolata, 1994). Masters and Johnson's (1970) criteria for PE stated that PE was present if the man ejaculated 50 percent of the time before his partner had an orgasm. Considering what is now known about the variety and range of female orgasmic response during intercourse, it appears remarkable that a man could be diagnosed with PE based on the orgasmic response of his female partner.

Men complaining of PE usually have no difficulty in obtaining an erection, although some cases of ED can result from the anxiety and frustration that can accompany rapid ejaculation. The time to ejaculation can vary from one sexual experience to another. Complaints about PE range from the man ejaculating even before or immediately after attempting intercourse to less than a minute to a few minutes after penetration. The current definition of premature ejaculation (*DSM-IV*) does not include a specific time factor. Most sex therapists and counselors now recognize that men can vary in their time to ejaculate just as women vary in their time to reach orgasm.

There also may be constitutional differences between men, which may contribute to ejaculatory control. While the notion that men can vary naturally in their ejaculatory response seems to be obvious, past treatment for PE focused on behavioral interventions rather than a biopsychosocial model. The common experience with PE is that the man feels an impending ejaculation and has no control over stopping or slowing down the ejaculatory reflex. The reflex is not under voluntary control, and once a point of no return (ejaculatory inevitability) is reached, the man cannot stop the process. One of the emotional consequences of PE is for the man to feel that he is cheating his partner of pleasure. Very often, the sexual partner makes that complaint loud and clear, adding to his anxiety about performance. We know that performance anxiety only makes matters worse.

As with erectile dysfunction, PE can be a recent or long-term problem. It can be related to some sexual activity (such as intercourse) and not others (oral sex or masturbation). It can also be partner and situation related. Abstinence from sexual activity and heightened excitement with a partner can result in episodes of PE. This is an example, which is often explained by the circumstances, and the PE episodes may not develop into an ongoing concern. Estimated causes of PE range from a physical problem (neurological, medical illness, bodily injuries, medication side effects) to psychological and interpersonal issues, which may include anxiety, stress, conflict, personality issues, and sexual skill deficits (Metz & McCarthy, 2003).

Case Example: Rob had recently experienced loss of his job when the plant in which he was working closed. At age 40, with limited skills, he went through a period of unemployment before again finding work. During the time between jobs, Rob's self-esteem took a beating. Even his sex life changed. Rob began experiencing difficulty controlling his ejaculation. It was just like when he was young and becoming sexually active. Back then he often "came too quickly," and the problem cost him a few relationships. Now, 10 years into his marriage, the problem surfaced again. Despite his wife's patience, his anxiety grew. He realized from past experience that worrying only made matters worse. He recognized that life stress and worry were contributing to the problem. He resumed doing self-stimulation exercises to better control his ejaculation. These had worked before when a therapist had coached him about using special masturbation techniques. Rob's confidence returned, his anxiety diminished, and both he and his wife were again enjoying satisfactory sexual relationships.

Rob was greatly assisted by his partner's participation in the so-called homework. Although he could do the penile stimulation exercise by himself, his wife often provided the stimulation. She felt she was helping by participating in the exercises, and Rob's anxiety about being sexual with her was at the same time greatly lessened. Having the active cooperation of one's sexual partner speeds the recovery as well as brings the partners closer together.

Rob was helped in gaining ejaculatory control by using traditional non-pharmacological treatment techniques. Men dealing with difficulties of ED or PE have something in common: their anxiety about sexual response and performance interferes with their ability to function sexually.

In addition to the therapist teaching a man how to cope with anxiety though the use relaxation techniques, specific homework assignments can be made to deal directly with the problem and help increase a man's sexual confidence. For example, let's consider a man complaining of ED who has no physical or relationship issues that may contribute to his problem. He is capable of getting an erection in nonsexual situations. However, when he is with a partner, he may either have difficult in getting or maintaining his erection. Fear of failure becomes his opponent. Dealing with this fear is where the start-stop exercise can help.

STOP-START EXERCISE

Stop-start means what it says. The man is first asked to self-stimulate until he gets an erection. He is then told to stop the stimulation and let the erection subside. Then he again stimulates himself until he regains the erection. Engaging in stop-start practice demonstrates to the man that he can regain an erection even if there is a loss of the initial erection. He can repeat this masturbation exercise either by himself or with his partner. Practice will go a long way in restoring sexual confidence.

After sufficient practice there will come a time when the man and his partner may wish to attempt intercourse. It is usually easier for the man to maintain his erection during initial attempts at intercourse by having his partner face him in a female-on-top position. She can help stimulate him to erection, guide his erect penis into her vagina, and come to rest in that position. Therapists call this the "quiet vagina" exercise. The man can just focus on the sensation of vaginal containment. If he should begin to lose his erection, she can move gently to restimulate him to hardness. She can even get off and stimulate him orally, manually, or with a vibrator—whichever they prefer as partners. Once erection is maintained with the quiet vagina technique, intercourse can move to gentle nondemand thrusting, again with the female on top. When the partners feel confident in him keeping the erection, the couple can move to other positions of intercourse as they wish.

Back to Rob and his PE concerns. The stop-start technique can also be used in treating rapid ejaculation. In the case of PE, it is not the erection that is the focus, but rather it is paying attention to the impending sense of ejaculation. Either by himself, or with his partner's assistance, he is stimulated to the point where he feels an ejaculation is approaching. Stimulation is then stopped, and the urge to ejaculate is allowed to diminish. The exercise is repeated again and again, with the goal being to help a man to gain a better sense of ejaculatory control. With practice, he can learn to adjust the amount of stimulation needed to maintain control without needing to stop the stimulation. These techniques take practice, and the degree of success may vary depending on other factors. However, many men and their partners have enjoyed success without requiring medical intervention (Metz & McCarthy, 2003, 2004; Milsten & Slowinski, 2000; Zilbergeld, 1992).

DELAYED EJACULATION

Some men have difficulty ejaculating even with sufficient stimulation. These men may take a long time to ejaculate or may not ejaculate at all during sexual activity. The commonly used term is delayed ejaculation (DE). Retarded, inhibited, and inadequate ejaculation are also terms used to describe the complaint. The incidence of occurrence of DE is difficult to describe in a normal population of men. While the complaint has in the past been considered rare, sex therapists report treating more men with DE.

There is a normal increase in time to ejaculation as men age, but this is not what men complaining of DE are describing. In these cases, they can often thrust or masturbate for an extended time period without ever reaching a point of ejaculatory release. Again, as in other male dysfunctions, the complaint can be related to the partner or a particular sexual activity (such as intercourse, masturbation, oral sex, etc.). The origins—just as in other male dysfunctions—seem to be a mix between several potential organic and psychosocial factors (Perelman, 2004). Only little evidence points to psychological causes with certainty. Clinicians have observed that DE has occurred in some men who have difficulties with intimacy. It is not unusual to see anxious men who experience DE having difficulty letting go sexually when with new partners.

Some men are used to a particular type of stimulation during their masturbation techniques, which is difficult to duplicate when having sex with a partner. Or the real-life situation with a partner may not match the fantasy world he experiences when alone. These men are not getting sufficiently aroused to reach the point of ejaculation. Finally, the experience of retrograde ejaculation occurs when the ejaculate is expelled into the bladder instead of out through the penis. It is an organic condition which is often caused by surgery (e.g., prostatectomy) or long-term diabetes, which interferes with the nerves controlling the bladder neck.

Case Example: Stan was an anxious man by nature. He had little dating experience since a troublesome divorce. Then he met Helen. She had been divorced for years, and had spent her time raising her children. Helen had many of the personal qualities that his previous wife lacked. Stan and Helen were a good match and grew to deeply love each other. Helen was open sexually. Stan was anxious about sex and intimacy, and it showed. Most striking was his inability to ejaculate during intercourse. At first she tolerated his difficulty, but it eventually led to her dissatisfaction with sex. The couple sought counseling. Stan responded well to medication for his general anxiety, and worked hard on exploring his sexual attitudes and narrow sexual script. He eventually felt free enough to begin to let go sexually. Ejaculation gradually became more frequent during intercourse, much to the relief of both partners.

PEYRONIE'S DISEASE

One other male condition deserves to be mentioned. Peyronie's disease is a condition involving scarring of the *tunica albuginea*, which is the tough connective tissue capsule that encloses the *corpora cavernosa*, enabling the penis to become rigid when the *corpora cavernosa* becomes engorged with blood. Peyronie's disease is characterized by the formation of a plaque of fibrous tissue in the tunica albuginea and is often accompanied by penile pain and deformity on erection. There may be difficulty with penetration as a result of the curvature, and the condition may be accompanied by some impairment of erectile capacity (Lue et al., 2004). Various treatment options are available and need to be determined by a urologist.

CONCLUSION

This chapter has outlined various common male sexual problems and dysfunctions. None of these exist in isolation, and they always have an impact on the person himself and/or on his relationships. This will be discussed in more detail in the following chapter, "Psychological and Relationship Aspects of Male Sexuality," also by this author. Treatment of sexual dysfunction is briefly mentioned in chapter 2 but is more thoroughly discussed in the chapter 3, "Pharmacological Treatment of Male Erectile Dysfunction," and chapter 4, "Devices Used for the Treatment of Sexual Dysfunctions in Men."

REFERENCES

American Psychiatric Association. (1994). *Diagnostic and statistical manual of mental disorders* (4th ed.). Washington, DC: Author. Feldman, H. A., Goldstein, I., Hatzichristou, D. G., Krane, R. J., & McKinlay, J. B. (1994). Impotence and its medical and psychosocial correlates: Results of the Massachusetts Male Aging Study. *Journal of Urology, 151*(1), 54–61.

Kinsey, A., Pomeroy, W., & Martin, C. (1948). *Sexual behavior in the human male*. Philadelphia, PA: Saunders.

Laumann, E. O., Paik, A., & Rosen, R. C. (1999). Sexual dysfunction in the United States: Prevalence and predictors. *Journal of the American Medical Association, 281* (6), 537–544.

Lief, H. (1981). Classification of sexual disorders. In *Sexual problems in medical practice.* Monroe, WI: American Medical Association.

Lue, T. F., Giuliano, F., Montorsi, F., Rosen, R. C., Andersson, K. E., Althof, S., Christ, G., Hatzichristou, D., Hirsch, M., Kimoto, Y., Lewis, R., McKenna, K., MacMahon, C., Morales, A., Mulcahy, J., Padma-Nathan, H., Pryor, J., Saenz de Tejada, I., Shabsigh, R., & Wagner, G. (2004). Summary of the recommendations on sexual dysfunction in men. *The Journal of Sexual Medicine, 1,* 6–23.

Masters, W., & Johnson, V. (1970). *Human sexual inadequacy.* Boston: Little, Brown & Co.

Masters, W., & Johnson, V. (1966). *Human sexual response.* Boston: Little, Brown & Co.

Metz, M., & McCarthy, B.(2004). *Coping with erectile dysfunction.* Oakland, CA: New Harbinger.

Metz, M., & McCarthy, B. (2003). *Coping with premature ejaculation.* Oakland, CA: New Harbinger.

Michael, R., Gagnon, J., Laumann, E., & Kolata, G. (1994). *Sex in America: A definitive survey.* Boston: Little, Brown & Co.

Milsten, R., & Slowinski, J. (2000). *The sexual male: Problems & solutions.* New York: W. W. Norton.

Perelman, M. (2004). Retarded ejaculation. *Current Sexual Health Reports, 1*(3). Philadelphia, PA: Current Science Inc..

Zilbergeld, B. (1992). *The new male sexuality.* New York: Bantam Books.

Chapter Two

PSYCHOLOGICAL AND RELATIONSHIP ASPECTS OF MALE SEXUALITY

Julian Slowinski

In the previous chapter we have described common male erectile problems such as erectile dysfunction (ED) and ejaculation problems (premature ejaculation, or PE, and delayed ejaculation, or DE). This chapter will focus on the psychological components of those types of dysfunction with a discussion of how relationships and partners are often affected. Even though the chapter focuses on men, many factors, such as the importance of sexual scripts and the impact of a person'wws life history, apply to women as well. Heterosexual and homosexual couples are affected by the same interpersonal dynamics, and whenever heterosexual couples are mentioned in this chapter, those scenarios apply just as well to homosexual relationships. Case examples are presented throughout the chapter; these case examples are fictional.

ED and other male sexual dysfunctions can be caused or influenced by a number of biopsychosocial components. It was not too long ago, and with little proof, when professionals felt that as many as 90 percent of cases of male erectile dysfunction had their origin in psychological issues and conflicts. The pendulum has shifted today to placing greater emphasis on exploring biological causes for sexual dysfunctions. Steady progress is being made in this area as new diagnostic techniques and medical treatments are becoming more successful.

Despite the progress in medical diagnosis and pharmacological intervention, practitioners continue to be aware of the important role that psychological and relationship issues play in the development and continuance of sexual dysfunctions. This is true even if the dysfunction is caused by medical conditions. There is considerable emotional impact on the man and his relationships even if the sexual dysfunction has a direct biological cause. Regardless of the roots of the problem, male sexual functioning is closely aligned with self-identity. The personal impact of sexual dysfunction is real. Any discussion of sexual dysfunction must keep in mind the interplay between the man and his life experience as a male. Before I go on to explain this in more detail, an important concept will be introduced: the sexual script.

SEXUAL SCRIPT: THE LENS THROUGH WHICH WE VIEW SEXUALITY

The concept of the sexual script was introduced into the sex therapy field by sociologists, William Simon and John Gagnon (1986) and is useful in understanding how each person views and expresses his or her sexuality. Everyone has a sexual script. It describes the whole range of a person's sexual experiences, attitudes, behaviors, and feelings. Everyone brings their sexual script into their relationships. Couples develop and expand their mutual sexual script. Sexual scripts are formed early in life and are influenced by messages received from families, peers, culture, and religion. Some scripts are narrow and rigid, while others are open and flexible. Progress in treatment is often related to a person's willingness to explore and expand their sexual script.

Sexual script is neither a good nor a bad thing. It just is what it is. However, scripts can influence and limit how one deals with one's sexual partner; how sex is negotiated; and how sexual behavior is perceived, valued, and even judged. A behavior or attitude that is viewed as normal sexual behavior by one partner can be seen as "weird, kinky, or perverted" by the other. Such difference can become the reason for sexual discord, difficulties, and even dysfunction in the sexual relationship.

Sexual script influences attitudes about others and oneself. The messages received about sex are reflected in attitudes about the body, sexuality, feelings, behaviors, intimacy, gender, and sex roles. These messages are internalized and can influence—positively or negatively—the response to sexual factors for the rest of a person's life. Unfortunately, some sex-negative messages interfere with a person's ability to enjoy adult sexual experiences. Sexual health is often the casualty, and dysfunction the result when guilt, misinformation, and inhibition accompany sexual experience.

For example, therapists often see clients who are trying to live their adult sexual lives guided by a narrow understanding of themselves as sexual beings. Messages such as "sex is dirty; save it for someone you love" can result in confusion. How one experiences sexual desire can serve as an example. Sexual desire is a fundamental experience of being human. Sexual feelings are biologically programmed, but in real-life experience, they are also influenced by cultural messages. These values influence the experience, acceptance, and expression of sexual feelings. If the internal psychological meaning of sexual desire represents a sex-negative message, then the experience of sexual desire can lead to much confusion, anxiety, and guilt. The result is that both sexual performance and subjective experience can be distressed.

Case Example: Mark was becoming increasingly concerned about his erectile difficulties. He and Eve had decided to wait until marriage before having intercourse. Even a year after their wedding, the couple had been unable to consummate their marriage (for discussions on unconsummated marriage see chapter 7 by Rosenbaum in this volume and chapter 10 by Ghanem et al. in *Sexual Health: Vol. 3*. Each attempt at intercourse ended in erectile failure and growing anxiety and frustration. It was clear that this sexually inexperienced couple were stuck in a cycle of performance anxiety and despair. The sex therapist Mark and Eve began seeing discovered that Mark was very uncomfortable with feelings of sexual arousal and desire. The sex-negative messages he had received while growing up in a conservative religious home ("if you touch yourself, you will go to hell") led him to fear and repress his natural sexual feelings. Even though their marriage had given them permission to be sexual, Mark couldn't get over the guilt, shame, and fear of giving in to and enjoying a married sexual relationship with Eve. His sexual script was narrow and ridden with guilt and fear. While it took time, counseling allowed him to be more accepting of his sexuality and eventually to function in a happy and guilt-free way.

THE ROLE OF LIFE HISTORY: IMPORTANT QUESTIONS

Every man brings his own personal history to his sexual relationships, as does every woman. Concurrent with his personal history is his own unique sexual script. His attitudes about being sexual have been formed by the messages he received from family, friends, culture, and even religious teachings. The family within which he was raised has also influenced his ideas about relationships and intimacy. What follows is a list of questions, which can elicit important information that can be relevant to understanding current sexual functioning.

What type of role model did his parents and family present to him about sex, intimacy, affection, love, sharing feelings, and what it means to be a male?

Was sexuality ever discussed at home? If so, did he feel comfortable asking questions? If he has a sexual partner, that partner is also bringing to the relationship a personal set of attitudes, assumptions, and sense of self as a sexual person. What were his early experiences of being a sexual person? Were there any sexual traumas, negative experiences, or repeated sex-negative messages that are presently a negative influence on his sense of self as a sexual person or on his sexual functioning? How were puberty and the sexual unfolding of adolescence experienced? How did he feel about his body, especially the size and shape of his penis? Was he prepared for the changes in body and emotional feelings that arise during puberty? Were natural sexual fantasies welcomed or feared? Was he comfortable with private sexual thoughts and feelings? If not, what was their nature? Was masturbation a positive or negative experience?

Are his attitudes and expectations about sex influenced by sexual myths, misinformation, and ignorance? Was there a concern about sexual orientation? If so, is he comfortable now? What were early dating and sexual experiences like? Were attempts at sexual activity with a partner pleasurable or fearfully approached and filled with shame and doubt? Were there any failures or disappointments in sexual functioning with a partner that led to future worry and continued failure? Does he use pornography or other erotic material? If so, how frequently? If so, does he need porn or sexual props in order to become aroused and function sexually with his partner? Does he practice safe sex?

Has he had any sexually transmitted infections? If so, what were the circumstances, and what is the present status? Have there been any unwanted pregnancies or abortions? Is so, what were the circumstances, and how does he feel about it now? If in a committed relationship or marriage, has he been sexually faithful to it? If he was not faithful, what are his feelings about the infidelity now? Does his partner know? How has the man reacted to changes in health and aging and their impact on his sexual functioning? Has he become insecure about himself as a sexual male?

How is his general health? What type of medicating is he taking and for what condition? Are either health conditions or medication affecting sexual functioning? Has there been or is there currently conflict in his imitate relationships? Is there a history of divorce, separation, or death of a spouse or partner? What role is sexuality playing in his present relationships? Is there stress in his everyday life with health, work, colleagues, family, elderly parents, children, a partner, or finances? Are there any past or current legal concerns? Is there use of tobacco, alcohol, or illegal drugs? Is there any history of mental health treatment? Is there a personal or family history of anxiety, depression, or other mental health difficulties? The following detailed case example serves to demonstrate how many of the above questions are helpful in clarifying presenting problems.

Case Example: Harry is a 35-year-old married man and father of two young children. He was referred by his physician whom he had initially visited with the complaint of gradual erectile failure, which started about a year ago. He had no complaints about ejaculation difficulties or of any pain or discomfort during sex.

Harry was in good general health, exercised regularly, and maintained a healthy diet. He did not smoke, and his use of alcohol was moderate. There was no family history of depression, heart disease, stroke, or diabetes. His parents, who were retired, enjoyed good health and were quite independent of requiring assistance from Harry or his older sister. He and his wife, Nancy, were on good terms with his parents and extended family. The same was true of his relationship with Nancy's family.

Harry worked long hours for an engineering firm, was well compensated, and enjoyed his work. Nancy was a schoolteacher who enjoyed her work and valued the time with her children and family that her teaching schedule allowed. The couple had recently moved into a new home, which was within their ability to afford. Other than the sexual complaint, Harry's life was fine.

Harry's physician took a complete medical history and performed lab tests, which showed that Harry's testosterone level was well within the normal range for someone his age. There was no evidence of neurological or vascular problems that might impede sexual functioning, and he was on no medication that could contribute to the ED. Harry was a healthy male, and he was referred for counseling to a clinical psychologist who specialized in sex and couples therapy.

Harry presented himself to the therapist as a bright, verbal, and somewhat anxious man who was eager to get help. He described his gradual loss of erections as taking place over the past year. At first, Harry noticed that his erections where not quite as firm as usual. He thought it was due to being tired. He reported having good morning and nocturnal erections. He rarely masturbated, but when he did, his erections were firm. He began to notice that he would lose his erection during intercourse. Sometimes, with Nancy's help, he could regain his erection; but by then, the "fun was out of it." Then there were the times when he couldn't get an erection at all. He found himself worrying ahead of time about whether he would fail, and that just made matters worse. His difficulty got to the point where he was actually avoiding being sexual so as not to have an embarrassing erectile failure. His worrying about erectile failure only made matters worse.

(Continued)

(Continued)

Harry had no previous erectile failures in his seven-year marriage to Nancy. They were still affectionate in a nonsexual way but lately had not attempted intercourse or any of their usual sexual playfulness. He reported that Nancy was also concerned about his problem and had supported his seeking assistance. She remained willing to join him in future sessions if recommended.

Harry gave the following family and sexual history He grew up in an intact family in a Midwest suburb and went to neighborhood schools. He got along well with his sister who was two years older. He described his parents as loving but quite socially and politically conservative. His father was a lawyer, and his mother worked in the local bank. Both parents were active in the local Protestant church, and Harry regularly attended religious instruction as a youngster and accompanied his family to Sunday services until he left for college. Both at home and at church, Harry learned the virtues of respect for authority, proper living, self-denial, and good citizenship. He could not recall anything about sex being discussed at home. The message at church was of respect and abstinence until marriage but never presented the pleasure of sexuality as anything joyful.

Harry had no one to turn to as a teen when he began to experience sexual feelings. He felt his parents were loving but unapproachable. His sister was as naïve about sexual matters as he was. His friends were of little help, as they believed the many myths about sex and "being a man." Their bragging only made him more confused because their boasts contrasted so much with the way he had been raised. He occasionally gave in to sexual fantasies and even tried masturbation but always felt there was just "something not right" about the being sexual.

Harry was a good student and was popular at school. He dated some in high school, engaged in some exploratory sex play with several girls, but never attempted intercourse. That happened during his third year of college with a girl from a similar background. They both were "scared to death," but managed to get through it. In fact, Harry dated that same girl until his senior year when they parted "as friends."

Harry didn't meet Nancy until he was already working as an engineer. While she came from a similar socioeconomic background as Harry, Nancy was raised with a more open acceptance of her sexuality. She had moved though her adolescent years with a healthy sense of her body and an appreciation for her feminine sexuality. When it came to sex, she was open and nonjudgmental. She was more sexually experienced that Harry but was patient with him. For Harry, Nancy's openness was a new discovery. He enjoyed being sexual with her. They were engaged and married within two years of meeting.

Once in counseling, Harry became aware that while he loved Nancy very much and wanted to stay married to her, there were times when her openness about sex made him a bit uncomfortable. She seemed to have a stronger sex drive than he did, and Nancy often initiated sexual activity. He said that many men would welcome such a sexy wife, but there were times when he felt pressure to perform. Nancy was quite responsive sexually and could really "let go" when she had an orgasm. He said that part of him enjoyed this, while another part experienced that old feeling that nice girls shouldn't enjoy sex too much. He began to be a bit judgmental about her sexual appetite and felt some anxiety and guilt about the enjoyment that he had with her. He became a little conflicted about his own level of desire and began to wonder if he could "really please her."

Harry said that about a year ago, Nancy brought up the topic of using sex toys to add a little spice to their love life. Some of her friends were saying vibrators and erotic videos were quite mainstream now and were enjoying introducing them into their lovemaking. She wanted to give it a try. Harry agreed, but part of him was somewhat uncomfortable. Nancy really enjoyed the freedom and new pleasures that were added to their sexual repertoire.

Harry found himself a bit taken aback by Nancy's new sexual enthusiasm. He kept telling himself that as consenting adults, they were not engaging in any activity that was uncommon to many other couples. Still, he felt a bit uncomfortable. It was shortly after this that he began to experience the onset of his erection problems.

When the erectile difficulties began, Harry did not make a connection between his discomfort and the changes in the marital sexual activity. He focused, as many men did, on worrying about getting and keeping an erection. When he did have an erection, he found himself "watching himself have sex." He began to monitor the status of his erection. Harry was experiencing two of the classic problems that contribute to causing and maintaining sexual difficulties. He was experiencing *performance anxiety*—would it work this time? (and if not, that would be awful)—and was *spectatoring*, watching himself have sex, instead of focusing on the pleasure of being with his wife.

Through treatment, and with the cooperation of Nancy, Harry was able to explore his attitudes about sexuality and respect how he and his wife came to the marriage with two different sexual scripts: his narrow,

(Continued)

(Continued)

and hers open and flexible. It was not a choice of good or bad, but just different. Nancy was not some sort of "loose woman" or "nympho," but just a woman who could embrace her sexuality and share it with her husband. Harry learned to deal with his discomfort and understand the source of his anxiety about changing and expanding his sexual repertoire. He learned how to focus less on sexual performance and more on the pleasure of being with his wife, learning to use her enjoyment as a means to enhance his sexual experience rather than feeling threatened by it.

PERSONALITY AND RELATIONSHIPS

A man's basic personality is reflected in how he interacts with the world and his relationships. Individual personality and mental health issues can play a very important role in sexual functioning. Personality traits or styles need not be dramatic or involve serious mental illness to influence sexual functioning. Personality characteristics reflect how a man deals with stress and conflict, as well as the positive aspects of intimacy, sharing, and pleasure. Some men live out their personality issues in their intimate and sexual relationships. They can exhibit individual and relationship conflicts such as anger, resentment, or disappointment in passive-aggressive ways that channel negative feeling to their partner through sexual dysfunction. There are times when a man or his partner are quite aware of negative, conflicted, or ambivalent feelings that are being expressed sexually through a variety of behaviors, including actual sexual dysfunction. At other times, there is little insight into what the basis of his difficulty is.

There are many personality variables frequently seen by sex therapists and counselors. Some men are chronic worriers and perfectionistic about many things. When they worry about sexual performance, they can do so to the point of developing erectile failure or ejaculation difficulties. There are self-centered men, some would call them narcissistic, who may interact with others only as a means to meet their own pleasure and prove their sexual self-worth. Since sexual functioning is a way of proving himself, any failure, including his partner's lack of sexual responsiveness, is unwelcome and potentially troublesome for him and the relationship. Depression can also be both a cause of and an effect of sexual dysfunction. Reduced interest in sex is a common complaint seen in depression. In fact, one of the difficulties in treating depression is the incidence of negative sexual side effects experienced by patients taking antidepressant medications. It can be a catch-22.

COUPLE SYSTEM

One approach that sex therapists take is to view sexual complaints as serving some purpose. This view was introduced by sex therapist Dr. Joseph LoPiccolo (1992), who suggested that just focusing on eliminating sexual symptoms missed the larger picture of the role of sexuality in the relationship. There are times when the couple's complex relationship system is maintained by the very presence of the sexual problem. The dysfunction may be a symptom of other relationships problems. Considering the emotional pain, embarrassment, and frustration that accompanies sexual dysfunction, what possible purpose could the problem serve? For a man experiencing a sexual dysfunction, he may feel that the only purpose the problem serves is to make him more miserable and provide more stress and frustration for him and his partner.

There are times in a relationship where problems can really represent an adaptation to other problems. When it comes to sex, a dysfunction can serve as a way of protecting the partners from dealing with other personal aspects such as passion, intimacy, and the exploration of sexual potential. In men, for example, ED or PE can serve as a means to avoid sexual contact and having to deal with "real" sexual and interpersonal issues. The man whose partner is a sexually uninhibited may feel threatened by her openness and the pressure on him to perform for her. Developing ED provides him a way out of having to deal with trying to please her. The failure of his penis to function is, in a way, protecting him from another type of fear and failure. From his partner's perspective, his dysfunction can also serve as a convenient excuse to also avoid dealing with her own uncomfortable issues of intimacy and sexual expression. Thus a balance is maintained in the relationship.

Nonsexual concerns can also interfere with sex and intimacy and should not be overlooked. The whole notion about what causes and maintains sexual dysfunction provides a window into seeing how personal sexual development plays its role in adult sexual functioning. There are times when the reason for the male dysfunction lies beyond the penis. This notion also explains why some men still have ongoing sexual and relationship difficulties even after the initial sexual complaint is cured. Modern treatment advances, including the current use of medication for ED, may eliminate the sexual difficulty while not at all addressing the complex relationship issues. This serves as a reminder that a man's sexuality is lived out in his intimate and sexual relationships.

SEXUALITY RESIDES IN THE RELATIONSHIP: WHAT MEN BRING TO THE RELATIONSHIP

What does a man bring to his relationships? We mentioned how sexual attitudes and opinions are formed, learned, and internalized into a man's sense of a sexual self. The results range from a healthy, positive sexual confidence and self-regard to one characterized by insecurities, misinformation, insufficient lovemaking skills, and inner discomfort with all matters sexual.

Many men are under the influence of sexual myths, which can even promote sexual dysfunction through their presentation of unrealistic and even false expectations about male sexual functioning. Many men, and their partners, have been influenced by embracing myths pervasive in many cultures: men are always ready for sex, foreplay must lead to sex, erections should be automatic, men are responsible for what goes on in sex, real sex requires a good erection, and penile length is a measure of masculinity (Milsten & Slowinski, 2000). This all relates to what sex therapist Bernie Zilbergeld (1999) refers to as the fantasy model of sex. He sums it up as "It's two feet long, hard as steel, and will knock your socks off" (p. 15). What a daunting expectation for men who are influenced by this myth.

Even if men view this fantasy characterization of male sexual prowess as humorous, they may believe the notion that sexual performance is what sex is all about. Believing this and other myths can lead not only to sexual dysfunction but also to sexual dissatisfaction, even if "the plumbing is working."

What does this fantasy model, which fosters that sex is a way of proving oneself as a man, imply about sexuality and relationships? It implies that sex is about performance, not about experiencing pleasure, not about love, not about enjoyment and fun, and not about having joy and satisfaction in pleasing a partner. Rather, the fantasy model focuses on doing, measuring up, and "knocking your partner's socks off." This is not to say that sexual passion is not to be enjoyed, but rather that enjoyment is more than pure performance. For men and their partners, a pleasurable and satisfying experience is really about how they feel about what they just shared. In other words, good sex is how the partners feel about the experience. Pleasure is not just about performance (see also chapter 5 in this volume, by Ellison). Sexual satisfaction and pleasure is also about a subjective experience. Partners know what feels good to them. The myths and experts can stay out their bedroom. Sex resides in the relationship.

WHAT ABOUT RELATIONSHIPS?

Most men's sexual lives are played out in their sexual relationships. In other words, relationships are where sexuality finds its home. All sexual relationships, even casual ones, are intimate at some level. Sex involves intimate sharing of self, not just the body, with another person. Some men function fine in casual sexual relationships but have difficulties in ongoing and committed relationships. Let's focus on the sexual relationship with a regular partner.

We have noted that partners bring themselves to any relationship, and certainly to the sexual expression within those relationships. There are many issues in the shared intimacy of daily life together that influence sexual functioning, even if the concerns about the partner are not about sex. All interactions, verbal and nonverbal can influence how partners feel about one another. Interactions generate feelings about the partner and oneself. They can be carried over into the sexual relations as well. These feelings become part of how partners respond sexually to each other. Some relationship issues are discussed and resolved, while others are not. Some unresolved issues and differences about expectations of one's partner could lead to feelings of resentment or even anger.

While some men function sexually despite negative feelings about their partners, others cannot. These men find that negative nonsexual feelings about the relationship can interfere with sexual functioning. It is hard to get erect if a man is feeling anger, frustration, or being taken for granted. Of course, these same feelings can interfere with sexual response in women. Men may experience decreased sexual desire for their partners and difficulty becoming aroused when with them, and may even develop dysfunctions with erection or ejaculation.

Some therapists remind clients that there is no political correctness in the deep feelings that develop in intimate relationships. Despite wanting to be sensitive to a partner's feelings, some personal tastes and aesthetic preferences can affect sexual functioning. For example, some men avoid sex or experience difficulty because of characteristics or changes in their partner, perhaps because of weight gain, surgery or medical conditions, personal hygiene, or just normal aging. They may be embarrassed to admit it, but men can't fake or pretend to themselves how they feel. Their lack of interest in sex or poor sexual performance can speak for itself. They just feel "turned off." The same can be true for women.

Many sexual complaints reflect differences in the couple's sexual script. Sexual scripts reflect and determine what type of sexual activities will be included and under what circumstances the couple will be sexual. Some examples would be choosing when to have sex; introducing new lovemaking techniques, sexual positions, or oral or anal sex; the use of sex toys or other erotic materials such as adult videos; frequency of sex; disagreement on sexual habits or practices; length and types of foreplay; too little tenderness after intercourse; family planning choices (Milsten & Slowinski, 2000). These and many other difficulties are often at the basis of many couples' sexual problems. A published report of married couples found that sexual difficulties and disagreements caused more marital unhappiness and stress than did actual sexual dysfunction (Frank, 1978).

Sexual relationships can suffer in a busy world where multiple demands and role stresses are placed on both partners. One could even say the modern life conspires against our sex lives. Often, a busy and tired partner can be annoyed at what is perceived as a sexual advance even if her mate was just being playfully affectionate. As a result, the man may feel rejected, while the partner thinks he is being inconsiderate.

Case Example: Nick was a fun loving guy who enjoyed sex. When he arrived home from work one day, he found his wife, Joanne, in the kitchen busily preparing dinner for the three kids and them. Nick was in a playful mood, came up behind Nancy, and began to fondle her breasts. Instead of responding with interest to his playfulness, an angry Joanne complained, asking how he could think about sex at a time when she was so stressed and busy. Nick stormed out of the kitchen. He was just being playful. She thought that he wanted sex and was being selfish and inconsiderate. Both remained angry for days. Their sex life suffered because of mutual resentment and misunderstanding, which could have been avoided if they had practiced better communication skills.

LIFESTYLE FACTORS AND GENERAL HEALTH

Lifestyle also has an impact on sexual functioning. Personal habits involving smoking, alcohol use, eating habits, sleeping, recreation, and exercise patterns all have an influence on a man and his general health. Healthy sexual functioning depends on a healthy body and good general health. It is important to remember that whatever health factors negatively affect the heart, blood vessels, and nervous system also affect and influence sexual functioning. For example, smoking is not only detrimental to the heart, but the effect of nicotine is also seen in the nerves and blood vessels, which serve the penis and genital organs. Health practitioners are also aware that ED can be an early warning sign for the possibility of future heart attacks or strokes. Healthy sexual functioning requires healthy body systems.

TIME, PLACE, AND PERSON

Some professionals say that the penis doesn't lie. What is erectile failure (or PE/DE) telling a man and his partner? Is the penis protecting the man from a real or potential risk or troubled relationship? Is his penis in some way protecting him from emotional harm or perhaps a bad decision? The erectile failure could give the man pause to think about what is happening. Some men experience sexual dysfunction because they try to be sexual at the wrong time, wrong place, or even with the wrong person. *Time, place,* and *person* are important ingredients in determining adequate sexual functioning. Often, it just takes common sense to see what the problem is. But some men aren't thinking about this when they are interested in, or think they should be interested in, being sexual just because the opportunity presents itself (remember the myth that a man should be always ready and always interested in sex?).

For many men, erectile failure is linked to particular circumstances. Perhaps they tried to be sexual when they were too tired or stressed, had just had a heavy meal or too much to drink or were going through a particularly stressful life phase. They may not have really felt like being sexual but suddenly had the opportunity or their partner requested it. For them, it was not the right *time* to have sex.

Timing is important in life, especially when it comes to being sexual. There are additional circumstances when timing may contribute to sexual failure. This includes coping with sex during pregnancy or a partner's illness or following the birth of a child. There are also normal developmental and adjustment situations, which may prove to be influential in interfering with adequate sexual functioning. A partial list includes the adjustment to children leaving home, the serious illness or death of a spouse or family member, the loss of a job or beginning new employment, moving to a new area, or separation or divorce. These stressors are frequently an unavoidable part of life. Yet stress has an impact on the body and especially influences sexual desire and functioning.

Case Example: John was a college sophomore who was really enjoying the freedom of living away from home and having an active social life on campus. He met an attractive girl at a fraternity party that featured all the beer they could drink. He and the girl ended up in bed after the party, and John was devastated when he cold not get an erection. His sexual reputation would be all over if word of his failure got out to the guys. John failed to appreciate that even a healthy young male could experience an episode of ED after too much alcohol. After having so much to drink, he failed because he tried to have sex at the wrong *time.*

The *place* where one has sex is also important. Many men and women need to be in comfortable and safe surroundings in order to function sexually and enjoy sex. Privacy is a big issue. One should not be rushed, either.

Case Example: Sid and Nancy loved raising their three kids and still found time to have an enjoyable sex life. But now the kids were teenagers and "knew all about sex." Sid noticed that his erections were not as hard and he was having trouble delaying his ejaculation. In a consultation with a sex therapist, he realized that he was worried that their teenage

(Continued)

(Continued)

children would know what was going on behind their parent's closed bedroom door. Sid was not comfortable in his own bedroom. His *place* had become unsafe. His anxiety about the kids knowing or hearing that he and Nancy were having sex had affected his sexual performance.

The *person* a man is having sex with is also important. This relates not only to a man who is experiencing a sexual dysfunction with a long-term partner, but also to a sexual encounter with someone other that his regular partner. A sexual partner can be inappropriate for a man for a number of other reasons. He can experience sexual difficulties because of a partner's age, religion, race, body type, reputation, career, or socioeconomic status. If a man is confused about his sexual orientation, he may experience dysfunction while attempting to be sexual with a partner of the wrong gender. Sex is never simple. Many variables can inhibit sexual response.

Case Example: Dave was a happily married executive who traveled extensively on business. On a recent trip to a foreign country, his hosts offered and provided him with female companionship in an exotic setting. Dave had never been unfaithful to his wife but felt he couldn't pass up this opportunity in a distant land, where no one would know anyway. Dave was surprised when he couldn't get an erection. There was nothing wrong with his penis. He just was not with the right *person.*

PERFORMANCE ANXIETY

There are times when a man experiences sexual dysfunction when the issue is not the person per se, but the fact that it is sex with a new person. It is true that for many men, sexual activity with a new partner is usually exciting and satisfying. Sexual performance is certainly not a problem, and even if there is some initial performance anxiety, adequate sexual functioning is experienced. However, being with a new partner can also be charged with anxiety and sexual inhibition. An initial failure, whether it is ED, PE, or DE, can lead to what therapists call *anticipatory anxiety.* In other words, the man develops performance anxiety and starts worrying about what will happen next time. He is anticipating failure.

The anxiety may increase, and the problem gets worse. When he does engage in sexual activity, he may engage in spectatoring, which is watching himself have sex. Thus he worries about his performance and critically monitors how he is doing. The building anxiety only serves to inhibit his sexual response even further. The result ranges from outright sexual failure to an unsatisfying diminished sexual response. He critically evaluates his performance and himself in a negative way that can eventually result in avoidance of sexual activity out of fear of failure. If his partner is overtly critical or unsupportive, it only makes matters worse. This scenario applies to all men, regardless of whether they experience difficulty with an established partner or a new one. The mental mechanisms and response to anxiety are the same. Only the circumstances make it different. Not satisfying a long-term partner on occasion is one thing. It is another to fail with a new person and perhaps jeopardize the future of the new relationship.

The personal dynamics in meeting and establishing a sexual relationship with a new partner can be influenced by a significant set of circumstances. Some men may be coming out of a painful divorce, a breakup of an important relationship, or even the death of a spouse. This history may make a man cautious about becoming involved with another partner. For such men, the prospect of intimacy might be perceived as a threat rather than a welcomed opportunity. What is happening?

There are times when a man in a new relationship is still dealing with feelings and unresolved issues about his previous partner. These feeling can interfere with his sexual response to his new partner. For example, his normal desire and arousal patterns may be interrupted by ambivalent feelings about becoming involved again or feeling unfaithful to the memory of a deceased or former lover. If there is remaining anger toward the former partner, or toward women in general, this can interfere with sexual response. A new partner may be much more sexually responsive than he was used to, perhaps making him uncomfortable or even a bit threatened about whether he is capable of pleasing her. Fear of failure with her can signal concerns about repeating the rejection he may have previously experienced. He might even be experiencing discomfort with his own positive sexual response and inadvertently short-circuit a natural reflex. He is contributing to the problem by focusing on the past to the detriment of staying focused on the pleasure of the moment of being with his partner. He cannot be in two places at once (Milsten & Slowinski, 2000).

PROBLEM AREAS IN RELATIONSHIPS

Relationships are marked by expectations. Some expectations are conscious and verbalized between partners. For example, there may be clear understanding of expectations about what roles and responsibilities each partner has in maintaining a household. Yet, other expectations may never be addressed openly, and a partner can be held in judgment for not meeting those expectations. That is, one partner has an expectation of the other, while the other does not know about it. For example, a man may have expected his partner to be more open sexually once they were married. Unmet expectations, particularly about sex, can cause problems in relationships, even to the point of contributing to sexual dysfunction. Often, these expectations only come to light in the course of counseling.

Case Example: Phil and Paula came for counseling complaining about "poor communication about everything, especially sex." Phil had shown a recent disinterest in sex with Paula. When they had been sexual in the past, Paula complained that Phil did not satisfy her anyway.

After discussing it they discovered that Phil was "turned off" by Paula's lack of sexual response, which he presumed would get better after marriage. Paula complained that it was Paul's responsibility to know what to do to please her sexually. Each had assumptions about the other that were never verbalized. Had these expectations been discussed earlier in their marriage, they could have examined their assumptions and possibly avoided this present dissatisfaction.

WHERE PROBLEMS RESIDE

When couples present with relationship and sexual difficulties, they learn to explore the essential ingredients of relationships that influence their lives together: *power, trust,* and *intimacy.* How couples deal with these three areas greatly influences how they feel about one another, the relationship, and their attitudes toward being in an intimate sexual relationship. Psychological causes for sexual dysfunctions that are related to the primary relationship are often played out in these three dimensions.

Power is not just about who is in control. It also refers to how a person feels valued and respected in a relationship. Does the other take the person's feelings into consideration? Does the person feel taken into consideration in decision making, even when it comes to the choice to be sexual or not? Is the relationship respectful?

Case Example: Steve treated Joan as if he was the boss. While she had a say in running the daily managing of the household, it was he who made major decisions, rarely consulted her, and didn't give much weight to her opinions or wishes. This information was obtained in counseling when Steve and Joan sought help for Joan's lack of interest in sex. Her lack of sexual desire was directly related to her not feeling respected as an equal partner in the marriage.

Trust refers to more than trusting a committed partner to be sexually faithful. Trust also means having a comfort level that a partner can be relied on to be responsible in financial matters, respect personal and relationship boundaries, and accept responsibilities for parenting and household issues. It means being dependable.

> **Case Example:** Nick and Michelle came into counseling because of Nick's recent ED, which was most likely related to current medication. He also was extremely angry with Michelle for sharing their sexual problems with her mother and sister. Because of her family knowing "his and their marital business" Nick felt uncomfortable and embarrassed around her family during their regular Sunday afternoon visits. Michelle thought it was "normal" and even "expected" to share with her family. Nick disagreed. He considered her sharing to be a violation of their marital boundaries. His sexual problems were compounded by his anger and by feeling betrayed that his wife shared such a sensitive male problem. Nick felt he couldn't trust Michelle.

Intimacy involves the ability to share, hear, respect, and communicate what is important in an honest and open fashion. Intimacy extends to both sexual and nonsexual matters in the life of a relationship. It also involves being in touch with oneself in an intimate way. By achieving this personal intimacy, one is better able to share oneself and also be more in tune with the partner's feelings, needs, and expectations.

> **Case Example:** Norman and Estelle had been married for 10 years before they realized that their sex life was going nowhere. After an early honeymoon phase of regular and enjoyable sex, they began to drift apart, and sexual contact became minimal. Norman had "no desire" and Estelle "couldn't care less." In the course of counseling, it became apparent that neither Norman nor Estella shared much about their daily lives, interests, and expectations of life in general. Both had come from a family where their parents showed little emotion or affection toward one another. Norman and Estelle were replicating the absence of intimacy of their parents' marriages. While they cared about one another, they failed to share so many things. Their sexual life together had become a casualty of the inability to be and deal with intimacy.

THE IMPACT OF MALE SEXUAL DYSFUNCTIONS

It is common for men to feel that their sense of male identity is closely related to their sexual functioning. Society greets his birth with the proclamation "it's a boy." His maleness sets in motion a host of cultural and family expectations. Being born male places significant expectations and obligations on a child. He receives many messages and myths about what it means to be a man. Unlike his sisters, the mark of his maleness, his genitals, is external and prominent. His penis is a constant and daily companion. As an infant, he fondled his penis in an innocent response to the pleasure brought by its stimulation. His penis had been responding with erections since he was in the womb, and erections would continue automatically throughout his years while he slept, as nature's way of assuring that the genitals would stay healthy and prepared for their reproductive function. A man's penis just cannot be ignored.

The nocturnal erections that a male experiences coincide with a phase of deep sleep characterized by rapid eye movement (REM). Varying with the age of the man, REM sleep cycles occur about every 90 minutes and can last for over an hour. At times, erotic dreams may accompany the erection phase of REM. Men are used to waking up at night or in the morning with a so-called REM erection. For a man concerned about having ED, having a good REM erection is a reassuring sign that his penis is working. While the REM erection may be firm, the man may still not have the usual experience of internal arousal and excitement, which accompanies erections during regular sexual activity. Because of this, some men may experience erection loss when trying to be sexual with a REM erection. While it may sound like a contradiction, having an erection may not mean that they were internally or emotionally "turned on."

As a male matures and sexual feeling and thoughts flood him during puberty, his penis becomes a focal point of pleasure, especially if masturbation is part of his experience. But this same focus on his genitals might also provide conflict. Shame and guilt may become familiar emotions to him if family, cultural, and religious taboos and restrictions label genital pleasure and self-stimulation as something to be avoided or even sinful. Myths about male potency and sexuality are part of his peer experience as boys incorporate misinformation and falsehoods about sex into their own view of themselves in a male role. If he is fortunate enough to live in a family that provides a healthy notion about sex or has access to appropriate and comprehensive sexuality education in his school or community, he may emerge from his youth with a healthy understanding of his sexuality and its place in his life. Whether he does develop healthy attitudes or not, the male is not indifferent to his penis. Penile functioning is a part of a man's sense of self. When things do not work as they should, or at least as expected, there are personal consequences.

When something adverse happens to a person, it does not happen in isolation. The event is superimposed on his basic personality functioning. His history, his personal strengths and weaknesses, will in effect influence and even determine his response to a disappointment. Therefore, when a man experiences a sexual dysfunction, especially erectile difficulties, it has the potential to affect him in many ways, both in and outside of the bedroom. In addition to experiencing a general sense of personal disappointment about himself as a sexually adequate male and his possible failure to meet his obligations to his partner, a man may question his sense of self-worth and his relationship with his partner. Old insecurities can resurface. He may react with anger, self-doubt, depression, and withdrawal from sex with his partner. Personal disappointment and preoccupation with failure may carry over into the workplace and affect work productivity. Some men engage in self-defeating behaviors, including acting out through drinking or getting involved with other partners as a way of trying to prove themselves or to find solace in attention from other women.

Women also experience feelings in response to their male partner's sexual dysfunction. It will depend on whether the sexual failure occurred in a committed long-term relationship or in a casual "one-night stand." It will depend on how important a functioning sexual relationship is to her. What was the reason for the dysfunction? Was it illness or just stress and circumstances like being rushed, anxious, stressed, or having too much to drink? What is the quality and history of the overall relationship? Very often, blame is a common response, whether directed at herself or him. Was she part of the problem? Was she no longer desirable to him? Had she aged or put on weight (remember, there is no political correctness here, just dealing with what people are feeling). Was there someone else? Does he still love her? Is she angry and resentful for being denied rightful sexual pleasure from him? Will she avoid being sexual with him as a way of sparing him further failure and embarrassment? Will a conspiracy of silence develop between them if they choose to avoid speaking of the problem and refrain from sexual activity, in an attempt to avoid sexual failure? Are or were there other problems in the relationship that might resurface at this is time, causing further stress? Perhaps working together on his sexual problem will serve as a reason for them to grow closer. Perhaps it will leave them further apart.

THERE IS ALSO A SHIFT IN THE RELATIONSHIP . . .

Self-confidence can be a tenuous feeling. Sexual dysfunction, especially erectile difficulties, affects self-confidence to the point where there can be subtle shifts in the relationship. No longer confident, a man can find himself being a bit unsure and passive and can place himself in a more dependent position with his partner. He may not even be aware of this shift, as it is not always recognized on the conscious level.

The same dynamics can be present in the partner. Having once been confident in his sexual performance, she can no longer take him for granted. She may also receive much of her esteem as a sexual partner based on his sexual response to her. That, too, is now threatened. The more she worries about his sexual difficulty, the more anticipatory anxiety she feels about future sexual encounters. In turn, she may inadvertently communicate her hesitancy, which can play into his growing performance anxiety. They both suffer. Finally, and as a consequence of his sexual difficulty, she may also experience sexual difficulties and dysfunction.

For some couples, their sexual contact consists of little more than having intercourse. For them, ED presents a significant challenge. Couples who have a varied sexual script that allows for other means of giving and receiving pleasure and achieving satisfaction are apt to cope much better when dealing with sexual dysfunctions. The man who knows that he need not have a good erection in order to please his partner has an advantage. He can still enjoy intimacy with his partner at the same time he is working on overcoming his sexual difficulty.

> **Case Example:** Bill and Helen were extremely anxious about his recent erectile difficulties. By the time they sought professional assistance they had stopped having sexual contact. The couple did report that they had a varied sexual script, which afforded them much joy and pleasure. They related that they were comfortable masturbating in each other's presence and stimulating each other's genitals manually, orally, or with a vibrator. The therapist explained that their lovemaking practices were an asset. They were encouraged to engage in their usual forms of satisfying sexual activity and not worry about whether Bill had an erection. Furthermore, they were to avoid even thinking about attempting intercourse. This helped the couple overcome their anxiety about sexual performance and became the foundation for more rapid success in treating his ED.

SELF-ASSESSMENT: HOW TO KNOW THAT YOU HAVE A PROBLEM

Many men and their partners are confused about whether they already have or are developing a sexual dysfunction. A self-assessment is the initial step in obtaining a better sense of the sexual complaint. Self-assessment involves reviewing past and current sexual functioning, life stresses, relationship issues, past and present medical history, and personal history. Information from these categories will help understand where the difficulties lie.

Overview of the Difficulty

In the previous chapter, we presented the DAVOS model of the sexual response cycle. One of the first questions to ask when someone is affected by sexual problems is which of the areas of desire, arousal, vasocongestion (erection), orgasm, and satisfaction may be affected. Once the category of the sexual problem is narrowed down, the male himself or a sex therapist or counselor can then ask more specific questions:

- *Desire:* Low desire in general or for the partner or for a particular situation
- *Arousal:* Not feeling turned on; in general, to a partner, or to a particular situation
- *Vasocongestion:* Not getting erections sufficient for intercourse; not keeping an erection
- *Orgasm:* Ejaculating too quickly; being aroused but not having an orgasm; having an orgasm but only after much time and stimulation; feeling like having an orgasm but not ejaculating; having a painful orgasm
- *Satisfaction:* Whether having a sexual difficulty or not, is there satisfaction with the sexual experience? If not, why?

SELF-ASSESSMENT: ERECTION DIFFICULTIES

Is there a previous history of similar sexual problems? Is there sufficient physical and/or psychological stimulation to cause an erection? Is the achieved erection firm enough to accomplish penetration? Is the difficulty getting and maintaining an erection related to all sexual activity or just related to a specific type of sexual activity (i.e., intercourse, masturbation, or oral sex)? Are there erections present upon awakening in the morning or during the night? Is the erection difficulty a general problem, or is it related to a specific partner or situation?

Health and lifestyle issues include the following: Is he taking any drugs or medications? Does he have any health conditions related to sexual functioning? Is there related personal or relationship stress? How confident is he about getting and keeping an erection? Is any significant anxiety currently interfering with his performance? Has he developed other sexual difficulties as a result of ED? Are there any current difficulties with anxiety, depression, or other mental health issues that could account for sexual dysfunction?

SELF-ASSESSMENT: EJACULATION DIFFICULTIES

The questions are similar to those about erectile functioning. They relate to the circumstances under which the difficulty may or may not be present, as well as medical, lifestyle, personal, and relationship stress.

Rapid Ejaculation (PE)

How long has he had the difficulty? How frequently is he able to control his ejaculation? Is it inadvertent and rapid? Does the time to ejaculation vary greatly? How often is he able to control his ability to ejaculate? Does PE occur even with minimal stimulation? Is it more likely to occur after periods of sexual abstinence? Does ejaculation time vary with the type of sexual stimulation received (e.g., intercourse, oral, or manual stimulation)? Is he focusing on genital pleasure in order to gain ejaculatory control? Attempts at distracting oneself from experiencing sexual feelings is a common mistake men make and does not lead to ejaculatory control. After all, how sexually pleasurable is thinking about baseball or doing times tables during sexual activity? Is the difficulty causing distress for the man or his partner?

Delayed Ejaculation (DE)

Is there a pattern of a delay of orgasm following a reasonable period of stimulation and arousal? Is the delay limited to specific sexual activities, partners, or situations? Are there any special or favorite types of penile self-stimulation and arousal practices that are not being duplicated when with a partner? Is he taking any current medications that might interfere with orgasm and ejaculation? Does the difficulty cause distress for the man and/or his partner?

SEEKING PROFESSIONAL ADVICE

Many men and their partners do not know where to turn for assistance with sexual problems. The causes and continuation of sexual difficulties may be related to a combination of physical, psychological, relational, medical, and lifestyle issues. When attempting to sort out these possible factors, a good place to begin is with an informed health provider who can rule out any medical conditions and medication side effects. Not all practitioners are comfortable asking questions and giving advice about sexual concerns. However, with the advent of new medications for ED and the attention that sexual dysfunctions are getting in the media, today's health practitioners are used to hearing about the sexual complaints of their patients.

A more detailed explanation about treatment will be presented in other chapters in this volume. Basic intervention will involve the primary physician or urologist taking a history of the sexual complaint. Additional information may be obtained thought tests (e.g., hormone levels). An initial intervention may involve using a sample of or prescription for one of the new oral agents for ED. A trial on ED medication will provide a diagnostic clue and may be all the patient needs to resume sexual functioning. It is worth mentioning that it is helpful to involve the partner in the discussion of treatment options.

Even if the health provider makes the correct diagnosis and provides the correct medication, the intervention may not be sufficient. Many men and their partners require further intervention beyond prescribed medication in order to improve sexual functioning. Relationship stress, which either may have caused or resulted from the sexual problem, may still be a source of discord, even if sexual functioning is improved. It may be incomplete treatment to provide medication to a man who has had a sexual dysfunction for years and remains quite anxious about his lovemaking skills or perhaps doesn't get along with his partner. In such cases, a referral to a licensed mental health therapist trained in sexual counseling is wise. The health practitioner may regularly refer to a therapist trained in treating sexual and relationship matters, or one can be found through national professional organizations, who certify the specialty. A reliable source of referral for names of certified sex therapists is the American Association of Sexuality Educators, Counselors and Therapists (AASECT; www.aasect.org).

Case Example: Tom and Dianne had endured his chronic erectile problems for years. He was embarrassed to speak to his doctor but was motivated to do so by a television commercial for a new impotence drug. Following an evaluation after which no physical cause was found, his doctor gave him a sample of the new medicine. But it didn't work. When Tom told his doctor, he was referred to a clinical psychologist who specialized in sex therapy. After a few visits, it became apparent that it was Tom's anxiety about performance that was overriding the effects of the medicine. With further counseling, he restored his confidence to the point that medication was no longer needed.

COMPREHENSIVE TREATMENT: DEALING WITH PERFORMANCE ANXIETY AND SPECTATORING

Sexual problems take their toll on each partner and the total relationship. In order for treatment to be comprehensive, thorough, and unlikely to be followed by future relapse, a cooperative approach between professionals is often indicated. If there are no medical causes or complications, then referral to a sex therapist may be the treatment of choice. If there are medical conditions or medications that need to be monitored, then the therapist and health provider can collaborate in treatment. Let's examine the role of the therapist.

The therapist can assist with identifying the personal and interpersonal variables that contribute to the development and continuation of the sexual dysfunction. This would include explaining what behaviors, emotions, feelings, types of negative thoughts, upsetting images, relationship issues, and life stresses were and still are involved as a negative influence on sexual functioning. These usually involve thoughts and feelings about sexual failure and disappointment that generate considerable anticipatory anxiety about future performance.

The self-doubt and shame that results from sexual dysfunction results in and can be further exacerbated by performance anxiety. If we use ED as an example, performance anxiety can increase with each potential sexual encounter. If failure is the result, the anxiety intensifies, even to the point of panic. This pattern may continue until he withdraws from sexual activity as a way of avoiding failure. Performance anxiety is a powerful mechanism that can affect men and women and can interfere with all levels of the sexual response cycle. Its presence and influence should not be underestimated.

Automatic negative thinking about imagined failure leads to becoming a spectator to one's own sexual activities. A man may begin to critically watch his performance during sex, instead of participating in the flow of enjoyment with his partner. He may be wondering, "How am I doing? Am I hard enough? What is my partner thinking? I better hurry up before I lose it. What if I come too soon?" Engaging in spectatoring is completely counterproductive and like its twin, performance anxiety, needs to be tamed in order to return to healthy functioning. It leads to catastrophizing (e.g., Wouldn't it be awful if I failed again? etc.). Fortunately, these worrisome barriers to sexual performance can be addressed through relaxation exercises to cope with anxiety, the use of positive

---

Case Example: Mike was an intelligent man, except when it came to his understanding of sexual performance. He had been under significant stress lately in his work as a trial lawyer. Sex had always been a good outlet for him to release the tension. Recently, he had an erection failure that took him by surprise. His wife understood that he was under pressure at work, but he did not accept this fact as an excuse. He began to worry about what would happen the next time. In fact he thought about it during the day. Sure enough, it happened again. Now he was really worried. The more he tried not to worry, the more anxious he became. He was in good health, so his erection problems were self-generated. It was as simple as that. He needed help and would seek it.

self-talk to counter the negative thinking that accompanies spectatoring, and the practice of using corrective imagery practice to see oneself functioning well instead of failing.

There are times when just the intention of enjoying being sexual is not enough. We have mentioned how a man's past personal and sexual history serve as a foundation for his later sexual behavior and functioning. Even in otherwise emotionally healthy men, negative and unresolved attitudes about sexuality, experiencing sexual feelings, and engaging in sexual behavior may be at the basis for a current sexual difficulty. In other words, sexual shame, guilt, and ambivalence are often at odds in a man trying to let go and enjoy natural sexual feelings and arousal. These underlying feelings can be dealt with in counseling, as can negative attitudes and anger or resentment about women, and the confusion of sexual passion with aggression. A history of having been physically or sexually abused may serve as a cause for sexual dysfunction. There may be other potential causes, many of which can be addressed once they are made known.

We said that sexuality resides within the relationship. Oftentimes, discoveries are made in the course of counseling that many nonsexual issues may have contributed to a problem. Therapists often state that sexual dysfunction is a couple's issue. There is no such a thing as an uninvolved partner. Again, the spouse of a man with a sexual dysfunction can be affected in various ways. Even the most loving and supportive partner has strong feelings about the problem and will react to them. These factors must be given respectful consideration, especially if an actual relationship conflict is present. Unmet expectations and residual anger from nonsexual events and issues in the marriage are often a component of the sexual complaint and must be addressed in the healing process. Nothing is more helpful to a successful treatment outcome than a cooperative and supportive partner. Conversely, an angry partner can present a barrier to sexual recovery. Sexual pharmacology has no cure for that. Rather, counseling offers the opportunity for growth and mutuality.

Finally, it is important to keep in mind that restoring healthy sexual functioning is not the same as fixing the relationship. A man may have a renewed ability to get an erection or have better control of ejaculation, but he may still have issues with his partner that interfere with relating to her as a sexual partner. The same can be said for his partner's feelings about him. She may not be very pleased at all that she must now be available to him and to his renewed potency. Relationship conflict issues often escape the awareness of health care providers whose main interest is the restoration of healthy physical functioning. It is important to attend to both the sexual problems and the relationships issues. It is wise to include professional sexuality and couples counseling as part of a comprehensive treatment approach.

Case Example: Joe was hard to get along with. He had a drinking problem and was at times verbally abusive to his wife, Helen. Their sex life was not satisfying to Helen. In fact, she was a bit relieved that his drinking was affecting his potency. But a visit to his doctor changed that. The new erection drug enabled him to be his old potent self again. He was happy, but Helen was less than pleased. His drinking and verbal abuse continued. But his erections were now reliable. Was this couple really helped by the simple intervention of providing medication?

RELATIONSHIP BUILDING AND AVOIDING RELAPSE

Sexual health usually flourishes in healthy relationships. We live out our sexual lives in partnership, even if partners come and go. With each new relationship, we bring ourselves and our own style along. Not only our sexual scripts but also the patterns of relating that we observed in our family of origin, as well as experiences gained from earlier relationships, affect who we are and how we relate to a partner. Men are not always the best judges as to what makes a relationship work. As a generalization, many women would say that men remain clueless about intimacy. To some extent, male culture does not sufficiently prepare men to deal with intimate relationships and communicate well, either as a giver or receiver. Miscommunication and being or feeling misunderstood is one of the biggest minefields in stressed intimate relationships. Good intentions are not enough. Effective communication is a skill, and skill building takes practice . . . for both partners. Chapter 7, volume 1 discusses effective communication skills.

Intimacy means different things to different people. For some, intimacy is understood as a total togetherness, an absolute overlap. This idealized notion can leave little freedom for the self and can be smothering for either or both partners. On the other hand, too much distance can lead to feeling disconnected from one's mate. As with many things in life, a balance between the two extremes seems to provide the environment needed to grow in a relationship, both as individuals and as committed partners. Couples need to work this out, because dissatisfaction in understanding what constitutes intimate living together is often reflected in sexual ways. An unhappy partner is not a very sexy partner.

Sexual expression in a relationship is a way partners connect and can be an expression of passion, love, recreation, indifference, mutual consent, or even exploitation. Emotions are also released or demonstrated in sex. Joy, anger, sadness, grief, or fear of loss or separation may be commonly expressed over

Case Example: Matt and Ellen were a happily married couple, at least until the first baby was born. With a two-career household and a baby, Ellen felt pressure to keep the household going. Matt was not too concerned about Ellen's dealing with the many demands of so-called women's work. He had seen his mom juggle the same responsibilities when he was at home. Like his dad, he enjoyed fishing and hunting and had plenty of tickets to sporting events. He was unprepared for Ellen's complaints about his lack of sharing in family responsibilities. He didn't get it. She became moody and not much fun. Sex became routine, and he noticed that he had trouble keeping an erection during sex. He blamed Ellen for not being exciting enough. He stayed out even more. Things did not get better between them.

the course of a sexual relationship. And it will mean different things over the course of a relationship. Again, the quality of the sexual experience will depend on the quality of the relationship.

What makes a good relationship? Following are some guidelines for relationships that respect the rights of both partners and that serve as a foundation for further growth. Not every relationship will have all these characteristics, but they are all possibilities one should consider. Is the relationship, in both its sexual and nonsexual aspects:[1]

- Consensual (Are both partners willing participants?)
- Non-exploitive (Is the relationship at the expense of another?)
- Honest (Is it an open and honest sharing?)
- Mutually pleasurable (Is it gratifying for both partners?)
- Other-enriching (Is the genuine well being of the partner being considered?)
- Self-liberating (Is genuine growth and spontaneity possible?)
- Sexually and socially responsible (Is it protecting one another's sexual health and avoiding sexually transmitted infections?) (adapted from Milsten & Slowinski, 2000, p. 278–279)

KEEPING THE EROTIC RELATIONSHIP STRONG

Keeping a relationship healthy takes time and effort. Yes, some may call it work. In this final section, we will address the reader directly with suggestions on how to keep a relationship strong.

Relationships are built on trust, respect, and effective communication. But when it comes to the sexual part of the relationship, couples are always looking for the recipe for good sex. Popular magazines and television shows are filled with tips for hot sex and advice from so-called experts on how to spice up a love life. There is no recipe except to find out what works for each partner. As we said before, good sex is what you and your partner feel good about afterward. You decide. Knowing what is "normal" and how the body functions is fine, but it is the subjective feeling of satisfaction about one's sex life that is the final judge. That does not mean that it is not helpful to increase sexual knowledge and enhance lovemaking skills. Those efforts often do result in mutual enjoyment along the way. Fortunately, there are accurate and helpful educational materials available today that have helped many men and women enhance their sexual experience. But trying to live up to standards of unrealistic performance, such as the exploits of actors in porn videos or erotic literature, can not only be frustrating but also unfair to men and their partners.

How does one keep the "erotic pot bubbling" in a relationship that is stressed by the many demands of family and professional life? We know that little things mean a lot in a relationship. A surprise gift of flowers or an occasional gentle touch or an affectionate word can go a long way in communicating that we care.

There are some essential ingredients in keeping a relationship going and creating an environment that nurtures an intimate and sexual relationship. The four ingredients are *time, talk, trust,* and *touch.* We have already mentioned the need for *trust,* and that trusting relationship goes beyond sexual fidelity. Relationships need *time* in order to stay connected. Men may feel that they can still have a good sexual relationship in spite of a busy schedule. They just do it when they can. Many women, on the other hand, complain that they need more general time with their partners in order to enjoy sex "when they get around to it." They don't like feeling they have a stranger in their bed.

Perhaps you have read the reports about how little time contemporary couples spending *talking.* "Don't forget to pickup the dry cleaning" doesn't count. Talking keeps couples connected, especially when it involves sensitivity and intimate topics. Set time (there is that word again) aside for one another. Your love life may start improving.

The importance of *touch* cannot be underestimated (see chapters 3 and 4, volume 1). Infants and mothers know the importance of intimate and loving touch. It bonds them together. The same is true for adults. Unfortunately, many men limit their touching to attempts at being erotic. It can give the impression to their partners that touching for sexual contact is all men are about. While women may enjoy erotic attention, they know there is more to being touched than initiating sexual contact. Nonerotic touching, even small affectionate gestures, keep partners connected. These touches also serve to keep the pot bubbling for future lovemaking when the time is right.

STAYING SEXUALLY HEALTHY AND AVOIDING DYSFUNCTION

We have stressed that sexual health is an integration of the mind, body, and relationships. How men think about their sexuality will in part determine their attitudes about performance and inadvertently influence the creation of sexual difficulties. Our thinking about something influences how we feel about it. There are times when "feeling bad" is directly related to "thinking bad." For example, having negative thoughts about performance can lead to feeling anxious and fearfully avoidant.

This relates to what we stated earlier, that sexual functioning and relationships are negatively influenced by fear, shame, false beliefs, ignorance, and unrealistic expectations. The stresses of modern life as well as unhealthy lifestyles can also have an impact on sexual functioning.

Some men aren't sure what turns them on or how they feel, and many of those who do know have trouble expressing it. Self-awareness and communication are never out of fashion in maintaining a good sexual relationship. Some men know what they like and want sexually but are hesitant to say or ask because they are embarrassed that their partner may not agree. A trusting relationship with the partner includes being able to discuss sexual interests and preferences. Good sex flourishes in a trusting relationship.

Case Example: Tim was raised in a conservative home and married Cindy, who came from a similar background. Neither came into the marriage with much sexual experience. They enjoyed sex, but Tim came to see it as "plain vanilla" sex. He had recently been exposed to adult erotica while visiting a couple with whom had had been close friends in college. To his surprise, the couple openly shared with him their enjoyment of watching adult videos together. They said he and Cindy should try it. It would spice up their sex life. Tim really wanted to tell Cindy about it but felt embarrassed and concerned that she might think "he was some sort of a pervert." Tim never asked, and he never knew what Cindy thought about it. The so-called plain vanilla sex did continue, and with it, his dissatisfaction.

What leads to sexual satisfaction? Is it performance or pleasure? Some would say performance leads to pleasure. It is not always the case. Performance, in terms of rock-hard erections and excellent ejaculatory control may be a goal for many men, but that alone does not guarantee sexual satisfaction. Men could avoid considerable unhappiness with their sex lives if they focused on the pleasure of being with their partners rather than a standard or goal that they must achieve in order for sex to be considered good or satisfying. Focusing on "successful" intercourse as the goal in sex has led to disappointment for many men and their partners. If performance is what sex is all about, then these men are missing out on the joys of *outercourse*, the focus on just plain pleasure and enjoyment. *Outercourse* is a term used by sex therapist Marty Klein and relationship expert Riki Robbins in their book *Let Me Count the Ways* (1998). It avoids the race to intercourse and the focus on partner orgasm. There is no goal but to share mutual pleasure. For some men, foreplay is becoming a lost art. Just ask their partners.

If a man has successfully been treated for a sexual dysfunction, he must be cautious about repeating a pattern that contributed to his initial sexual problems. If there were active health concerns, he should continue to follow medical advice. Lifestyle changes, (e.g., quitting smoking) should be maintained. Relationship problems should be attended to before they fester. Finally, there is a need to remain realistic about his sexual behavior and expectations. He knows that there are times when it is unwise to attempt being sexual. He learned what being too tired or too stressed could to do his functioning. A failure under those circumstances should not surprise him. It may result in a dent in his ego but is not a problem.

If a man experiences a single episode of difficulty, be it erectile failure or ejaculation difficulty, he should not panic. These things happen from time to time and are not a big deal. He has not lost all that he has gained. He should avoid panic and not get into a frenzy of performance anxiety. His penis will work again, if he lets it. A supportive partner will be a great benefit at these times. If the sexual difficulty is more than occasional, he may benefit from a booster session with his therapist or a visit to his doctor to check if a recent organic problem has developed. If he had an organic basis to his original problem, an adjustment in his medication might be all that is needed to restore both confidence and functioning.

Case Example: Jim had successfully dealt with a bout of premature ejaculation. He had consulted an excellent sex therapist who conducted a detailed evaluation on him and taught him techniques to control both his anxiety and ejaculation. Treatment was so successful that he was able to discontinue the medication that was prescribed to aid in inhibiting his ejaculation. Both Jim and his wife were pleased. He was unprepared for the rapid ejaculation that occurred one weekend. He began to panic, and the problem became worse with each intercourse attempt. He knew what he was doing wrong but did not know why it happened.

He returned to his therapist, who reassured him this was a temporary setback. Jim had been enjoying sex so much recently that he failed to continue to monitor his arousal level as he had been instructed to. The situation improved, and Jim learned a valuable lesson.

FINAL TIPS

Here is some advice that a man can follow to obtain and maintain a healthy outlook. This advice will help him to relax and enjoy his sexuality and reduce the chance of sexual performance problems (Milsten & Slowinski, 2000, p. 268):

- Be realistic about expectations for yourself and your partner.
- Be aware of distortions in your thinking about making love and about being open to sexual pleasure.
- Examine any unresolved notions about sex being bad, dirty, or sinful, and how these attitudes may reflect on your feelings about women and their enjoyment of sex.
- Look for ways that might be distracting yourself during sexual activity, and inn the process reducing your arousal level.
- Beware of rushing through foreplay just to get to the main event. You could be missing meaningful pleasure and arrive at attempting penetration while insufficiently aroused. In other words, enjoy the pleasures of "outercourse" before moving to intercourse.
- Examine feelings about the partner that might be acting as a turn-off.
- Finally, and generally, examine your sexual script for messages, attitudes, and behaviors that need attention and changing.

CONCLUDING THOUGHTS

The trend today is to initially manage male sexual dysfunction from a medical perspective. Often, that is all that is needed to resume satisfactory functioning. It is true that advances in medical treatment have been an enormous benefit to millions of men and their partners. But in order for treatment to be comprehensive, attention must still be paid to the various psychological and relationship aspects of male sexuality. Sexual behavior does not occur in a vacuum. Each man brings his own learning as well as behavioral and emotional history into his sexual life. The same is true of a man's sexual partners. Sex is not simple. The path to maintaining sexual health begins with prevention. Enjoy the journey.

NOTE

1. Another recommended resource is Gottman and Silver (2000).

REFERENCES

Frank, E. (1978). Frequency of sexual dysfunction in normal couples. *New England Journal of Medicine,. 299,* 111–115.

Gottman, J., & Silver, N. (2000). *The seven principles for making marriage work.* New York: Crown Publishers.

Klein, M., & Robbins, R. (1998). *Let me count the ways.* New York: Tarcher/Putnam.

LoPiccolo, J. (1992). Postmodern sex therapy for erectile dysfunction. In R. Rosen & S. Leiblum (Eds.), *Erectile disorders, assessment and treatment* (pp. 171–197). New York: Guilford Press.

Milsten, R., & Slowinski, J. (2000). *The sexual male: Problems & solutions.* New York: W. W. Norton.

Simon, W., & Gagnon, J. (1986). Sexual scripts, permanence & change. *Archives of Sexual Behavior, 15,* 99–120.

Zilbergeld, B. (1999, revised edition). *The new male sexuality.* New York: Bantam Books.

Chapter Three

PHARMACOLOGICAL TREATMENT OF MALE ERECTILE DYSFUNCTION

Tarek Anis, Rany Shamloul, and Hussein Ghanem

This chapter will describe the pharmacological treatment options for erectile dysfunction (ED) currently available or under development. We will start by going over peripherally acting drugs, since these are usually the options one would first consider. Then we will describe centrally acting (in the brain) drugs, followed by those that act both peripherally and centrally. The chapter ends by summarizing recent research that focuses on developing novel ways of treating ED.

PERIPHERALLY ACTING DRUGS

PDE 5 Inhibitors

Since the introduction of sildenafil (Viagra) in 1998, the first marketed phosphodiesterase 5 (PDE5) inhibitor, treatment of ED has been dramatically transformed. Vardenafil (Levitra) and tadalafil (Cialis) are now also available, and other PDE5 inhibitors are in various stages of development. Novel administration methods of approved PDE5 inhibitors are also under development (e.g., nasal inhalation).

Mechanism of Action

Erectile function is dependent on the normal hemodynamic processes that are mediated by the integration of the central and peripheral nervous systems (see Volume 2, chapter 5). For smooth muscle relaxation and vasodilation of the *corpus cavernosum* to occur, nitric oxide must be released by both the endothelium and nerves supplying the cavernous tissue (Kandeel, Koussa & Swerdloff, 2001). The release of nitric oxide via the cytosolic enzyme, guanylate cyclase, catalyzes the production of cyclic guanosine monophosphate (cGMP). This results in decreased intracellular calcium levels, thereby promoting relaxation of cavernosal smooth muscle. Increased penile blood flow ensues, sinusoidal spaces expand, and venous outflow is occluded, resulting in erection.

There are currently 11 different families of PDE isoenzymes that have been identified (Rosen & Kostis, 2003). PDE5 is the isoenzyme primarily responsible for the degradation and inactivation of cGMP. Inhibition of this enzyme increases cavernosal cGMP, which further augments smooth muscle relaxation and vasodilation, thus potentiating penile erection (Corbin, 2004). Sildenafil, tadalafil, and vardenafil selectively inhibit PDE5, thereby contributing to the induction and/or persistence of erection.

Although all three agents are highly selective for PDE5, they inhibit PDE5 activity at different plasma concentrations, have different duration of enzyme inhibition, and vary in their degree of selectivity toward other PDE isoforms. This degree of varying selectivity for other isoforms assists in explaining some of the adverse effects associated with PDE5 inhibitors (Gresser & Gleiter, 2002). For example, visual disturbances are related to the inhibition of PDE6, which is located in the retina, and the inhibition of PDE11 is theorized to be responsible for myalgia (muscle pain) and back pain (Meueleman, 2003). The duration of action is, respectively, 4–8 hours (sildenafil), 2–8 hours (vardenafil), and 24–36 hours (tadalafil) (Gresser & Gleiter, 2002).

Contraindications

When taking PDE5 inhibitors, it is important to avoid drugs (such as nitroglycerin, isosorbide dinitrate, and isosorbide mononitrate) or other agents (such as amylnitrate or poppers) that contain nitrates. This is due to the fact that these drugs would interfere with each other, resulting in a potentially dangerous drop in blood pressure. Therefore, at the present time, the use of organic nitrates (including only occasional short-acting sublingual nitroglycerin) is an absolute contraindication to the prescription of the PDE5 inhibitors.

Some patients with a diagnosis of coronary artery disease (CAD) who do not develop ischemia (often they have had revascularization procedures such as percutaneous coronary interventions or coronary artery bypass grafting) continue to carry nitroglycerin, when it may not be needed. If these patients have ED, it may be worth evaluating their true need for nitrates, which may include an exercise stress test. If it is deemed that nitrates are not needed, these agents could be discontinued, and a trial of PDE5 inhibition initiated.

In the event that a man develops angina during sexual activity after having taken a PDE5 inhibitor, he should stop sexual activity, and if the pain does not resolve in a few minutes seek emergency care. It is crucial that he communicates to his care providers that he has taken a PDE5 inhibitor so that nitroglycerin or other organic nitrates would not be given for anginal relief (Jackson, Rosen, Kloner, & Kostis, 2006). If the chest pain is angina, then nonnitrate antianginal/anti-ischemic agents (beta-blockers, calcium channel blockers, aspirin, oxygen, morphine, heparin, statin, others) may be administered (Cheitlin et al., 1999).

If a PDE5 inhibitor has been taken, when is it safe to readminister nitrates? If the patient has taken a short-acting PDE5 inhibitor (sildenafil or vardenafil—half-life about 4 hours) nitrates can be restarted 24 hours after the last PDE5 dose (Cheitlin et al., 1999). As tadalafil is a long half-life agent (17.5 hours), a study suggests that at least 48 hours should elapse between the last tadalafil dose and readministration of a nitrate (Kloner et al., 2003). Obviously, each case should first be evaluated individually by the health care provider to assess the risk-benefit for each particular patient.

If a patient develops an acute myocardial infarction while taking PDE5 inhibitors, then the usual therapies such as aspirin, thrombolytics, percutaneous coronary intervention, and antiplatelet agents may be administered; however, organic nitrates should not be given (Kostis et al., 2005)

Side Effects

When treating ED with PDE5 inhibitors, sometimes some of the other 11 types of PDEs (PDE1 to PDE11) are activated, resulting in side effects. Sildenafil and vardenafil cross-react slightly with PDE6, which is expressed in the retina. This may explain the complaint of some patients that sildenafil causes visual disturbances. Back pain is associated with tadalafil, perhaps via cross-reaction with PDE11. Except for visual disturbances, the other reported side effects of PDE5 inhibitors (headaches, flushing, slight lowering of blood pressure) are likely caused by PDE5 inhibition in smooth muscle tissues outside the penile *corpus cavernosum* (Padma-Nathan et al., 2004).

Precautions

Recently, the prescribing information for both vardenafil and tadalafil that addresses the use of these agents in combination with α-adrenergic antagonists (used in the treatment for enlarged prostate) was updated. Prior to this revision, the use of vardenafil in combination with α-adrenergic antagonists was contraindicated. Similarly, the administration of tadalafil in patients taking α-adrenergic antagonists, other than tamsulosin (0.4 mg once daily), was also contraindicated. The revised package insert for both vardenafil and tadalafil now recommends caution during coadministration with α-blockers due to the possible occurrence of symptomatic hypotension (low blood pressure).

For patients currently stabilized on α-adrenergic antagonist therapy, it is advised that vardenafil or tadalafil be initiated at the lowest recommended starting dose. Likewise, when initiating α-adrenergic antagonist therapy in patients whose vardenafil or tadalafil therapy is already stabilized at a specific dose, the lowest possible starting dose should be prescribed, and dosage titration should be closely monitored. Recommendations regarding the coadministration of sildenafil with α-adrenergic antagonists remains unchanged. Specifically, the administration of sildenafil in doses greater than 25 mg should be postponed for at least 4 hours after taking any α-adrenergic antagonist.

Drug Interactions

The PDE5 compounds also are susceptible to pharmacokinetic interactions caused by drugs that induce or inhibit their metabolism. The PDE5 agents all appear to be primarily metabolized in the liver. Drugs that interfere with PDE5 metabolism include cimetidine, erythromycin, the HIV protease inhibitors saquinavir and ritonavir, as well ketoconazole or itraconazole. While all of these drugs increase plasma levels of PDE inhibitors, the reverse (decreased plasma levels) are found when the drug rifampicin has been taken.

When sildenafil or vardenafil is taken with a high-fat meal, the rate of absorption is delayed. Men also should be warned against consuming alcohol in large quantities, as the potential for additive hypotensive effects may be of concern for some patients. Tadalafil pharmacokinetics are not affected by the presence of food or alcohol, and the pharmacokinetics of alcohol are not affected by tadalafil. However, patients should be cautioned not to consume excessive quantities of alcohol in combination with tadalafil as this can increase the potential for orthostatic signs and symptoms including increased heart rate, decreased standing blood pressure, dizziness, and headache.

New PDE5 Inhibitors

Two novel PDE5 inhibitors are currently under development. Prince, Campbell, and Tong (2005) recently reported the results from a multi-institutional, study of the preliminary safety and tolerability of SLx-2101, a new long-acting PDE5 inhibitor. The other drug is avanafil, a new, highly specific and rapidly metabolized PDE5 inhibitor with an ultrashort duration of action (Kaufman and Dietrich 2005).

Local Treatment of ED

The concept of local treatments of ED is found far back in history in the Arabian, Greek, and Roman worlds when all sorts of ointments, herbs, and medications were applied locally to the genitals to enhance so-called vigor. The modern era started with the development of artificial erection as a tool for the diagnosis of ED. Virag (1985) reported improvements after sessions of provoked erections with saline in patients with arterial impotence (arterial impotence means that the ED is due to impaired blood supply to the penis, as opposed to venous leakage, for example).

Artificial erections were first used therapeutically by injection of mixed saline and vasoactive agents (papaverine and saline) to enhance natural erections. Then emerged the concept of self-injection therapy (Zorgniotti & Lefleur, 1985). Several drug combinations have increased the overall efficacy rate of injection therapy to as high as 90 percent of the ED population. Automatic injection improved the acceptance of the technique. The use of adrenergic agents to reduce the risk of priapism and a better knowledge of the medications and their dosage have made the technique safer and more effective (Virag, 1985).

Finally, until the recent appearance of effective oral medications, intracavernous injection therapy (ICI) was the most frequently used treatment for ED. Its long-term use is challenged by a high drop-out rate, whose reasons have never been fully explained.

Intracavernosal Injection Therapy (ICI)

Patients with either failed or contraindicated oral therapy for ED (e.g., patients already taking nitrates, or those with heart failure) should be offered the second-line treatment of ED, intracavernosal vasoactive drug injection (also known as ICI). The characteristics, potential limitations, and adverse effects of the treatment should be explained to the patient (Montorsi et al., 2002). The patient is asked to read and sign an informed consent form. Patients with a history of hemoglobinopathy, bleeding diathesis, Peyronie's disease, or idiopathic priapism are excluded from treatment. In addition, patients with poor manual dexterity (use of their hands), poor visual acuity, or morbid obesity or those in whom a transient hypotensive episode may have a deleterious effect (for example, unstable cardiovascular disease and transient ischemic attack) are not ideal candidates for this treatment (Montorsi et al., 2002). Finally, patients with serious psychiatric disorders or patients who might misuse or abuse this therapy should be excluded from treatment.

The first phase of the program consists of the dose titration of the drug or mixture used for injections. Since individuals respond differently to these injections, the exact dosage needs to be determined in each case. Patients are placed in the sitting position on the examination couch during each injection and kept in this position for 30 minutes. Systemic blood pressure is recorded at baseline in the event of syncope (fainting) and to check for hypertension. The right side (lateral aspect) of the penis is cleansed with an alcohol swab. The first injection is then performed with a very small amount of either the drug or the mixture. The needle is inserted by a quick jab up to the hilt of the needle so that the tip of it reaches the center of the right *corpus cavernosum*. Injections must not be performed on the dorsal and ventral aspects of the penis to avoid damage to the dorsal neurovascular bundle of the penis and urethra, respectively (to review the anatomy of the male reproductive organs, see volume 2, chapter 6).

Immediately after injection, the base of the penis is squeezed firmly between the right thumb and index finger, while the accessible portion of the penis is massaged for up to 5 minutes by squeezing it laterally along the length of the shaft between the left thumb and index and middle fingers, thus distributing the drug throughout the pendulous shaft. Patients are then left alone to watch an erotic video, and they are invited to masturbate without ejaculation to optimize sexual stimulation. The erectile response is then assessed by the physician and patient.

The dose of the injected drug or mixture is considered adequate when it produces an erection that is equal to 50 to 75 percent of the maximal erectile response reported by the patient. If a patient reaches a maximal rigid erection during the titration phase in the clinic, a lower dose is suggested for home use since the erectile effect induced by the drug or mixture during sexual activity is usually greater than that observed under laboratory conditions (Montorsi et al., 2002). If the first injection does not produce a satisfactory erectile response (that is, less than 50% of the maximal potential response), the patient is reinjected after at least 24 hours, and the dose is slightly increased. The titration process proceeds until the optimal dose is identified or the maximal injected volume (at our clinic, 0.5 mL) is reached. If after the injection a full rigid erection persists for longer than 1 hour, 20–40 mg of adrenaline are injected intracorporeally to obtain complete detumescence. Appropriate electrocardiographic and blood pressure monitoring is used during this procedure.

Patients are contacted by telephone the next day to verify persistence of detumescence. They are instructed to limit injection use to three times a week, with no more than one injection in any 24-hour period. They are also taught to inject the right and left cavernous body alternatively. Patients are then warned to return immediately to the emergency department if erection persists for longer than 3 hours. This condition is called priapism.

Patients are also told to refrigerate the drug or mixture if it contains prostaglandin E1 (PGE1) and to examine the drug or solution for changes in color or the formation of a precipitate. Patients are reassessed once a month for the first two months and subsequently every three months. At each follow-up visit, injection frequency, duration and consistency of erections, and patient satisfaction are recorded. The penis is carefully examined for nodules, hematomas, or areas of induration. Liver function test results are assessed every six months.

The follow-up of approximately 4,000 patients treated worldwide with papaverine alone or in combination with phentolamine has been previously published (Zentgraf, Baccouche, & Junemann, 1988); in addition, long-term results with intracavernous injection therapy based on PGE1 have been reported (Linet & Neff, 1994; Porst, 2000). Reported adverse effects have included hematomas; burning pain after injection; urethral damage; caverno-sitis or local infections; fibrotic changes of the *corpora cavernosa;* curvature; and prolonged erections, or priapism. The two most important complications are prolonged erections and localized fibrotic changes of the *corpora cavernosa.*

Prolonged erections are usually encountered during the dose titration. The development of painless fibrotic nodules within the *corpora cavernosa* may lead to penile curvature. This problem has been reported in 1.5 to 60 percent of patients treated for one year (Zentgraf, Baccouche, & Junemann, 1988).We believe that most of the fibrotic nodules occur in patients who inject them-selves very frequently (multiple traumas to the corporeal tissue) and who do not compress the injection site for a sufficient amount of time, with the sub-sequent development of intracavernous hematomas.

The increase in the frequency of spontaneous erections and the decreased need for treatment are common findings during follow-up of intracavernous vasoactive injection therapy. It has been suggested that the long-term use of PGE1 intracavernous injections is able to markedly improve cavernosal artery function as shown by color Doppler sonography (Wespes, Sattar, Noel, & Schulman, 2000). The improved hemodynamic response seen in patients inject-ing themselves regularly may be explained on a microvascular level. It has been shown that the long-term administration of vasoactive agents in monkeys causes hypertrophy of sinusoidal smooth muscle at the ultrastructural level. Both papaverine and PGE1 lead to a hypertrophic response, but papaverine results in a combination of hypertrophy, atrophy, and fibrosis, whereas with PGE1, the normal cellular architecture is preserved. With the sinusoidal muscle "toned up" after long-term self-injection with PGE1, the efficiency of sinusoidal smooth muscle action may improve, leading to the observed increase in caver-nosal artery flow. In addition, it has been shown that PGE1 may improve the hemodynamic response partly by promoting neovascularization, which means the growth of new blood vessels (Wang & Large, 1991). This issue remains controversial because Wespes and co-workers were unable to demonstrate any significant changes of the intracavernous structure following long-term treat-ment with intracavernosal alprostadil.

Many drugs have been used for intracavernous injection. In the following few paragraphs, we discuss the main characteristics of the most widely used ones. Readers less interested in specific details may want to skip ahead to the next section on intraurethral therapy.

Papaverine

Papaverine hydrochloride is an opium alkaloid that results in intracellular inhibition of phosphodiesterase, which in turn interferes with the calcium ion mobilization, thus facilitating relaxation of smooth muscles in the sinusoids and dilation of helicine arteries (Wang & Large, 1991). In short, it causes erections when injected into the *corpus cavernosum*. Doses ranging from 10 to 60 mg are usually given when papaverine is used as a single agent or in combination with phentolamine alone or with phentolamine and PGE1. Intracavernous injections of papaverine may induce corporeal fibrosis. This is thought to be due to the acidity of papaverine solutions (ranging from 3 to 4 pH).

Reported efficacy rates with doses between 30 and 110 mg varied between 27 and 78 percent and were dependent on dosage and the patient population investigated (Wespes, Rondeux, & Schulman, 1989). A literature analysis of 19 publications that included 2,181 patients overall demonstrated that papaverine produced an average response rate of 61 percent in in-office testing (Porst, 1996). The most important adverse effect was priapism in 3 to 18.5 percent, which mostly occurred during the titration phase. Fibrotic alterations were seen in 5 to 30 percent of patients, with an average of 5.7 percent in 15 retrospective studies (Porst, 1996).

Papaverine is extensively metabolized in the liver, and papaverine-induced hepatotoxicity in the form of increase of liver transaminases and drug-induced hepatitis has been reported (Andersson, Holmquist, & Wagner, 1991). Because of safety concerns, monotherapy with papaverine has been discontinued in most industrialized countries. However, because of its considerably low cost, self-injection monotherapy with papaverine still continues in many developing countries.

Phentolamine and Papaverine-Phentolamine Combination

Phentolamine mesylate is an α1- and α2-adrenergic receptor blocking agent that dilates arterial vessels and abolishes sympathetic inhibition of erection. Lack of effect on venous return by intracavernous phentolamine has been demonstrated both in animal and human studies (Wespes, Rondeux, & Schulman, 1989). Since a single intracavernous phentolamine injection does not produce a satisfactory erectile response, the drug is not used alone but in combination with papaverine and PGE1 (Montorsi et al., 1993).

The most common adverse effects observed after intravenous administration of phentolamine are orthostatic hypotension and tachycardia. Combining the cyclic nucleotide cAMP and cyclic guanosine monophosphate (cGMP) accumulating effects of papaverine and the α-adrenoceptor blocking effects of phentolamine results in an increased average response rate of up to 60 to 70 percent observed during in-office testing. In other words, the two drugs act in separate ways but facilitate each other, both resulting in increased blood flow into the *corpus cavernosum* (i.e., causing erection). With home use, response rates as high as 90 percent have been reported (Montorsi et al., 1993). The global efficacy rate of this combination as evaluated in large retrospective studies is 68.5 percent (Porst, 1996). Frequent adverse effects were similar to those of papaverine. Priapism was reported in 6 to 15 percent, and fibrosis in an average of 12 percent of patients treated.

PGE1 (Alprostadil)

PGE1 has α1-blocking (antagonist) properties mediated through a membrane receptor and relaxes the cavernous and arteriolar smooth muscle while causing restriction of venous outflow. PGE1 produces full erections at doses as low as 2.5 mg. When used as a single agent, the maximal injected dose usually ranges from 30 to 40 mg. PGE1 is the most widely used component of multidrug vasoactive mixtures, which permit a reduction in the doses of the single agents, thus reducing adverse effects (Montorsi et al., 2002). The most frequently reported adverse effect of PGE1 intracavernous injections is local corporeal pain, which occurs in 13–80 percent of the patients and is dose related (occurring more frequently at doses greater than 15 mg).

A review of large studies shows that the efficacy rate of alprostadil during in-office titration varied between 70 and 75 percent in more than 10,000 patients (Wespes, Rondeux, & Schulman, 1989). In a variety of prospective self-injection trials, the success rates (defined as successful vaginal penetration per injection) varied between 89 and 96 percent; this is higher than any reported efficacy rate among all the available marketed vasoactive drugs (Porst, 1996). The positive effect of alprostadil injections on quality of life has been demonstrated (Willke et al., 1997). Clinical and self-reported measurements were used to assess physiological and psychological status at baseline and at 3, 6, 12, and 18 months for 579 patients who entered the self-injection phase of an open-label, flexible-dose clinical trial. It was clear from this study that clinical improvements in erectile function due to alprostadil therapy were associated with improvements in sexual activity, sexual satisfaction, and overall mental health.

Adverse effects seen with alprostadil treatment include the above-mentioned penile pain; priapism, which is seen during the dose titration phase; and corporeal fibrosis, which is encountered in 7.5–11.7 percent of patients during the four to five years of long-term follow-up. Between 33 and 47 percent of penile fibroses healed spontaneously, suggesting that the incidence of persistent penile fibroses in patients undergoing long-term self-injection therapy is between 5 and 7 percent (Porst, 1996).

Moxisylyte

Moxisylyte is known to be a competitive norepinephrine antagonist, acting on postsynaptic α-receptors. (Receptors are located either presynaptically on the nerve ending or postsynaptically on the smooth muscle cell).

In vivo it clearly decreases the spontaneous activity, amplitude, and tone of the contractions of cavernous smooth muscle in dogs, and it relaxes in vitro norepinephrine-contracted corporeal smooth muscle strips (Imagawa, Kimura, & Kawanishi, 1989). The most interesting characteristic of this drug is its very low rate of adverse effects, including priapism (<1%) and fibrosis (<2%). However, in all published moxisylyte trials, clinically relevant drops in blood pressure accompanied by orthostatic symptoms and dizziness were described in 5–8 percent of patients.

Vasoactive Intestinal Polypeptide—Phentolamine Combination and Other Options

Because vasoactive intestinal polypeptide (VIP) injected alone intracorporeally in volunteers did not result in rigid erections, a combination of VIP and phentolamine was developed for self-injection therapy (McMahon, 1996). In a large prospective trial with 289 patients, 77 percent responded with erections considered by the investigators to be sufficient for intercourse (Hackett, 1998). In this study, two cases of priapism (0.6%) were observed. In a large, multi-center study from the UK, an efficacy rate consistently higher than 80 percent was seen in all patient categories, irrespective of the origin of the disease; however, the total drop-out rate was 65 percent, which is considerably higher than in all other alprostadil injection trials.

Calcitonin gene-related peptide (CGRP) relaxes smooth muscle cells by hyperpolarization via potassium channel opening and cAMP stimulation. In patients, intracavernous injections of CGRP induced dose-related increases in penile arterial inflow, cavernous smooth muscle relaxation, cavernous outflow occlusion, and an erectile response.

Linsidomine chloridrate is the active metabolite of the antianginal drug molsidomine, and it is believed to liberate nitric oxide nonenzymatically (nitric oxide donor), which in turn stimulates guanylate cyclase, leading to an increase in the intracellular concentration of cGMP. The injection of 20 mg of PGE1 produced greater erectile effects than 1 mg linsidomine in most patients. The drug safety profile and its low cost make linsidomine an appealing drug for patients responding to the papaverine-phentolamine combination.

Sodium nitroprusside, a nitric oxide donor was evaluated in a comparative trial with alprostadil. In a total of 95 patients, 49 percent responded with partial rigidity and 15 percent with complete rigidity to 300–400 mg doses of nitroprusside, compared with 54 percent and 20 percent, respectively, after 20 mg of alprostadil. With nitroprusside doses of 600 mg, global response rates of 84 percent were achieved. Because alprostadil produced better response rates, and sodium nitroprusside was incriminated with hypotonic blood pressure reactions in up to 15 percent of the patients, this compound did not enter the phase of multicenter trials (Martinez-Pineiro, 1995).

Intraurethral Therapy

Intraurethral therapy is another second-line treatment of ED administered for the same reasons as intracavernosal treatment. Transurethral drug delivery allows the transfer of drugs from the urethra directly into the *corpora cavernosa*. All intraurethral drugs for the enhancement of erections are postulated to work by diffusing from the *corpora spongiosa* (urethra) to the cavernosal spaces. Intraurethral alprostadil has been developed and marketed by Vivus (Menlo Park, CA). The Medicated Transurethral System for Erection (MUSE) consists of a polypropylene applicator with a hollow stem 3.2 cm in length and 3.5 mm in diameter. The tip (measuring 3 or 6 mm in length) contains a semisolid pellet of medication that is available in four dose strengths: 125, 250, 500, and 1000 mg.

Alprostadil is administered while the male is in a sitting or standing position by fully inserting the stem of the applicator into the distal urethra. A button is depressed to deposit the pellet. A gentle rocking of the applicator from side to side will separate the medicated pellet from the applicator tip. The patient should urinate immediately before administration, because the medicated pellet has been developed specifically to dissolve in the small quantity of urine that remains in the urethra after urination. After removing the applicator, massaging the penis for 30–60 seconds allows the compound to spread out and be absorbed fully. Most studies show limited efficacy and patient satisfaction. Discomfort, pain, and burning associated with treatment, as well as cost, made more than 80 percent of patients to discontinue MUSE at home.

Topical Pharmacological Therapy

This group of drugs is uncommonly prescribed as evidence is lacking about their effectiveness. If an effective form is introduced, it would be beneficial particularly to patients who are candidates for second-line treatment of ED but are not comfortable with intracavernosal injection or intraurethral application. This group of medications includes nitroglycerin, minoxidil, papaverine, and PGE1.

CENTRALLY ACTING DRUGS

Apomorphine

Physiological erections are initiated, in large part, by central stimuli. Depending on the type of stimulus, various areas of the cortex are involved, like the occipital region for visual, the rhinencephalic region for olfactory, the thalamic region for tactile, and the limbic region for imaginative stimuli. These and other stimuli from higher centers are sending inputs to hypothalamic nuclei—medial preoptic area (MPOA) and paraventricular nucleus (PVN). PVN is believed to be the nucleus where apomorphine acts as a dopaminergic substance. From the PVN, signals are then transmitted to the brainstem nuclei and then to the periphery of the erectile axis (Bancila et al., 2002).

Apomorphine acts in the PVN of the hypothalamus as a dopamine (D2) receptor agonist. It works as a proerectile conditioner at that level to increase the responses of the erectile pathway following appropriate sexual stimulation.

Apomorphine SL (sublingual) has been approved for marketing in Europe at the doses of 2 and 3 mg. The erectogenic effects are usually seen within 20 minutes its administration; provided there is the presence of an adequate sexual stimulation. The main side effect is nausea, but over time and repeated dosages, it rapidly dissipates. Other side effects with Uprima include headache, dizziness, and flushing.

Contraindications with apomorphine include heart medications (particularly those for hypertension) and, because of potential synergy, any other dopamine agonists such as bromocriptine, hydergine, deprenyl, and L-dopa. Apomorphine has not been FDA approved in the United States.

Trazodone

Trazodone, a serotonin reuptake inhibitor, is a nontricyclic antidepressant that has been associated with prolonged erection and priapism when administered orally in depressive patients. In healthy volunteers, trazodone dose dependently increased nocturnal penile tumescence (NPT) following rapid eye movement (REM) related erections and blocked the detumescence phase of erection, which is under sympathetic control, thereby prolonging the erection (Saenz de Tejada et al., 1991).

Melanotan II

Melanotan II is a synthetic nonselective analog of α-melanocyte–stimulating hormone (α-MSH). α-MSH and adrenocorticotrophin, known as the melanocortins, are implicated in the regulation of sexual behavior including penile erection and sexual motivation (Giuliano, Clement, Droupy, Alexandre, & Bernabe, 2005).

Melanotan II delivered subcutaneously has been reported to initiate penile erection in men without erectile problems as well as men with psychogenic and organic ED (Wessells et al., 1998). It is also noted to significantly increase sexual desire (Wessells, Levine, Hadley, Dorr, & Hruby, 2000). The frequent side effects associated with melanotan II administration are nausea and yawning (Wessells et al., 2000).

Delequamine

Delequamine is a selective α2-adrenoceptor antagonist. α2-adrenoceptors are present on the noradrenergic cell bodies in the locus coeruleus and their pre-synaptic terminals throughout the brain. The central effect of α2-adrenoceptor blockade by delequamine leads to an increased noradrenaline level at the synapse by blocking reuptake into the presynaptic terminal, leading to sexual arousal (Bancroft, Munoz, Beard, & Shapiro, 1995).

During the waking state, normal controls reported significantly higher subjective ratings of sexual arousal before erotic stimulation and increased likelihood of spontaneous erections or significant prolongation of erectile response to visual erotic stimuli following high dose of delequamine (Munoz, Bancroft, & Turner, 1994).

CENTRALLY AND PERIPHERALLY ACTING DRUGS

Yohimbine

Yohimbine is an indole alkaloid from the cortex of the Coryanthe yohimbe tree, which has been claimed to have aphrodisiac activity. The principal pharmacological action of yohimbine is as an α2-adrenoceptor antagonist. α2-adrenoceptors are located both peripherally and centrally, especially in the *locus coeruleus* neurons, which are associated with sexual arousal and response.

Peripherally, pre- and post-junctional α2-adrenoceptors are present in the human penile erectile tissues. Activation of presynaptic α2-adrenoceptors in erectile tissue inhibits the release of noradrenaline at the sympathetic nerve endings, hence reducing the sympathetic transmission (Molderings, Engel, Roth, & Gothert, 1989).

When given orally, yohimbine reaches peak levels in 10–15 minutes, and the half-life is 0.6 hours. The efficacy of yohimbine on sexual function has been questioned, perhaps because of early questionable multidrug preparations. Yohimbine has been shown to have some effect on psychologic ED. However, the value of yohimbine in the treatment of erectile failure has been carefully assessed in two separate, systematic reviews and meta-analyses of randomized clinical trials.

The first included four independent but convergent meta-analyses integrating results of trials using yohimbine alone or in combination with other drugs. This extensive and in-depth review, together with a sophisticated statistical evaluation, found a consistent positive effect of yohimbine alone or in combination with other drugs relative to placebo (Carey & Johnson, 1996). The second meta-analytic report focused exclusively on the controlled, randomized studies that used yohimbine alone. In this assessment, the superiority of yohimbine was clearly demonstrated (Ernst & Pittler, 1998).

Side effects include nausea, vomiting, diarrhea, trouble sleeping, and head-ache. Very unlikely side effects include tremor, dizziness, nervousness, anxiety, irritability, fast heartbeat, and painful prolonged erections.

Phentolamine

Phentolamine is a nonselective α-adrenoceptor antagonist with similar affinity for α1- and α2-adrenoceptors. Phentolamine mesylate induced relaxation of *corpus cavernosum* erectile tissue is thought to occur by direct antagonism of α1- and α2-adrenoceptors, as well as by indirect functional antagonism via a nonadrenergic, endothelium-mediated mechanism, sug-gesting nitric oxide synthase activation (Vemulapalli & Kurowski, 2001). The clinical utility of phentolamine is presumably a reflection of the contribution of adrenergic neurotransmission to the maintained flaccidity of the penis, and thus, inhibition of α-adrenoceptor activity alone may be sufficient for erection to commence. Oral / intracavernosal phentolamine may therefore facilitate penile erection by inhibiting the functional predominance of α1-adrenoceptor activity that maintains erectile tissues in a nonerect state. Attenuation of the opposing adrenergic contractile response enhances nitric oxide-mediated *cor-pus cavernosum* relaxation. Furthermore, phentolamine may delay detumes-cence, which is mediated by noradrenaline, contributing to the maintenance of penile erection.

OTHER OPTIONS

L-Arginine

Nitric oxide (NO) is derived from l-arginine by nitric oxide synthase (NOS). L-arginine was found to augment endothelium-dependent vasodi-lation in hypercholesterolemic rabbits and humans (Girerd, Hirsch, Cooke, Dzau, & Creager, 1990). The rationale for l-arginine therapy is related to the supposition that dietary supplementation with NO-precursor l-arginine may normalize endothelium-dependent vasodilation and have a benefi-cial effect on erectile function (Ito, Kawahara, Das, & Strudwick, 1998; Padma-Nathan et al., 2004).

Gene Therapy

The common aim of gene therapy is to introduce new or lost genetic mate-rial into the cells of the target tissue in order to recover the organ's function. Initially, gene therapy was addressing diseases that had an underlying genetic component, trying to repair this primary genetic defect. Meanwhile indica-tions for gene therapy, at least theoretically, have been extended to almost all diseases where a therapeutic gene is identified that is able to restore or support a lost or reduced cellular function.

The penis, or to be more precise the *corpus cavernosum,* as the main effector organ for erection, is a perfect target for gene therapy. It has an anatomically favorable external location with a mainly separated blood circulation system well suited for periodic injections of specific genetic material. A needle-free gene gun has been suggested recently for transcutaneous high-pressure delivery of plasmid DNA to the penis. Additional temporary compression of the penile root to a great extend avoids early entry of the gene products into the systemic circulation. This minimizes unwanted systemic side effects and results in excellent uptake into cavernosal endothelial and smooth muscle cells.

This type of treatment is currently under development, and research focuses on developing gene therapy targeting NOS (Chancellor et al., 2003; Christ, 2003; Magee, Davila, Ferrini, Raijfer, & Gonzalez-Cadavid, 2003).

General concerns with NOS gene therapy are the relatively short duration of the physiological effect, the unknown side effects of long-term overexpression of NO, and, finally, the potential of priapism (Christ, 2003). Other researchers are targeting potassium channels (Christ, 2003). This approach looks very promising and safe for clinical application and is currently awaiting FDA approval for phase I clinical trials. Finally, Rho-kinase (Chitaley et al., 2002), which affects smooth muscle contractility; as well as growth factors (Rogers, Jou, Guo, & Lipschutz, 2003); neurotrophic factors (Park, Ahn, Kim, Kim, & Ryu, 2003); and stem cells (Bochinski et al., 2004; Deng et al., 2003) are currently being investigated for gene therapy.

In the last decade, pharmacological approaches for treatment of erectile dysfunction have revolutionized our understanding of the physiology of erection. Drugs like sildenafil, tadalafil, and vardenafil have to a great extent helped improve the sexual lives of many men who otherwise had no option but invasive surgeries for their erectile dysfunction disease. Not very long ago, an effective scientific-based therapy for erectile dysfunction seemed rather unattainable. Now, with the advent of new pharmacological agents and the very rapid development in genetic therapeutic approaches, the long-awaited cure of erectile dysfunction seems, at least, imaginable.

REFERENCES

Andersson, K. E., Holmquist, F., & Wagner, G. (1991). Pharmacology of drugs used for treatment of erectile dysfunction and priapism. *International Journal of Impotence Research, 3,* 155–172.

Bancila, M., Giuliano, F., Rampin, O., Mailly, P., Brisorgueil, M. J., Calas, A., & Verge, D. (2002). Evidence for a direct projection from the paraventricular nucleus of the hypothalamus to putative serotoninergic neurons of the nucleus paragigantocellularis involved in the control of erection in rats. *The European Journal of Neuroscience, 16*(7), 1240–1248.

Bancroft, J., Munoz, M., Beard, M., & Shapiro, C. (1995). The effects of a new alpha-2 adrenoceptor antagonist on sleep and nocturnal penile tumescence in normal male volunteers and men with erectile dysfunction. *Psychosomatic Medicine, 57,* 345–356.

Bochinski, D., Lin, G. T., Nunes, L., Carrion, R., Rahman, N., Lin, C. S., & Lue, T. F. (2004). The effect of neural embryonic stem cell therapy in a rat model of cavernosal nerve injury. *BJU International, 94,* 904–909.

Carey, M. P., & Johnson, B. T. (1996). Effectiveness of yohimbine in the treatment of erectile disorder: Four meta-analytic integrations. *Archives of Sexual Behavior, 25*(4), 341–360.

Chancellor, M. B., Tirney, S., Mattes, C. E., Tzeng, E., Birder, L. A., Kanai, A. J., de Groat, W. C., Huard J., & Yoshimura, N. (2003). Nitric oxide synthase gene transfer for erectile dysfunction in a rat model. *BJU International, 91,* 691–696.

Cheitlin, M. D., Hutter, A.M.J., Brindis, R. G., Ganz, P., Kaul, S., Russell, R. O. Jr., & Zusman, R. M. (1999). Use of sildenafil (Viagra) in patients with cardiovascular disease. Technology and Practice Executive Committee, *Circulation 99*(1), 168–177.

Chitaley, K., Bivalacqua, T. J., Champion, H. C., Usta, M. F., Hellstrom, W. J., Mills, T. M., & Webb, R. C. (2002). Adeno-associated viral gene transfer of dominant negative RhoA enhances erectile function in rats. *Biochemical and Biophysical Research Communications, 298,* 427–432.

Christ, G. J. (2003). Frontiers in gene therapy for erectile dysfunction. *International Journal of Impotence Research, 15*(Suppl. 5), S33–40.

Corbin, J. D. (2004). Mechanisms of action of PDE5 inhibition in erectile dysfunction. *International Journal of Impotence Research, 16*(Suppl. 1), S4–7.

Deng, W., Bivalacqua, T. J., Chattergoon, N. N., Hyman, A. L., Jeter, J. R., Jr., & Kadowitz, P. J. (2003). Adenoviral gene transfer of eNOS: High-level expression in ex vivo expanded marrow stromal cells. *American Journal of Physiology. Cell Physiology, 285*(5), C1322–1329.

Ernst, E., Pittler, M. H. (1998). Yohimbine for erectile dysfunction: A systematic review and meta-analysis of randomized clinical trials. *Journal of Urology, 159,* 433–436.

Girerd, X. J., Hirsch, A. T., Cooke, J. P., Dzau, V. J., & Creager, M. A. (1990). L-arginine augments endothelium-dependent vasodilation in cholesterol-fed rabbits. *Circulation Research, 67*(6), 1301–1308.

Giuliano, F., Clement, P., Droupy, S., Alexandre, L., & Bernabe, J. (2006). Melanotan-II: Investigation of the inducer and facilitator effects on penile erection in anaesthetized rat. *Neuroscience, 138(1),* 293–301.

Gresser, U., & Gleiter, C. H. (2002). Erectile dysfunction: Comparison of efficacy and side effects of the PDE-5 inhibitors sildenafil, vardenafil and tadalafil—review of the literature. *European Journal of Medical Research, 7*(10), 435–446.

Hackett, G. (1998). The results of a 6 month multi-center placebo-controlled study of InvicorpTM in the treatment of nonpsychogenic erectile dysfunction. *Journal of Urology, 159*: 240. Imagawa, A., Kimura, K., Kawanishi, Y. (1989). Effect of moxisylyte hydrochloride on isolated human penile corpus cavernosum tissue. *Life Sciences, 44,* 619–623.

Ito, T., Kawahara, K., Das, A., & Strudwick, W. (1998). The effects of ArginMax, a natural dietary supplement for enhancement of male sexual function. *Hawaii Medical Journal, 57*(12), 741–744.

Jackson, G., Rosen, R. C., Kloner, R. A., & Kostis, J. B. (2006). The second Princeton consensus on sexual dysfunction and cardiac risk: New guidelines for sexual medicine. *Journal of Sexual Medicine, 3*(1), 28–36.

Kandeel, F. R., Koussa, V. K., & Swerdloff, R. S. (2001). Male sexual function and its disorders: Physiology, pathophysiology, clinical investigation, and treatment. *Endocrine Reviews, 22*(3), 342–388.

Kaufman, J., & Dietrich, J. (2005). Safety and efficacy of avanafil, a new PDE5 inhibitor for treating erectile dysfunction [Abstract]. *Program and abstracts of the Sexual Medicine Society of North America Fall Meeting, New York, NY.* Abstract 68.

Kloner, R. A., Hutter, A. M., Emmick, J. T., Mitchell, M. I., Denne, J., & Jackson, G. (2003). Time course of the interaction between tadalafil and nitrates. *Journal of the American College of Cardiology, 42*(10), 1855–1860.

Kostis, J. B., Jackson, G., Rosen, R., Barrett-Connor, E., Billups, K., Burnett, A. L., et al. (2005). Sexual dysfunction and cardiac risk (the Second Princeton Consensus Conference). *The American Journal of Cardiology, 96*(12B), 85M–93M.

Linet, O. I., Neff, L. L. (1994). Intracavernous prostaglandin E1 in erectile dysfunction. *The Clinical Investigator, 72,* 139–149.

Magee, T., Davila, H. H., Ferrini, M. G., Raijfer, J., & Gonzalez-Cadavid, N. F. (2003). Gene transfer of antisense PIN (protein inhibitor of NOS cDNA) ameliorates aging-related erectile dysfunction in the rat. *Journal of Urology, 169*(4), 305.

Martinez-Pineiro, L. (1995). Preliminary results of a comparative study with intracavernous sodium nitroprusside and prostaglandin E1 in patients with erectile dysfunction. *Journal of Urology, 153,* 1487–1490.

McMahon, C. G. (1996). A pilot study of the role of intracavernous injection of vasoactive intestinal peptide (VIP) and phentolamine mesylate in the treatment of erectile dysfunction. *International Journal of Impotence Research, 8,* 233–236.

Meuleman, E. J. (2003). Review of tadalafil in the treatment of erectile dysfunction. *Expert Opinion on Pharmacotherapy, 4*(11), 2049–2056.

Molderings, G. J., Engel, G., Roth, E., & Gothert, M. (1989). Characterization of an endothelial 5-hydroxytryptamine (5-HT) receptor mediating relaxation of the porcine coronary artery. *Naunyn-Schmiedeberg's Archives of Pharmacology, 340*(3):300–308.

Montorsi, F., Guazzoni, G., Bergamaschi, F., Ferini-Strambi, L., Barbieri, L., & Rigatti, P. (1993). Four-drug intracavernous therapy for impotence due to corporeal venoocclusive dysfunction. *Journal of Urology, 149,* 1291–1295.

Montorsi, F., Salonia, A., Zanoni, M., Pompa, P., Cestari, A., Guazzoni, G., Barbieri, L., & Rigatti, P. (2002). Current status of local penile therapy. *International Journal of Impotence Research, 14*(Suppl. 1), S70–81.

Munoz, M., Bancroft, J., & Turner, M. (1994). Evaluating the effects of an alpha-2 adrenoceptor antagonist on erectile function in the human male. 1. The erectile response to erotic stimuli in volunteers. *Psychopharmacology (Berl), 115*(4), 463–470.

Padma-Nathan, H., Christ, G., Adaikan, G., Becher, E., Brock, G., Carrier, S., et al. (2004). Pharmacotherapy for erectile dysfunction. *Journal of Sexual Medicine, 1*(2), 128–140.

Park, K., Ahn, K., Kim, K. K., Kim, M. K., & Ryu, S. B. (2003). Effects of intracavernosal IGF-1 gene delivery on erectile function in the aging rat. *International Journal of Impotence Research, 15,* S35.

Porst, H. (2000). Current perspectives on intracavernosal pharmacotherapy for erectile dysfunction. *International Journal of Impotence Research, 12*(Suppl. 4), S91–S100.

Porst, H. (1996). The rationale for PGE1 in erectile failure: a survey of world-wide experience. *Journal of Urology, 155,* 802–815.

Prince, W. T, Campbell, A. S., Tong, W., et al (2005). SLX-2101, a new long-acting PDE5 inhibitor: Preliminary safety, tolerability, PK and endothelial function effects in healthy subjects [Abstract]. *Program and abstracts of the Sexual Medicine Society of North America Fall Meeting, New York, NY,* Abstract 50.

Rogers, K. K., Jou, T. S., Guo, W., & Lipschutz, J. H. (2003). The Rho family of small GTPases is involved in epithelial cystogenesis and tubulogenesis. *Kidney International., 63,* 1632–1644.

Rosen, R. C., & Kostis, J. B. (2003). Overview of phosphodiesterase 5 inhibition in erectile dysfunction. *American Journal of Cardiology, 92*(9A), 9M–18M.

Saenz de Tejada, I., Ware, J. C., Blanco, R., Pittard, J. T., Nadig, P. W., Azadzoi, K. M., Krane, R. J., Goldstein, I. (1991). Pathophysiology of prolonged penile erection associated with trazodone use. *Journal of Urology,* 145(1), 60–64.

Vemulapalli, S., & Kurowski, S. (2001). Phentolamine mesylate relaxes rabbit corpus cavernosum by a nonadrenergic, noncholinergic mechanism. *Fundam Clin Pharmacol, 15,* 1–7.

Virag, R. (1985). About pharmacologic induced prolonged erection. Lancet, Mar 2;1(8427), 519–520.

Wang, Q., & Large, W. A. (1991). Modulation of noradrenaline-induced membrane currents by papaverine in rabbit vascular smooth muscle cells. *The Journal of Physiology, 439,* 501–512.

Wespes, E., Sattar, A. A., Noel, J .C., & Schulman, C. C. (2000). Does prostaglandin E1 therapy modify the intracavernous musculature? *Journal of Urology, 163,* 464–466.

Wespes, E., Rondeux, C., & Schulman, C. C. (1989). Effect of phentolamine on venous return in human erection. *British Journal of Urology, 63,* 95– 97.

Wessells, H., Fuciarelli, K., Hansen, J., Hadley, M. E., Hruby, V. J., Dorr, R., & Levine, N. (1998). Synthetic melanotropic peptide initiates erections in men with psychogenic erectile dysfunction: Double-blind, placebo controlled crossover study. *Journal of Urology, 160*(2), 389–393.

Wessells, H., Levine, N., Hadley, M. E., Dorr, R., & Hruby, V. (2000). Melanocortin receptor agonists, penile erection, and sexual motivation: Human studies with Melanotan II. *International Journal of Impotence Research, 12* (Suppl. 4), S74–S79.

Willke, R. J., Glick, H. A., McCarron, T. J., Erder, M. H., Althof, S. E., & Linet, O. I. (1997). Quality of life effects of alprostadil therapy for erectile dysfunction. *Journal of Urology, 157,* 2124–2128.

Zentgraf, M., Baccouche, M., & Junemann, K. P. (1988). Diagnosis and therapy of erectile dysfunction using papaverine and phentolamine. *Urologia Internationalis, 43,* 65–68.

Zorgniotti, A. N, & Lefleur, A. (1985). Autoinjection of the corpus cavernosum with a vasoactive combination for vasculogenic impotence. *Journal of Urology, 133,* 39–41.

Chapter Four

DEVICES USED FOR THE TREATMENT OF SEXUAL DYSFUNCTIONS IN MEN

Rany Shamloul, Ahmed El-Sakka, and Hussein Ghanem

Over the years, several treatment options for persistent male sexual dysfunctions have been introduced. The use of various instruments during management of erectile dysfunction (ED) and delayed or lack of ejaculation dates back to the 1950s. Devices used during management of male sexual dysfunctions may be externally applied, such as vacuum constriction devices (VCDs), external penile splints, vibrators, and electroejaculators. On the other hand, penile implants or prostheses are primarily internal devices used to treat resistant cases of ED. All of these options will be discussed in detail in this chapter.

VCDs have been acceptable options for the conservative management of ED for a long time. They are the most commonly used devices to treat impotence when medical treatment is not effective or is contraindicated. VCDs are generally more acceptable to older men in steady relationships than to young newly married or dating men. Short-term side effects include numbness of the penis, hinged erection, trapped ejaculation, and pain.

External penile splints are usually used by a subpopulation of men with ED who find vacuum constriction devices or injection therapy unsatisfactory because of pain or because of their perceived unnatural approach (Levine and Dimitriou, 2001). These devices generally are not medically validated.

Urologists did not develop a significant interest in the treatment of ED until the introduction of the inflatable penile prosthesis in 1973 (Montague & Angermeier, 2001). Penile prostheses implantation has a high satisfaction rate regarding treatment options for ED according to published reports. Sexual satisfaction is defined as sexual pleasure reached by both partners during sexual intercourse and is strongly associated with the experience of orgasm during the encounter. However, due to the invasiveness of such procedure and its high cost, it is considered as the last option for patients with severe ED who failed to respond to less invasive treatment modalities such as oral or intracavernosal injection therapy.

Orgasmic and ejaculatory dysfunctions are best treated with medical devices for fertility, such as special vibrators and electrostimulators. While ejaculatory dysfunctions are uncommon causes of male infertility in the general population (Dubin & Amelar, 1971), they are the major cause of infertility in certain clinical situations, such as in men with spinal cord injury (SCI), multiple sclerosis, diabetic neuropathy, idiopathic anejaculation, or iatrogenic neurological lesions. Historically, the result of treating such individuals has been quite poor. More recently, in men with SCI, the development and refinement of penile vibratory stimulation (PVS) (Sønksen, Biering-Sørensen, & Kristensen, 1994) and electroejaculation (EEJ) (Halstead, VerVoort, & Seager, 1987) have greatly enhanced the prospects for treatment of ejaculatory dysfunction (Sønksen & Ohl, 2002). Both of these methods will be described later.

The introduction of all of the aforementioned devices undoubtedly has not only helped male patients with various sexual dysfunctions but also rescued many threatened sexual relationships. In this chapter, we will review the various devices used for treatment of male sexual dysfunctions.

VACUUM CONSTRICTION DEVICES (VCDs)

VCDs work by creating a negative (or vacuum) pressure, which increases the blood flow into the *corpora cavernosa*. This causes the penis to become erect, and the erection is maintained by trapping the blood in the penis by the use of a constriction ring at the base, restricting the venous outflow (Jonas et al. 1999). The erection produced by a vacuum device is different from a physiologic erection or one produced by intracavernous injection. The blood oxygen level in the *corpus cavernosum* is less, and the portion of the penis proximal to the ring (closest to the body) is not rigid, which may produce a pivoting effect. Nevertheless, this type of erection is usually sufficient for penetration and intercourse.

Experiments with vacuum air pumps were described by J. van Musschenbrack in Leiden in 1694. Illustrations of this are available at the Library of the State University in Leiden. An American, John King, is credited with the first clinical use in 1874 of a vacuum device (King, 1874), but compression was added in 1917 by Dr. Otto Lederer, who requested a patent for his surgical device to produce erections with a vacuum (Lederer, 1917). In 1960, Gedding Osbon, trying to improve his own sexual performance, developed a device that became commercially available in 1975; but it took him until 1982 to be granted permission to market the device because of concerns with both safety and efficacy. His device was called the youth equivalent device and is now called ErecAid (Osbon, 1985). Nadig, Ware, and Blumoff (1986) reviewed the use of the device in 35 men. And Nadig (1989) reviewed a total of 340 patients over 6 years, 83 percent of whom used the device. Witherington (1989) also described the ErecAid system and reviewed 1,517 users favorably. Turner et al. (1990) found that sexual satisfaction and self-esteem improved whilst psychological symptoms decreased.

In his early studies in 1986, Nadig found the device to be safe, provided that the negative pressure did not exceed 200 mm Hg and the constricting bands were not applied for longer than 30 minutes. However, others did not agree. Benson (1989) argued that it seems scientifically doubtful "that a non-physiological erection, predicated upon trapping blood in the penis, with proximal crural flaccidity, urethral compression hindering ejaculation and general cooling of the phallus should elicit such a high favorable response rate" (p. 141).

The vacuum devices are made of a clear plastic cylinder with either a battery or hand pump attachable and a collection of sizes of rings. The rings and applicator are also available separately, without the cylinder (Jonas et al., 1990). Correctaid, a reinforced semi-rigid condom with a mouth tubing to apply suction was available in the 1980s but fell out of favor. It was not effective and the silicon was too thick to allow much feeling. The rings are now made of soft latex and have side handles for ease of removal. Some manufacturers make a notch in the ring at the place over the urethral bulb to prevent trapping of the ejaculate (Jonas et al., 1999).

Vacuum devices require enthusiasm on the part of the male and a sympathetic partner. It is therefore less likely that single younger men are going to use them, but the middle and old age groups tend to choose this treatment modality (Soderhald et al., 1997). The patient requires manual dexterity and a penis that is large enough to fit into the plastic tubing (Turner et al. 1990). It is advisable to loan this device for one month or more so that the patient can practice peacefully in the leisure of his home at least daily. In order to use the device, the constriction rings are placed over the clear plastic tube with a loading device; choosing the size of the ring is done by guesswork, but most men start at the middle size. The inside of the plastic tube is liberally covered with lubricating jelly to get a seal, the flaccid penis is inserted, and the tube pushed against the pubic bone. The vacuum is then applied, by hand or by battery pump, and tumescence (or engorgement) occurs. This initial tumescence may make it easier to put the penis in the cylinder before proceeding to continue pumping, usually for up to 3 minutes, until a satisfactory erection is achieved. Then the ring at the base of the tube is slipped onto the penis to maintain the erection. The rings should only stay on for 30 minutes maximum (Jonas et al., 1999).

This will finally give an erection that is colder, slightly bluish, and hinged at the base where the ring is located, but many patients find it adequate for vaginal penetration.

Contraindications to use are almost none. Men with loss of sensation in their genitals (due to spinal cord injury, multiple sclerosis, or diabetic neuropathy) should be careful to not use VCDs for longer than 30 minutes and to closely monitor the integrity of the skin where the constriction device was applied. Nadig stated that patients with scarring and deformity of the penis due to Peyronie's disease or following penile implant removal for infection are not likely to attain rigidity (Nadig, 1996), but it is worth trying as others have had good results in this group especially in keeping penile length after explanted penile implant (Moul & Mcleod, 1989). Negative features of VCDs are that they can be fiddly and noisy, and that the constriction ring present makes the man continually aware that he has a problem. The device may be expensive for the patient to buy (prices range from $90 to $400), and the partner may dislike the look of the end result—a coldish, bluish erection.

Patient satisfaction varies enormously and is related to effectiveness. In one study, 94 out of 127 patients (74%) found the device straightforward, 12 needed to contact the manufacturer, and 14 patients not achieving good results or experiencing pain had an instructional session with the manufacturer. Five out of these 14 individuals later achieved satisfactory results (Sidi, Becher, Zhang, & Lewis, 1990).

Petechial skin bruising, especially at the site of the ring, occurs in 16 to 39 percent of men using VCDs (Baltaci et al. 1995). Patients on antiplatelet therapy or warfarin do not appear to have any increase in bruising or ecchymosis. Pain occurs at the site of the ring. This lessens with use and also when an appropriate size ring is selected, with only less than 3 percent of the patients stopping use of the device. Ejaculatory changes, including pain on ejaculation occurred in up to 16 percent of patients, and blocked ejaculation occurred in 25 percent (Cookson and Nadig, 1993). Numbness during erection was a problem in 5 percent of patients. Pivoting at the base occurred in 6 percent (Cookson and Nadig, 1993).

Satisfaction rate, both short- and long-term, varies considerably from as low as 27 percent to as high as 68 percent short-term (69% with 2-year follow-up) (Cookson and Nadig, 1993). The main reasons for patient dissatisfaction are the following:

- Inability to maintain full erection, 12 percent
- Pain, 4 percent
- Inconvenience/awkwardness, 4 percent
- Marital problems, 5 percent

Partner dissatisfaction with:

- Performance, 11 percent
- Penile temperature, 7 percent
- Appearance, 13 percent

In one study, only 20 out of 74 patients were satisfied with the erections they achieved. These, however, were patients who had all failed counseling and self-injection. All patients with psychological impotence failed. The authors did suggest that patient selection and lack of good initial instruction and lack of free phone help may have contributed to failure (Meihart, Lycklama, Nycholt, Kropman, & Zwartendijk, 1993).

In 1998, using penile plethysmography, the penile blood flow was measured before, during, and after the use of the ring (Marmar, Benedictus, & Praiso, 1998). There was a 70–75 percent decline in the amplitude of the pulse volume curve, but continuous blood flow was maintained in each case. In other words, the circulation did not stop completely. In 33 patients, after removal of the ring there was transient increased amplitude consistent with post-ischemic hyperemia (i.e., temporarily increased blood flow following a period of restricted circulation). These findings suggested an adequate penile blood flow and that the devices were safe. However, the 30-minute rule should be strictly adhered to, as the ring causes significant reduction in blood flow, and in one report complete cessation (Broderick, Mcgahon, Stone, & Whit, 1992). In 72 percent of patients with penile plethysmography, the pressure achieved was greater than 100 mm Hg buckling pressure. In addition, the mean increase in length was 3.7cm +/− 0.7, and the increase in circumference 3.5cm +/− 0.9. This compared favorably with the increase in length and width for normal erections (Marmar et al., 1998). The vacuum devices, which are available by prescription, are well tried and tested; the Food and Drug Administration approved these devices for sale as over-the-counter medical devices in the United States.

Vacuum devices, despite some shortcomings, have many potential advantages for a subset of patients, especially if the design and function of these devices continue to be improved.

EXTERNAL PENILE SPLINTS

External penile splints have been available since the early 1900s. Their use and acceptance by patients have been hampered by their design as unnatural "sleeves" that may partially or completely cover the penile shaft, resulting in reduced penile and vaginal pleasurable sensation (Levine & Dimitriou, 2001). Moreover, external penile splints with multiple components may separate during coitus, making intercourse uncomfortable and possibly painful. In general, the advantages of external splints are their noninvasiveness and relative inexpensiveness.

Recently, an external penile support device was developed and patented in an effort to provide an improved option. Using the suspension bridge design concept, two support rods made of stainless steel completely enclosed in medical-grade silicone tubing have at the distal end an integrated support loop that positions around the sub coronal sulcus, which is the area below the glans of the penis (for anatomical illustrations, please refer to chapter 6 of *Sexual Health: Vol. 2*). A retractable retaining bar maintains the loop around the corona once the glans is positioned in the device. Proximally, the rods are attached to one of three different-sized support rings positioned around the base of the penis. Once individually sized and placed on the flaccid penis, it allows complete exposure of the penile shaft and glans. It was designed to stretch the penis maximally without blocking or inhibiting orgasm or ejaculation. This device was found to be most stable on men capable of partial tumescence when compared with men with complete flaccidity (Levine & Dimitriou, 2001). Although the new device is an intriguing and potentially effective treatment option, the need to size each individual precisely has made its mass production rather difficult.

PENILE PROSTHESES

In contrast to other mammal species such as the whale, dog, bear, gibbon, or otter, the human male does not have a penile bone inside his penis to enforce erection. The earliest surgical efforts to treat impotence included resection of the dorsal vein of the penis. This method did not prove effective. It therefore seemed logical that Bogoras in 1936 used a piece of rib cartilage in order to reinforce rigidity in the penis. However, the rib cartilage and bone implants were reabsorbed after several months, and therefore the erection-producing effect was abolished (Bogoras, 1936; Furlow, 1981).

Today, there are basically three types of penile prostheses available: (1) malleable, (2) semirigid, and (3) inflatable devices. All of them have to be inserted surgically. The first alloplastic implants (i.e., made from nonhuman material) were described in 1952—according to unpublished data by Scardino—using acrylic prostheses. These devices were originally positioned between the *corpora cavernosa;* however, they were less successful than polyethylene prostheses, which were later implanted inside the *tunica albuginea*. Loeffler, Samegh, & Lash (1964) acknowledged the disturbance a patient may find if he chooses a penile implant, but also advised that patients with organic impotence did not have many other choices of management, at least during those days. In 1966, Beheri already reported on 700 penile implants. He used two polyethylene rods and placed each one inside the *corpora cavernosa* (Beheri, 1966). After having finally found the appropriate material (silicone rubber) and the exact implantation site (inside the *tunica albuginea*), prosthetic surgery for the treatment of erectile failure became more and more popular in the late 1960s. Scott, Bradley, & Tim (1973) described a completely new concept using inflatable silicone cylinders that could be filled voluntarily via a pump that became implanted in the scrotum, transporting fluid to the cylinders from a reservoir that was positioned behind the rectus muscle. In 1973, Small and Carrion designed a prosthesis that was much easier to implant and had fewer complications but that had the disadvantage of a more or less permanent erection due to rigid rods, which were positioned inside the *corpora cavernosa* (Scott et al., 1973). These two new types of devices started the development and design of numerous new prostheses throughout the following three decades (Jonas et al., 1991; Mulcahy, Krane, Lloyd, Edson, & Siroky, 1990).

In 1975, Small and Carrion's device consisted of a pair of silicone rod prostheses, which were implanted through a midline perineal incision. The prosthesis was available in 16 different lengths and 3 diameters, which already emphasized the inability to make a proper length determination prior to surgery. Therefore, different-sized prostheses had to be available in the operating room. In order to decrease hospital inventory, individual device trimming at the tails of all implants was finally introduced (Small, Carrion, & Gordon, 1975). By December 1977, a total of 260 patients worldwide had already received implants, and only 3 of 106 implanted patients had a poor result. However, due to the rigid characteristics of the device, a more or less permanent erection resulted, and the need for improvements became evident.

One solution was found by Subrini. This author used softer silicone-preparations positioned in the midpart of the device in order to avoid permanent erection in the resting position (Subrini, 1982). Subrini described his preliminary experience in 1974 (Subrini & Couvelaire, 1974). Between 1970 and 1982, he operated on a total of 283 impotent patients with an overall failure rate of only 1.7 percent. Success ranked as high as 95 percent after primary surgery and 98.3 percent if surgery had to be performed a second time. A different way of combining the features of malleability with simple design was done by Jonas, who in 1978 published a report on the silicone silver penile prosthesis. This device was characterized by silver wires embedded inside the silicone rubber to stabilize the penis in different positions: downwards or against the body during the resting position or upwards for intercourse. Despite the fact that the silver strands could break after numerous bendings (following approximately 5,000 double bendings at one specific point on a simulator) the silver never protruded the silicone rubber nor was the function inhibited by fractures of the silver wires (stability). In order, however, to avoid future discussions of whether broken silver strands could lead to negative results, since 1984 the individual silver strands have been embedded in thermoplastic Teflon, making further breakages impossible (Jonas, 1999). The original device (standard version) was manufactured in three different diameters (9.5, 11, and 13 mm) in lengths between 17 and 24 cm. A total of 22 different prostheses were available. In order to diminish costs, the "trimming-tip version" was introduced, a device which could be shortened at its proximal end making only two pairs of different lengths necessary in two different diameters.

The concept of a metal strand inside the malleable silicone prostheses for reliable and flexible stability was copied later in the 1980s in the *AMS Malleable 600* prosthesis in which a steel-capped, fabric-wrapped stainless steel core was used instead of Teflon-coated silver strands. Further features were the removable silicone jacket and the rear-tip extenders. The *AMS Malleable 600 prosthesis* has since been replaced by the *AMS Malleable 650 prosthesis*. The *Mentor* malleable penile prosthesis also contains a silver strand; however, this strand is coiled in a spiral, giving a corkscrew appearance. The silver strand is only positioned in the midportion of the device; therefore the proximal end can be trimmed to the exact length required (American Medical Systems, 1983). The *Duraphase* penile prosthesis is a device in which rigidity and flaccidity are controlled using articulating (joined by hinges) segments, a stainless steel cable, and a spring on each end of the central part. It consists of 12 rigid polysulfone articulated disks with a centrally placed stainless steel cable and 2 spring mechanisms. The maximal angle of all 13 disk interspaces is 220 degrees, which is the possible angle of the erection that can be mimicked by bending of the prosthesis. A new device (Duraphase), which was more recently introduced, showed fewer complications than with the inflatable devices and especially stressed the features of excellent bendability, superior concealability, and perfect rigidity. The original *Duraphase* prosthesis was later replaced by the *Duraphase II* prosthesis.

After the rather unsuccessful attempts prior to the 1970s, the tremendous breakthrough in alloplastic surgery for impotent men came in February 1973 when the first inflatable penile prosthesis was implanted by Scott et al. Already by 1979, 21 physicians had performed penile implantation in a total of 1,243 patients at different centers. The success rate was 91.5 percent; however, as stated by practically all authors in this period of time, there was a reoperation rate of around 30 percent. Reasons for reoperation are usually infection, malfunction, skin ulcers, implant extrusion, fibrosis, and lack of satisfaction.

From 1973 to the present numerous alterations and improvements of penile prostheses have been applied. Today's most popular device, the *AMS 700 CX* has apparently mastered the majority of problems, such as kinking of the tubings, cylinder wall aneurysms, and unequal filling of the device. The *AMS 700 CX* now has a three-ply (or three-layered) cylinder wall that minimizes the risk of cylinder bulging; the diameter of each cylinder can expand from 12 up to 18 mm, improving prosthetic erection in circumference; and tubing connectors allow easy handling and safe connection of the tubes to and from the cylinder (Fein, 1988). The smaller *AMS 700 CXM* prosthesis has a smaller reservoir, pump, and cylinders, which expand from 9.5 to 14.2 mm. This smaller inflatable prosthesis is especially useful in implant recipients who have fibrotic *corpora*. The *AMS 700 CX* was developed from the original inflatable Scott device and consists of three components: the cylinder, the pump, and the reservoir.

The concept of having a reservoir also was applied in the *Mentor* inflatable penile prosthesis, described for the first time in 1982 (Malloy, Wein & Carpeniello 1982). The essential difference between the very similar looking devices, however, is the material: the *Mentor* device is manufactured from *Bioflex* polyurethane, which was quoted to be more durable and less elastic than silicone. Such material should last longer and prevent cylinder aneurysms. In 1987, the results of 202 implantations were reported: Reoperation was necessary in 8 percent of implantations; of these, approximately 50 percent were due to technical problems. Later, the rate of complications dropped to 3.5 percent. Again, good results were obtained using this device in far more than 90 percent of implantations. The latest *Mentor* development is the *Alpha 1* inflatable penile prosthesis, which features cylinders and pump that are firmly connected, leaving only one connector between the pump and reservoir. This diminishes mechanical problems (Engel, Smolev, & Hackler, 1987).

The latest improvement in the three-component inflatable device is the *AMS 700 Ultrex* penile prosthesis, which expands in circumference from 12 to 18 mm and extends in length within the *corpora cavernosa* depending on tissue elasticity. This should give the patient a more natural prosthetic erection than before. The cylinders consist of an inner and outer silicone layer and a woven Lycra and Dacron middle layer. The two-way stretch of this middle layer permits girth expansion and length extension. Recent experience shows that the *AMS 700 CX* device has a five-year mechanical failure rate of 9.1 percent, while the *AMS Ultrex* device has a five-year mechanical failure rate of 35 percent (Daitch, Angermeier, Lakin, Inglebright, & Montague, 1997). Decreased cylinder survival is the primary reason for the increased failures seen with the *Ultrex* prosthesis. In 1993, the *Ultrex* cylinders were improved; the magnitude of improvement in survival with these modified cylinders remains to be demonstrated.

In order to reduce the possibility of mechanical failure, many attempts have been made to reduce components, connectors, and tubes in the concept of inflatable devices. Another consideration was the ease of surgical implantation, to offer a penile implant as pre-prepared as possible so as to reduce fitting, trimming, and fillings to an acceptable minimum. The *Mentor Mark II* prosthesis is an inflatable penile prosthesis that is preassembled and has no connectors, making any trimming and connecting procedures unnecessary. The device, however, has to be filled interoperatively by the surgeon.

Depending on the surgical approach, scrotal and infrapubic types are available for this kind of device. In this two-component device, pump and reservoir are combined as resipump. Twelve differently shaped devices are offered for individual length fitting. The *AMS Ambicor* prosthesis is a two-component prosthesis produced by American Medical Systems (see References). This device comes in 3 diameters (11, 13, and 15 mm) and lengths varying from 14 to 22 cm. Adjustments between lengths are made with the addition of rear-tip extenders. Experience with this new prosthesis at this time is still limited (Jonas et al., 1999).

The *AMS Hydroflex* self-contained penile prosthesis consists of two prefilled cylinders. In each cylinder, there is a reservoir at the rear end, an inflation pump and deflation valve, and finally an inflation chamber. Through repeated pumping close to the glans, the fluid moves from the rear reservoir into the inflation chamber, and the penis becomes erect. When continuous pressure is applied to the deflation valve, which is just behind the inflation pump, the fluid returns in the rear reservoir, and the penis becomes flaccid. The device comes in three different cylinder diameters, 11, 13, and 15 mm, and four different lengths, and all typical surgical approaches may be used for implantation. Preliminary clinical implantation results in 140 patients showed uncomplicated surgery with satisfactory results. The *Hydroflex* is no longer available; it has been replaced by the *AMS Dynaflex*. Mechanical device failure was seen in 7.5 percent of 120 recipients of the *Dynaflex* prosthesis who were followed for a mean of 42 months; however, further clinical experience has to provide proof of satisfactory function (Surgitek, 1987).

Today, the principle types of penile implants are the malleable, semirigid, and one-to-three-component inflatable devices. The continuing requests for further improvements are based on the patient's wish for a more and more normal and physiological sex life (Jonas et al., 1999). The postoperative complication rates as well as the chance for necessary repeated surgery should not be overlooked during success assessment.

The mechanical success rate following penile implant at around 95 percent is excellent, and more and more data are available indicating that patients and partners are handling their sex lives very well, even in cases where impotence due to spinal cord injury was treated with penile implantation. Still, more efforts should be devoted to the psychological impact for patient and partner, and sophisticated pre-, peri- and postoperative guidance for both partners is mandatory.

Prosthetic infection is the most disturbing complication following surgery. The coexistence of infection and foreign body requires immediate removal of the prosthesis; however, a reimplantation may be done after few months. Diabetic patients carry the highest risk of this complication, where additional special care must be provided in order to avoid wound healing problems. Our own experience has shown that once the device is infected, local or systemic antibiotic treatment has no effect. Therefore, especially when the device communicates through the open wound, removal is the only possible treatment in order to avoid septic exacerbation. If, especially in case of the diabetic patient, the infection is not controlled efficiently after removal of the device, necrosis of the *corpora* may develop (Jonas et al., 1999). This fact further backs the absolute need for removal of an infected device as soon as possible.

The postoperative complication rates due to infection described in the literature are seen to be as high as 8.3 percent (Carson & Robertson, 1988). This necessitates specific attention to preoperative preparation, intraoperative handling, and postoperative care. On the other hand, recent attention has been given to salvage procedures. In these procedures, the entire infected device is removed, and then the operative area is copiously irrigated with antibiotic solution and antiseptics. A new prosthesis is then implanted using fresh instruments. Using this protocol, Brant and colleagues were able to achieve success in 10 of 11 patients (91%) with mean follow-up of 21 months (Brant, Ludlow & Mulcahy 1996).

At all times all patients should receive information on how to use the prostheses optimally. They should especially be made aware that the friction during intercourse is an important factor that may provoke perforation of the prosthesis. If the partner has no or little vaginal secretion during sexual stimulation, a lubricant may be advisable.

Prosthesis reimplantation may be necessary for different problems. The data from the literature show that reimplantation may also lead to satisfying results (Jonas et al., 1999). However, due to scarring and fibrosis, the penis can shorten; therefore the first surgical attempt still offers the most promising results (Kaufmann 1982). Due to today's availability of alternative treatment modalities (such as oral medication and intracavernosal injections) that are noninvasive or minimally invasive, these modalities should be used before considering the implantation of a penile prosthesis (Jonas et al., 1999). Nevertheless, penile implants still offer the best rate of success, over 95 percent—inclusive of partner's satisfaction, independent of etiology or the type of prosthesis used. The inflatable devices are the most elegant ones, which best imitate physiological behavior; however, potential complications include the possibility of mechanical failure. It is the author's viewpoint that different types of devices should be presented to the patient prior to surgery, and he should decide what type of prosthesis he would like to have implanted after being fully informed of the advantages and disadvantages of the individual types. In general, the malleable devices last longer than the inflatable ones. Patients should be informed that a 5–15 percent failure rate is expected in the first 5 years and that the majority of devices will fail in 10–15 years and will need to be replaced. Potential complications include mechanical failures, cylinder leaks, tubing leaks, infection, perforation, persistent pain, and self-inflation.

In case of complications or after removal of the device, reimplantation is possible. This, however, requires a more difficult surgical procedure with a decreased chance of success. We do believe that with proper indication, careful patient selection, proper surgical technique, and adequate instructions for both partners about how to use the device correctly and what realistic expectations might be, penile prostheses can fulfill the couple's need for pursuing sexual satisfaction. It is particularly important to give the patients a realistic scenario of possible outcomes in order to bring their expectations into a down-to-earth range.

The past two decades have witnessed a phenomenal advance in the understanding of penile physiology and several revolutionary new treatments for patients with ED (see chapter 3 of this volume). It is now well accepted that the conservative and the less invasive interventions should be the primary solutions for treatment offered to ED patients. The long-term side effects and the interaction between the newly introduced medications and other commonly used drugs in old patients with ED will remain an interesting field for more research and investigation. We do believe that penile prostheses should only be considered when all other less invasive therapeutic modalities have failed or if the patient refuses those modalities.

ELECTROEJACULATION (EEJ) AND PENILE VIBRATOR STIMULATION (PVS)

Electroejaculation (EEJ)

Rectal EEJ has been one of the most frequently used treatments for ejaculatory dysfunction in men with SCI for many years. EEJ was first described in humans by Learmonth (1931). Horne, Paull, and Munro (1948) reported the first use of EEJ in SCI persons, resulting in successful ejaculation in 9 of 15 men. In the 1980s, Seager further refined the method of EEJ and developed several prototypes of equipment (Halstead et al., 1987). Electroejaculation is carried out with an electrical probe, which is inserted rectally and is positioned with the electrodes in contact with the anterior rectal wall in the area of the prostate gland and the seminal vesicles. The electrical stimulation is administered in a wavelike pattern with voltage progressively increasing in 1–2 V increments until ejaculation occurs (Halstead et al., 1987; Ohl & Sønksen, 1996). It is usually recommended that a low level of electrical baseline (100 mA) be maintained between voltage peaks and during ejaculation. However, in a recent study focusing on sphincteric events during EEJ and PVS in men with SCI, it was suggested that it would be optimal in EEJ procedures to discontinue electrical stimulation completely during ejaculation to allow greater relaxation of the external urethral sphincter, which may increase the percentage of semen ejaculated in the antegrade direction (Brackett et al., 2000; Ohl, Sønksen, & Bolling, 2000; Sønksen, Ohl, & Wedermeyer, 2001).

Antegrade ejaculate is not produced in a projectile fashion, but rather as an intermittent release of semen during the course of the procedure (Brindley, 1981a; Halstead et al., 1987). Between 15 and 35 stimulations are usually needed to ensure emptying of the semen (Halstead et al., 1987). The voltage and current that have been reported to successfully produce ejaculation range from 5 to 25 V and 100–600 mA, respectively (Ohl, Bennett, McCabe, Menge, & McGuire, 1989a). Prior to the EEJ procedure, the patient's bladder is catheterized to completely empty it of urine, because many individuals have a substantial portion of retrograde ejaculation (Ohl et al., 1989a). Because urine may adversely affect this retrograde ejaculate, a buffering medium (e.g. Ham's F 10 medium) can be instilled into the bladder before the EEJ (Ohl & Sønksen, 1997). After the procedure, the bladder is catheterized again to empty the retrograde fraction. Rectoscopy is performed prior to the procedure to confirm that there are no preexisting rectal lesions and after the procedure to exclude injury to the rectum. It should be noted that EEJ could cause significant discomfort in men with partly preserved sensation, and they may require either a spinal or general anesthesia before treatment (Brindley, 1981a; Ohl & Sønksen, 1997; Perkash, Martin, Warner, Blank, & Collins, 1985; Sarkarati, Rossier, & Fam, 1987). Blood pressure monitoring should be performed throughout the procedure; men who are susceptible to autonomic dysreflexia or who have experienced episodes with prior trials of EEJ may be premedicated with nifedipine (Steinberger, Ohl, Bennett, McCabe, & Wang, 1990).

Penile Vibratory Stimulation (PVS)

The first reported use of PVS in a man with SCI was with a massager (Comarr, 1970). The activated massager or vibrator is held at the base of the penis. A number of investigators have reported successful results in achieving ejaculations with PVS, but Brindley (1981b) has been credited with refining the technique most frequently used with PVS in men with SCI. In his initial studies, Brindley (1981b, 1984) reported successful ejaculation in 48 of 81 men with SCI. The PVS procedure is performed with the individual in the supine position or in a sitting position (Sønksen et al., 1994). The goal of PVS is to activate the ejaculatory reflex in the thoracolumbar area of the spinal cord. The afferent penile dorsal nerve stimulation is provided by application of a vibrating disc against the frenulum for periods of 3 minutes or until antegrade ejaculation occurs. If no ejaculation occurs, the stimulation period is followed by a rest period of 1–2 minutes and stimulation begins again. An antegrade ejaculation occurs as a pulsatile projectile ejaculation similar to normal ejaculation.

In contrast to EEJ, nearly all spermatozoa in PVS trials are ejaculated in the antegrade direction in SCI men (Ohl et al., 1997). The required time to induce ejaculation by PVS in SCI men ranges from 10 seconds to 45 minutes (Beretta, Chelo, & Zanollo, 1989; Brindley, 1981b; Szasz and Carpenter, 1989). During PVS, somatic reactions such as erections, abdominal muscle contractions and leg spasms may be seen (Szasz & Carpenter, 1989). In contrast to EEJ, PVS requires an intact spinal cord at the level of T11-S4 in order to induce antegrade ejaculation (Brindley, 1981b, 1984; Szasz & Carpenter, 1989). However, the data from Brindley's (1984) study concerning the exact level and completeness of spinal cord lesion in relation to the ejaculatory response is unclear. Szasz and Carpenter (1989) reported from their work that the level and completeness of the spinal cord lesion could not predict with certainty successful ejaculation by PVS in a group of 35 men with SCI. Furthermore, Brindley (1984) noted that the most important factor indicating whether an ejaculate could be obtained by PVS was the clinical presence or absence of the hip flexion reflex (L2-S1), which is elicited by scratching the soles of the feet. Ejaculation was obtained in 75 percent of men with SCI who had an intact hip flexion reflex and in no men who did not have the hip flexion reflex. However, it should be noted that 25 percent of men with SCI who had the clinical presence of hip flexion reflex failed to ejaculate by PVS. Szasz and Carpenter (1989) noted that the absence of bulbocavernous reflex (S2-S4) predicted no ejaculatory response by PVS in most men with SCI.

Although there are no clearly defined or standardized parameters for the application of PVS in men with SCI, it has been suggested that the output of the vibrators and, in particular, the amplitude might have some effect on the ejaculatory response (Brindley, 1984; Szasz & Carpenter, 1989). In fact, a wide range of ejaculation rates (19–91%) has been reported in the literature and may be the result of the fact that several nonmedical vibrators have been used and the output from these vibrators may vary widely and is not standardized (Beilby and Keogh, 1989; Beretta et al., 1989; Brindley, 1981b, 1984; Sarkarati et al., 1987; Szasz & Carpenter, 1989).

Sønksen et al. (1994) examined the ejaculatory response in men with SCI to varying amplitudes of PVS and found that the highest rates of ejaculation (antegrade plus retrograde) were seen with a vibrator amplitude level of 2.5 mm and a frequency of 100 Hz (96%), and low rates were seen when the amplitude was only 1 mm (32%), also at a frequency of 100 Hz. The effectiveness of the high amplitude vibration by obtaining an ejaculation rate of 83 percent in another comparable group of 41 SCI men with ejacu-latory dysfunction was also noted. Based on these results a medical grade vibrator (*Ferticare,* see References) for SCI men has been developed. In the same study (Sønksen et al., 1994), antegrade ejaculation was seen only in men with cord lesions above T10, and no other absolute predictors of the ejaculatory response were identified among patient characteristics related to reflexes, completeness of lesions, somatic reactions, age, and time since SCI. However, when the reflexes and/or somatic reactions such as erections, abdominal muscle contractions, and leg spasms were present during PVS, there was a significantly higher percentage of men with antegrade ejacula-tion compared with those men in whom none of the reflexes and/or somatic reactions were seen.

In general, PVS is a well-tolerated procedure with very few potential com-plications. Local skin abrasion may occur on occasions where the vibrator is applied, but no special treatment is usually required other than relief from further irritation.

In a review of the literature examining papers written on widely differing patient groups, the incidence of any retained ejaculatory function among SCI men was between 0 and 55 percent, with most studies showing numbers that approach 0 percent (Sønksen & Biering-Sørensen, 1992). EEJ may be suc-cessful in obtaining ejaculate from men with all types of SCI, including men who are missing major components of the ejaculatory reflex arc (Ohl and Sønksen, 1997). In a prospective study by Ohl et al. (1989a), predictors of suc-cess in relation to the response of 48 men with SCI to EEJ were studied. In relation to successful EEJ, they found no significant difference between men with SCI with high vs. low or complete vs. incomplete spinal cord lesions. Ejaculation was produced in 60 percent of cervical patients compared with 50 percent of lumbar patients. Ejaculation was seen in 71 percent of men with complete lesions and in 61 percent with incomplete lesions. However, more recent studies show that it is possible to induce ejaculation with EEJ in 80–100 percent of all men with SCI (Lucas et al., 1991; Matthews, Gardner, & Francois, 1996; Nehra, Werner, Bastuba, Title, & Oates, 1996; Ohl, McCabe, Sønksen, Randolph, & Menge, 1996; Ohl and Sønksen, 1997).

Multiple sclerosis and diabetes can also affect ejaculatory function through either a central or peripheral nerve disturbance. Electroejacula-tion has been successfully used to induce ejaculation and achieve pregnancy (Ohl et al., 1989b). Patients with diabetic neuropathy occasionally suffer from peripheral neuropathy, which may lead to ejaculatory dysfunction. Many diabetic men with ejaculatory dysfunction experience a relatively slow progression of their problem, with an initial phase of decreased ejaculate volume followed by retrograde ejaculation and then total absence of ejacu-lation. Some subjects can be treated with sympathomimetic agents in the initial phase of the dysfunction, but, once well established, total absence of ejaculation will require EEJ, which has been demonstrated to be successful in both sperm retrieval and in establishing pregnancies in this subpopulation (Gerig, Meacham, & Ohl, 1997).

Any other conditions that affect the ejaculatory mechanism of the central and/or peripheral nervous system, including surgical nerve injury, may be treated successfully with EEJ. In a recent study examining sperm retrieval and sperm cryopreservation before intensive anticancer therapy in pubertal boys, EEJ was successfully performed in two persons who failed to obtain ejaculation by masturbation (Müller et al., 2000). Approximately 80 percent of all SCI men with an intact ejaculatory reflex arc (above T10) can be managed with PVS to induce reflex ejaculation when using correct vibration output (amplitude 2.5 mm and frequency of 100 Hz) (Sønksen et al., 1994). Furthermore, PVS is very simple in use, noninvasive, does not require anesthesia, and is preferred by the patients when compared with EEJ (Ohl, Sønksen, Menge, McCabe, & Keller, 1997). Consequently, PVS is recommended to be the first choice of treatment in SCI men with ejaculatory dysfunction with EEJ reserved for PVS failures. Like EEJ, PVS has also been used successfully to induce ejaculation in pubertal boys who failed to obtain ejaculation by masturbation in order to cryopreserve sperm before anticancer therapy (Müller et al., 2000).

Penile vibratory stimulation and vaginal self-insemination performed by the couple at home is a viable option for those SCI men with adequate semen parameters (Brindley, 1984; Nehra et al., 1996; Löchner-Ernst et al., 1997; Sønksen et al., 1997). A non-spermicidal container is used for collection of the ejaculate and a 10-mL syringe is used for ovulation timed vaginal self-insemination. Brindley (1984) reported seven home pregnancies following PVS and vaginal self-insemination with delivery of five healthy babies (one ongoing/one spontaneous abortion). Recently, several pregnancies have been reported from PVS procedures combined with self-insemination at home (Dahlberg et al., 1995; Löchner-Ernst, Mandalka, Kramer, & Stöhrer, 1997; Nehra et al., 1996; Sønksen et al., 1997; Tepper, 1997). Most studies reported that multiple ovulation cycles were used to achieve home pregnancies, and the overall pregnancy rate per couple range from 25 to 61 percent.

The unique advantage of PVS is the possibility of home use. It will also allow the majority of SCI couples to perform the PVS procedure themselves at the hospital when a specimen is required in connection with assisted reproduction techniques. Furthermore, several successful pregnancies have been reported (Brinsden, Avery, Marcus, & Macnamee, 1997; Dahlberg et al., 1995; Hultling et al., 1997; Löchner-Ernst et al., 1997; Nehra et al., 1996; Ohl et al., 1995; Sønksen et al., 1997) using spermatozoa obtained by PVS or EEJ combined with assisted reproduction techniques such as intrauterine insemination or in vitro fertilization with or without intracytoplasmic sperm injection. The overall pregnancy rate per cycle from those studies (Brinsden et al., 1997; Dahlberg et al., 1995; Hultling et al., 1997; Löchner-Ernst et al., 1997; Nehra et al., 1996; Ohl et al., 1995; Sønksen et al., 1997) averages about 25 percent. It should be noted that this rate is similar to the pregnancy rate per cycle during natural procreation in healthy couples wanting to become pregnant (25–30%) (Spira, 1986), although assisted ejaculation procedures and reproduction techniques are required for SCI men and their partners.

If assisted ejaculation procedures fail or yield insufficient motile and/or viable spermatozoa for assisted reproductive techniques, surgical procedures of sperm retrieval are indicated. There have been several case reports of pregnancies obtained with sperm from surgical retrieval in SCI men (Dahlberg et al., 1995; Marina et al., 1999; Watkins, Lim, Bourne, Baker, & Wutthiphan, 1996). When sperm is surgically retrieved from this patient population, the couples are generally required to use in vitro fertilization with intracytoplasmic sperm injection. Many women are able to become pregnant with home insemination or hospital-based insemination, obviating the need for in vitro fertilization. If one adopts the procedure of direct sperm retrieval, the couple is usually committed to an invasive and expensive interventional procedure.

SUMMARY

Several instrumental devices have been implemented in the management armamentarium of male sexual dysfunctions. The use of various instruments in the management of ED and delayed or even lack of ejaculation dates back to the 1950s. In this chapter, we reviewed some important clinical aspects of various devices used in the treatment of male sexual dysfunctions. The vacuum constriction device (VCD) is the most commonly used device to treat impotence when medical treatment is not effective or contraindicated. VCD is an easy-to-handle and reasonably-priced instrument that depends on applying negative pressure to the penile tissue, resulting in suction of the blood in a sufficient amount into the penis to achieve an erection. The device is more acceptable to older men in a steady relationship than to young newly married or dating men. Side effects include numbness of the penis, hinged erection, trapped ejaculation, and pain.

Penile implants or prostheses are devices used to treat resistant cases of ED. The two main types are the malleable and the inflatable prostheses. The mechanism of action depends on surgical implantation of two synthetic rods (with or without a pump and a reservoir) in each erectile body in the penis (*corpus cavernosum*) to induce an artificial erection. The main complications are infection, persistent pain, tubing or cylinder leakage, and erosion.

Vibrators and electroejaculators are devices that can help treat cases of ejaculatory dysfunction through nerve stimulation, inducing ejaculation. In the era of effective oral drug therapy for male sexual dysfunctions, instrumental devices are becoming second-line and third-line treatment options.

REFERENCES

American Medical Systems Inc. (1983). AMS malleable 600. AMS product information.

American Medical Systems AMS 700 penile implant. http://www.visitams.com/prof_erectile_restoration_product_objectname_prof_male_700_inflatable.html.

American Medical Systems DURA II. http://www.visitams.com/prof_erectile_restoration_product_objectname_prof_male_DuraII.html.

American Medical Systems Malleable 600/650. http://www.visitams.com/prof_erectile_restoration_product_objectname_prof_male_malleable_650.html.

Baltaci, S., Aydos, K., & Anafartaka, K. (1995). Treating erectile dysfunction with vacuum tumescence device: A retrospective analysis of acceptance and satisfaction. *British Journal of Urology, 76,* 757.

Beheri G. (1966). Surgical treatment of impotence. *Plastic Reconstructive Surgery, 38,* 92–97.

Beilby, J. A., & Keogh, E. J. (1989). Spinal cord injuries and anejaculation. *Paraplegia, 27,* 152.

Benson, R. (1989). Editorial comment. *Journal of Urology, 141,* 322.

Beretta, G., Chelo, E., & Zanollo, A. (1989). Reproductive aspects in spinal cord injured males. *Paraplegia, 27,* 113–118.

Bogoras, N. (1936). Über die volle plastische Wiederherstellung eines zum Koitus fähigen Penis (Penisplasticatotalis). *Zentralblatt für Chirurgie, 63,* 1271.

Brant, M. D., Ludlow, J. K., & Mulcahy, J. J. (1996). The prosthesis salvage operation: Immediate replacement of the infected penile prosthesis. *Journal of Urology, 155,* 155–157.

Brindley, G. S. (1981a). Electroejaculation: Its technique, neurological implications and uses. *J Neuro Neurosurg Psych, 44,* 9–18.

Brindley, G. S. (1981b). Reflex ejaculation under vibratory stimulation in paraplegic men. *Paraplegia, 19,* 299–302.

Brindley, G. S. (1984). The fertility of men with spinal injuries. *Paraplegia, 22,* 337–348.

Brinsden, P. R., Avery, S. M., Marcus, S., & Macnamee, M. C. (1997). Transrectal electroejaculation combined with in-vitro fertilization: Effective treatment of anejaculatory infertility due to spinal cord injury. *Human Reproduction, 12,* 2687–2692.

Broderick, G., Mcgahon, J., Stone, A., & Whit, R. (1992). The hemodynamics of vacuum constriction erections: Assessment by colour Doppler ultrasound. *Journal of Urology, 147,* 57–61.

Carson, C. C., & Robertson, C. N. (1988). Late hematogenous infection of penile prostheses. *Journal of Urology 139,* 150.

Comarr, A. E. (1970). Sexual function among patients with spinal cord injury. *Urologia Internationalis, 25,* 34–168.

Cookson, M., & Nadig, P. (1993). Long-term results with vacuum constriction device. *Journal of Urology 149,* 290–294.

Daitch, J., Angermeier, K., Lakin, M., Inglebright, B., & Montague, D. (1997). Long-term mechanical reliability of AMS 700 series inflatable penile prostheses: Comparison of CX/CXM and Ultrex cylinders. *Journal of Urology 159,* 1400–1402.

Dubin, L., & Amelar, R. D. (1971). Etiologic factors in 1294 consecutive cases of male infertility. *Fertility and Sterility, 22,* 469–474.

Fein, R. L. (1988). Cylinder problems with AMS 700 inflatable penile prosthesis. *Urology, 31*(4), 305.

Ferticare Medical Vibrator. http://www.medicalvibrator.com/. $695.

Furlow, W. (1981). Sex prosthetics. In L. Wagenknecht, W. Furlow, & J. Auvert (Eds.), *Genitourinary reconstruction with prostheses.* Stuttgart, New York: Thieme.

Gerig, N. E., Meacham, R. B., and Ohl, D. A. (1997). Use of electroejaculation in the treatment of ejaculatory failure secondary to diabetes mellitus. *Urology, 49,* 239–242.

Halstead, L. S., VerVoort, S., & Seager, S.W.J. (1987). Rectal probe electrostimulation in the treatment of anejaculatory spinal cord injured men. *Paraplegia, 25,* 120–129.

Horne, H. W., Paull, D. P., & Munro, D. (1948). Fertility studies in the human male with traumatic injuries of the spinal cord and cauda equina. *New England Journal of Medicine, 239,* 959–961.

Hultling, C., Rosenlund, B., Levi, R., Fridström, M., Sjöblom, P., & Hillensjö, T. (1997). Assisted ejaculation and in-vitro fertilization in the treatment of infertile spinal cord-injured men: The role of intracytoplasmic sperm injection. *Human Reproduction, 12,* 499–502.

Jonas, U., Evans, C., Krishnamurti, S., Montague, D., Sarramon, J. P., Sohn, M., Wespes, E., & Wesseles, H. (1999). Surgical treatment and mechanical devices. *Proceedings of the International Consultation on Erectile Dysfunction.*

Kaufmann, J. J. (1982). Penile prosthetic surgery under local anesthesia. *Journal of Urology 128,* 1190.

King, J. (1874). *The American physician—domestic guide to health.* Indianapolis, IN: Streight & Douglas, 384.

Learmonth, J. R. (1931). A contribution to the neurophysiology of the urinary bladder in man. *Brain, 54,* 147–176.

Lederer O. 1917. Specification of letter patent. *U.S. Patent Office No. 1,225,341.* Washington, DC: U.S. Patent and Trademark Office. (Application filed November 29, 1913; serial no. 1917,803,853. Granted May 8, 1917.)

Levine, L. A., & Dimitriou, R. J. (2001). Vacuum constriction and external erection devices in erectile dysfunction. *Urology Clinics of North America, 28,* 335–341.

Löchner-Ernst, D., Mandalka, B., Kramer, G., & Stöhrer, M. (1997). Conservative and surgical semen retrieval in patients with spinal cord injury. *Spinal Cord, 35,* 463–468.

Loeffler, R., Samegh, E., & Lash, H. (1964). The artificial os penis. *Plast Reconstr Surg, 34,* 71.

Lucas, M. G., Hargreave, T. B., Edmund, P., Creasy, G. H., McParland, M., & Seager, S.W.J. (1991). Sperm retrieval by electro-ejaculation: Preliminary experience in patients with secondary anejaculation. *British Journal of Urology, 67,* 191–194.

Malloy, T. R., Wein, A. J., & Carpeniello, V. L. (1982). Improved mechanical survival with revised inflatable penile prosthesis using rear-tip extenders. *J Urol, 128,* 489.

Marina, S., Marina, F., Alcolea, R., Nadal, J., Pons, M. C., Grossmann, M., Exposito, R., & Vidal, J. (1999). Triplet pregnancy achieved through intracytoplasmic sperm injection with spermatozoa obtained by prostatic massage of a paraplegic patient: Case report. *Human Reproduction, 14,* 1546–1548.

Marmar, J., Benedictus, T., & Praiso, D. (1998). Penile plethysmography on impotent men using vacuum constrictor devices. *Urology, 32,* 198–204.

Matthews, G. J., Gardner, T. A., & Francois, E. J. (1996). In vitro fertilization improves pregnancy rates for sperm obtained by rectal probe ejaculation. *Journal of Urology 155,* 1934–1937.

Meihart, W., Lycklama, A., Nycholt, A., Kropman, R., & Zwartendijk, J. (1993). The negative pressure device for erectile disorders—when does it fail? *Journal of Urology 149*, 1285–1289.

Montague, D. K., & Angermeier, K. W. (2001). Penile prosthesis implantation. *Urology Clinics of North America, 28*, 355–361.

Moul, J., & Mcleod, D. (1989). Negative pressure devices in the explanted prosthesis population. Journal of Urology 142, 729–731.

Mulcahy, J. J., Krane, R. J., Lloyd, L. K., Edson, M., & Siroky, M .B. (1990). Duraphase penile prosthesis—results of clinical trials in 63 patients. *Journal of Urology 143*, 518.

Müller, J., Sønksen, J., Sommer, P., Schmiegelow, M., Petersen, P. M., Heilman, C., & Schmiegelow, K. (2000). Cryopreservation of semen from pubertal boys with cancer. *Medical and Pediatric Oncology, 34*, 191–194.

Nadig, P. (1989). Six years experience with the vacuum constriction device. *Int J Impot Res, 1*, 55.

Nadig, P. (1996). Vacuum erection devices: A review. *World Journal of Urology 8*, 114.

Nadig, P., Ware, J., & Blumoff, R. (1986). Non-invasive device to produce and maintain an erection-like state. *Urology, 27*, 126.

Nehra, A., Werner, M. A., Bastuba, M., Title, C., & Oates, R. D. (1996) Vibratory stimulation and rectal probe electroejaculation as therapy for patients with spinal cord injury: Semen parameters and pregnancy rates. *Journal of Urology, 155*, 554–559.

Ohl, D. A., Bennett, C. J., McCabe, M., Menge, A. C., & McGuire, E. J. (1989a). Predictors of success in electroejaculation of spinal cord injured men. *Journal of Urology 142*, 1483–1486.

Ohl, D. A., Grainger, R., Bennett, C. J., Randolph, J. F., Seager, S. W. J., & McCabe, M. (1989b). Successful of electroejaculation in two multiple sclerosis patients including a report of a pregnancy utilizing intrauterine insemination. *Neurology Urodynamics, 8*, 195–198.

Ohl, D. A., Hurd, W. W., Wolf, L. J., Menge, A. C., Ansbacher, R., Christman, G., & Randolph, J. F. (1995). Electroejculation and assisted reproductive techniques. *Fertility Sterility, 64*(Suppl.1), 138.

Ohl, D. A., McCabe, M., Sønksen, J., Randolph, J. F., & Menge, A. C. (1996). Management of infertility in SCI. *Topics in Spinal Cord Injury Rehabilitation, 1*, 65–75.

Ohl, D. A., & Sønksen, J. (1996). Sperm collection for assisted reproduction in ejaculatory dysfunctions. In A. A. Acosta & T. F. Kruger (Eds.), *Human spermatozoa in assisted reproduction* (pp. 455–472). Carnforth: Parthenon Publishing.

Ohl, D. A., & Sønksen, J. (1997). Current status of electroejaculation. *Advances in Urology, 10*, 169–189.

Ohl, D. A., Sønksen, J., & Bolling, R. (2000). New stimulation pattern for electroejaculation based on physiological studies. *Journal of Urology 163* (Suppl. 1), 1522.

Ohl, D. A., Sønksen, J., Menge, A. C., McCabe, M., & Keller, L. M. (1997). Electroejaculation versus vibratory stimulation in spinal cord injured men: Sperm quality and patient preference. *Journal of Urology 157*, 2147–2149.

Osbon, G. (1985). Erection aid device. *U.S. Patent No. 4,378,008*. Washington, DC: U.S. Patent and Trademark Office.

Perkash, I., Martin, D. E., Warner, H., Blank, M. S., & Collins, D.C. (1985). Reproductive biology of paraplegics: Results of semen collection, testicular biopsy and serum hormone evaluation. *Journal of Urology, 134*, 284–288.

Rejoyn Vacuum Therapy System http://www.rejoyn.com/RVTS.html; $129.99

Sarkarati, M., Rossier, A. B., & Fam, B. A. (1987). Experience in vibratory and electroejaculation techniques in spinal cord injury patients: A preliminary report. *Journal of Urology 138*, 59–63.

Scott, E., Bradley, W., Timm, G. (1973). Management of erectile impotence. *Urology, 2,* 80.

Sidi, A., Becher, E., Zhang, G., Lewis, J. (1990). Patient acceptance of and satisfaction with an external negative pressure device for impotence. *Journal of Urology* 144, 1154–1156.

Small, M. P., Carrion, H. A., & Gordon, J. A. (1975). Small-Carrion penile prosthesis. Urology, 5, 479.

Soderhald, W., Thrasher, J., & Hansberry, K. (1997). Intracavernosal drug induced erection therapy versus external vacuum device in the treatment of erectile dysfunction. *BJ. Urol., 79,* 952–957.

Sønksen, J., & Biering-Sørensen, F. (1992). Fertility in men with spinal cord or cauda equina lesions. *Seminars in Neurology, 12,* 106–114.

Sønksen, J., Biering-Sørensen, F., & Kristensen, J. K. (1994). Ejaculation induced by penile vibratory stimulation in men with spinal cord injuries: The importance of the vibratory amplitude. *Paraplegia, 32,* 651–660.

Sønksen, J and Ohl D(2002). Penile vibratory stimulation and electroejaculation in the treatment of ejaculatory dysfunction. *International Journal of Urology* 25: 324–332.

Sønksen, J., Ohl, D. A., Giwercman, A., Biering-Sørensen, F. and Kristensen, J. K. (1996) Quality of semen obtained by penile vibratory stimulation in men with spinal cord injuries: observations and predictors. *Urology* 48, 453–457.

Sønksen, J., Ohl, D. A., and Wedemeyer, G. (2001). Sphincteric events during penile vibratory ejaculation and electroejaculation in men with spinal cord injuries. *Journal of Urology 165,* 426–429.

Sønksen, J., Sommer, P., Biering-Sørensen, F., Ziebe, S., Lindhard, A., Loft, A., Nyboe Andersen, A., & Kristensen, J. K. (1997). Pregnancies after assisted ejaculation procedures in men with spinal cord injuries. *Archives of Physical and Medical Rehabilitation 78,* 1059–1061.

Steinberger, R. E., Ohl, D. A., Bennett, C. J., McCabe, M., and Wang, S. C. (1990). Nifedipine pretreatment for autonomic dysreflexia during electro-ejaculation. *Urology 36,* 228–231.

Subrini, L. (1982). Subrini penile implants: Surgical, sexual and psychological results. *European Urology, 8,* 222.

Subrini, L., & Couvelaire, R. (1974). Le traitement chirurgical de l'impuissance virile par intubation prothtique intravacerneuse. *Journal of Urology and Nephrology, 80,* 269.

Surgitek. (1987). SURGITEK R Flexi-Falte IL intracorporeal inflatable penile implant. *Surgical procedure guide,* USA.

Szasz, G., & Carpenter, C. (1989). Clinical observation in vibratory stimulation of the penis of men with spinal cord injury. *Archives of Sexual Behaviour, 18,* 461–474.

Tepper, M. S. (1997). Making babies: Vibrostimulation and insemination. *New Mobility, 8,* 18, 20, 22. (Also available online. Retrieved April 4, 2006, from http://sexualhealth.com/article.php?Action=readandarticle_id=2andchannel=3andtopic=71.)

Turner, L., Althof, S., Levine, S., Tobia, S., Kursh, E., Bodner, D., Resnick, M. (1990). Treating erectile dysfunction with external vacuum devices: Impact on sexual, psychological and marital functioning. *Journal of Urology 141,* 322.

Watkins, W., Lim, T., Bourne, H., Baker, H. W., & Wutthiphan, B. (1996). Testicular aspiration of sperm for intracytoplasmic sperm injection: An alternative treatment to electro-emission: case report. *Spinal Cord 34,* 696–698.

Witherington, R. (1989). Vacuum constriction device for management of erectile impotence. *Journal of Urology 141,* 320–22.

Chapter Five

WOMEN'S SEXUAL PROBLEMS AND CONCERNS

Carol Rinkleib Ellison

What is a sexual problem? Who defines it? Might what is labeled a "problem" sometimes be only a "concern," or even regarded as "just how it is"? Beliefs about doing sex and how we conceptualize and describe sexual problems and therapy issues shape how individuals experience them in their lives and how clinicians treat them.

In this chapter, I will discuss some of the cultural beliefs that lead to perceived sexual problems. I will provide examples from the research that underlies my book *Women's Sexualities: Generations of Women Share Intimate Secrets of Sexual Self-Acceptance.*

In 1993–1994, curious about what is typical in the sex lives of contemporary college-educated American women, Dr. Bernie Zilbergeld and I surveyed a nationwide sample of convenience, asking women how they experienced and expressed their sexualities. The 2,632 women who responded to our 16-page questionnaire were born between 1905 and 1977; 556 were age 50 or older. Thirty-two percent had some college or a two-year degree; 21 percent had a four-year degree; and 40 percent had done some graduate work or had a graduate degree. Although we had planned for and attempted to have greater ethnic diversity, 83 percent were Caucasian. With respect to sexual orientation, 7 percent described themselves as lesbian, 5.5 percent as bisexual, and the remainder as heterosexual. The survey was preceded by in-depth interviews of about 100 women, 72 done by me, the rest by others. For additional details of this research, see Ellison (2000) or www.womenssexualities.com. The survey questionnaire can be seen on the Web site.

MEDICAL MODEL

In the world of formal psychology and medicine, successful sex and sexual health are typically thought of in physical terms. The goals of treatment are usually that the patient or client achieve and maintain lubrication/erection; have intercourse or a same-sex equivalent; and achieve orgasm. Therapy success is defined in terms of enhanced or restored physical functioning. This is a sex-as-performance model.

Historically, no premium was put on women desiring sex. More recently, low desire has been labeled pathological, and increasing sexual desire has become a therapy goal. Desire is usually thought of in body/mind terms as a physical/psychological urge for sex. This author does not think of the body and mind as separate. Mental thoughts and images are expressed in the body.

The concepts and language of sex therapy as it is most widely practiced were formalized by William Masters and Virginia Johnson in their 1970 book *Human Sexual Inadequacy*. In their sex therapy, "normal" sex is considered to be sexual intercourse, and problems are called *dysfunctions,* defined by my dictionary as abnormal, impaired, or incomplete functioning of an organ or part. Those who do not function the right way—that is, according to their model of sexual responsiveness, the human sexual response cycle (excitement, plateau, orgasm, resolution)—are said to have a sexual dysfunction and to be *sexually inadequate.*

The language of this model contains nouns and adjectives that label conditions and individuals or imply mechanical performance requirements, such as *dysfunctions, sexual disorders, impotent, frigid, achieve erection, premature ejaculation, functioning,* and *sexual response cycle.*

Many people today think or say *achieve orgasm* as if those two words go together. The ubiquitousness of this phrase, which subtly implies that sex is a task with orgasm as its aim, demonstrates how pervasive what I call the *manufacturing orgasms* sexual script is.

The manufacturing orgasms script probably began before Sigmund Freud (1856–1939), but it was the emphasis on clitoral and vaginal orgasms that began with Freud and his followers that firmly rooted the ideas I call *manufacturing orgasms sex* into our collective consciousness. Few of us raised in this culture have escaped the influence of nearly a century of debate about clitoral and vaginal orgasms. The obsession with clitoral and vaginal orgasms started with Freud in the early twentieth century. In *A General Introduction to Psychoanalysis,* published in English translation in 1920, Freud wrote:

> We know that the little girl feels injured on account of her lack of a large, visible penis, envies the boy his possession, and primarily from this motive desires to be a man. . . . During childhood, the clitoris of the girl is the equivalent of the penis; it is especially excitable, the zone where auto-erotic satisfaction is achieved. In the

transition to womanhood it is most important that the sensations of the clitoris are completely transferred at the right time to the entrance of the vagina. In cases of so-called sexual anesthesia of women the clitoris has obstinately retained its excitability (p. 274).

In 1927 he added that "the abolition of clitoris sexuality is a necessary precondition for the development of femininity" (Freud, 1927, p. 139). And in 1938 he published: "If the woman finally submits to the sexual act, the clitoris becomes stimulated and its role is to conduct the excitement to the adjacent genital parts; it acts here like a chip of pinewood, which is utilized to set fire to harder wood. It often takes some time before this transference is accomplished, and during this transition the young wife remains anesthetic. This anesthesia may become permanent if the clitoric zone refuses to give up its excitability ..." (pp. 613–614).

Freud's *opinions* were cloned, expanded on, and repeated in the marriage manuals and medical textbooks of the 1930s through the 1950s as if they were scientific fact. Vaginal orgasms, a woman's orgasms through intercourse, were said to be a sign of marital maturity, and simultaneous orgasms through intercourse were touted as the ultimate in lovemaking. In his classic *Ideal Marriage, Its Physiology and Technique,* first published in 1926, T. H. Van de Velde wrote:

> ... in ideal communion the stimulation will generally be focused on and in the vagina.... And this will be fully adequate for such a variety and intensity of sensation as will culminate in the orgasm.
>
> In the normal and perfect coitus, mutual orgasm must be almost simultaneous; the usual procedure is that the man's ejaculation begins and sets the woman's acme of sensation in train at once (1968 edition, p. 165).

And in *Love without Fear*, a popular sex manual published first in 1947 and revised in 1957, Eustace Chesser advised his readers that both partners should, in coitus, concentrate their full attention on one thing: the attainment of simultaneous orgasm.

Manufacturing Orgasms Sex

These authors, much-read and influential in their time, specifically defined sexual success in terms of manufacturing orgasms to quite detailed specifications. They told their readers, many of whom were seeking to solve the mysteries of how to do sex, that orgasm is the goal of sex. To be sexually successful in this *manufacturing orgasms sex* script, you *must* have an orgasm. The orgasm *must* occur in intercourse.

And according to these prominent male physicians, the stakes are even higher: you and your partner *must* have not just any orgasms, but simultaneous orgasms. We recognize now that these are opinions, not truth, but they are opinions that still have influence. Some college-age women who participated in my interview/questionnaire research, for example, believed that to be good at sex they needed to aspire to vaginal and/or simultaneous orgasms.

As we grow up and find our way to understanding how we're supposed to have sex, we take in the cultural messages and expectations offered to our generation. "Emily" (the names of research participants have been changed), born in 1919, was one of the women I interviewed. Emily read marriage manuals available in this era. She described simultaneous orgasms as a regular part of her lovemaking.

Emily told me, "I had read some books and they all promoted simultaneous orgasms and I had them with no problem in the first year of marriage. I had learned on my own how to build arousal. During intercourse I would tell him to stop for a few moments and let the feelings subside and then start again. And then again. I had tremendous orgasms by prolonging the event this way. I had discovered when I masturbated that if I stopped right when I was starting to move that way and just let the buzzing and the feelings all calm down, and then I would go on, I would prolong the pleasure."

What Vera and Peg, born in the 1940s, first learned about orgasms was that they were supposed to have *vaginal* ones. And they did. Vera told me: "I've never had an orgasm with oral sex. My orgasms are brought on by something inside that gets hit and I feel 'boom.' It doesn't come from the outside." Peg said, "I really like vaginal orgasms. I am one of the rare birds for whom intercourse doesn't necessarily have to be preceded with clitoral stimulation. I have clitoral orgasms also."

But many women have experiences that do not fit the orgasmic fashions of their times. If they and their partners believe and then judge themselves by socially-imposed criteria about how they should be responding, they may think of themselves as sexually inadequate. That is what happened to this RN, born in 1940, who participated in the questionnaire survey: "A psychodynamic psychiatrist taught us medical-nursing students that clitoral stimulation/orgasm was immature. I felt inadequate and was unable to have intercourse orgasm (without manual stimulation, too) until my late 30s."

Freudian theorists and analysts, most of them male, labeled women who did not reach orgasm through vaginal penetration by a penis as *frigid, neurotic, infantile*, and *suffering from incomplete psychosexual development*. Long-term psychoanalysis was their treatment of choice for *frigid* women, although it often did little to improve sexual satisfaction. Another treatment, fortunately rare, for the so-called *problem* of clitoral sensitivity was to eliminate the clitoris and its surrounding structures entirely, supposedly to keep this source of pleasure from interfering with the vagina's sensitivity (Barbach, 1975, p. 30).

Better would have been to teach these women—and their partners—to be more skillful in their lovemaking. The problem was not clitoral sensitivity, of course, but beliefs. The potentially wonderful variety in sex and women's orgasms was being reduced to one right way. Opinions about how sex and orgasms should be were being taken as fact.

More History

The Freudian psychological interpretations of sexuality influenced sex research throughout the twentieth century. Even in Freud's time, not everyone agreed with him. Sexual literature and research were addressing such questions as, Are there distinctly different kinds of orgasms? If there are, is one kind more mature or better than another?

In the widely read *Sexual Behavior in the Human Female*, published in 1953, Alfred Kinsey and his colleagues (all men) wrote of research in which gynecologists stroked areas of the vaginas, labia, and cervixes of over 800 women with a Q-tip-like probe; these doctors also exerted pressure with a larger object. Since few of these women felt the touch when their inner vaginal walls were gently stroked or lightly touched and even fewer were conscious of a light stroke or pressure to the cervix, the Kinsey group concluded that vaginal sensation is limited to the outer third of the vagina, and "it is improbable that any area which is insensitive to tactile manipulation could be stimulated erotically" (Kinsey, Pomeroy, Martin, & Gebhard 1953, pp. 577–580). They thought, therefore, that women shouldn't be expected to have *vaginal orgasms.*

This statement planted an erroneous belief in our sexual mythology that still affects the way many people think about women's sexuality today: the idea that women's potential for vaginal/internal pleasure is quite limited. This myth was repeated in the 2005 film *Kinsey*. The Kinsey researchers were not considering, however, that the experience of a sexually aroused woman with full genital engorgement, actively engaged in intercourse, might be quite different from that of a woman, possibly anxious, on a gynecologist's examining table.

By the 1960s and 1970s, reactions against the Freudian dogma had swung the pendulum so far that some sex therapists, researchers, and feminists had replaced it with an equally dogmatic clitoral model (Ellison, 1979, 1980, 1981). At its extreme, the clitoral model position was the following: Women get little real stimulation from intercourse; orgasm is always due to clitoral stimulation in some form. This was a dominant theme, for example, in Shere Hite's 1976 *The Hite Report*. Even though some were as dogmatic as the Freudians had been, by the 1970s, more women were speaking out.

For example, the clitoral model also was a central theme in Lonnie Barbach's *For Yourself* (1975), an important contribution to the recognition of women's orgasmic potential. Barbach's term *preorgasmic* let women embrace their potential for orgasm. She taught many women to be orgasmic and inspired many feminist therapists to conduct preorgasmic women's groups. But the model epitomized the manufacturing orgasm script. Often, mutual enjoyment and pleasure were sacrificed so the woman could have her orgasm.

Masters and Johnson characterized the clitoris as the *center of female sensual focus* that acts as a *transformer* of all sexual stimulation (Masters & Johnson, 1966, p. 63). They described stimulation during intercourse as due to movement and tugging on the clitoral hood rather than accepting that a woman might experience other movement and sensations from deeper within her vagina. They introduced a new medical diagnosis, *masturbatory orgasmic inadequacy,* for women who could have intercourse orgasms but could not have clitoral ones through partner or self-manipulation (Masters & Johnson, 1970, p. 240).

When we name an experience, we impose values and judgments on it. By coming up with this label, Masters and Johnson gave a new group of women, most of whom probably thought they were just fine the way they were, the message that they should consider themselves "inadequate." Experiencing orgasm in one way but not in another need not be a problem. There is infinite variety in women's orgasmic experiences. What is a problem is to feel judged and inadequate because someone else is telling you what your experience should be instead of validating the experiences you are having.

A 1980–1981 study of my own revealed distress due to clitoral model thinking. A woman who was then 32 told me: "When I took a human sexuality course, I was too embarrassed to speak up and say I don't turn on by being manually stimulated. I don't even particularly like it. My clitoral area is too sensitive or something. But I'm almost 100 percent orgasmic in intercourse. I really turn on to my husband, his body, the way he smells. Sex is good for us, and we have a lot of fun together."

Whichever way the pendulum was swinging, there were dissenting views. Germaine Greer noted in 1971 that we had been infected by a *veritable clitoromania* and went on to say:

> It is nonsense to say that a woman feels nothing when a man is moving his penis in her vagina: the orgasm is qualitatively different when the vagina can undulate around the penis instead of vacancy ... Real satisfaction is not enshrined in a tiny cluster of nerves but in the sexual involvement of the whole person. If we localize female response in the clitoris we ... (substitute) genitality for sexuality (Greer, 1971, pp. 36–37).

In the male-centered Freudian image, the orgasm is produced by the thrusting penis. Greer gave us a woman-as-equal image. The man is *moving* rather than *thrusting* his penis, and the vagina is *undulating* around the penis. The woman is involved, rather than being "done to."

The clitoral-vaginal orgasms issue was not exclusively heterosexual. In *The Joy of Lesbian Sex,* for example, Emily Sisley and Bertha Harris wrote of how the term *frigidity* had "taken on the cultural meaning of being incapable of achieving vaginal orgasm with a penis" and said of the impact on lesbians of this way of thinking:

> Lesbians, of course, suffered even more (than heterosexual women) from Freud's disqualification of the clitoris as a socially approved site of orgasm, and, even while the steam was pouring from their eyeballs from clitoral orgasm, believed in their heads that "mature womanhood" would be forever denied them until their vaginas could somehow make friends with a penis (1977, pp. 80–81).

A SATISFACTION—SELF-ESTEEM MODEL

What happens when we change criteria for being successful in sex? How does our perception of sexual problems and concerns change if we define success in a sexual interlude not in terms of physiological functioning, but in terms of creating erotic pleasure with outcomes of intimacy, satisfaction, mutual pleasure, and self-esteem?

My answer to the *manufacturing orgasms sex* script was to come up with a new definition of sexual success that does not define success in a sexual interlude in terms of physical functioning. I define success, instead, in terms of creating erotic pleasure with outcomes of intimacy, satisfaction, mutual pleasure, and self-esteem. This redefinition of success in sex has become the cornerstone of the intimacy-based sex therapy I practice.

In my view, a couple is sexually successful when they create erotic pleasure, to whatever level and in whatever form they desire on that particular occasion, if each ends up feeling good about him/herself and the other, and they have a good time.

To facilitate such experiences is the guiding intention of the therapist; enhanced physical functioning is likely but not considered necessary for sexual success. Intercourse and orgasms are choices, not requirements for successful lovemaking. Variety in orgasmic experiences is welcomed. There is no one right way. Individuals are encouraged to focus attention on "Am I enjoying what's happening right now?" rather than on "How am I doing?"

My definition of sexual success includes the word *create*, but not the word *achieve*. It says nothing about having intercourse or how stimulation occurs, nor does it mention lubrication, achieving erections, lasting longer, achieving orgasms, or any other particular aspect of physical responsiveness.

From my perspective, the Freudians took a narrow view of the glorious potential of a woman's sexual responsiveness. Focusing in on one way of having sex as the so-called right way or even considering a question like, "Is it okay if there is clitoral stimulation during intercourse?" reduces sex from a dynamic interaction between two people to the rubbing of a magic button or two to mechanically reach a goal.

The language of an intimacy/experiential model labels difficulties with phrases that describe process or experience and includes such words and phrases as *create pleasure; create orgasm; erotic experience; enhance self-esteem; experiencing erectile problems; having orgasmic difficulties; ejaculating sooner than he (or his partner) would like; optimize physical responsiveness; conditions for pleasure;* and *continuum of erotic possibilities.* Sex need not be desired; the idea that one would like to engage in sex is sufficient. Sexual pleasure can be reached via interest and consent.

The model acknowledges the tremendous variability in how individuals experience and express sexual pleasure. For example, a woman for whom intercourse is painful would not initiate intercourse but might be very interested in and consent to other forms of mutual erotic pleasure. Her conditions for pleasure would be very different from those of a woman who tremendously enjoys sexual intercourse.

THE NEW VIEW

The *New View of Women's Sexual Problems* was written by the Working Group for A New View of Women's Sexual Problems, 12 clinicians and social scientists concerned with the increasing medicalization and pharmacologicalization of women's sexual problems and concerns. This author was a member of that group. The document was first released at a press conference on October 25, 2000, and copublished simultaneously in 2001 in the journal *Women and Therapy*, Vol. 24, Nos. 1/2 and as a book edited by Ellyn Kaschak and Leonore Tiefer.

> The first part (of *The New View*) criticizes current American Psychiatric Association nomenclature for women's sexual problems because of false equivalency between men and women, erasing the relational contact of sexuality, and ignoring differences among women. The second part offers guidance for new nomenclature from international sexual rights documents. The third part offers our new classification system (p. 1).

The New View's women-centered definition of sexual problems is "discontent or dissatisfaction with any emotional, physical, or relational aspect of sexual experience," which "may arise in one or more ... interrelated aspects of women's lives" (p. 5). These aspects, in four categories, include sociocultural, political, or economic factors; partner and relationship factors; psychological factors; and medical factors.

ELLISON/ZILBERGELD SURVEY

Results from the Ellison/Zilbergeld survey of 2,632 women support New View thinking. There is tremendous variability in how women experience and express their sexualities. Experiences of sexuality are multidimensional.

Aspects of Sexual Expression Experienced in the Previous Year

Our questionnaire asked those of the 2,632 respondents who had had a sexual partner in the previous year to respond to a series of questions on "some aspects of sexual expression you may have experienced." We presented the following list of 23 sexual circumstances and asked the respondents to indicate if they had experienced each in the previous year not at all, rarely, sometimes, often, or all the time.

Under the heading "I have experienced the following in the last year" were the following: (1) difficulty finding a partner I wanted to be sexual with; (2) lower sexual desire than I wanted to have; (3) being too tired to have sex; (4) being too busy to have sex; (5) not feeling sexually satisfied; (6) my partner not as interested in sex as I was; (7) my partner less interested in closeness after sex than I; (8) my partner choosing inconvenient times for sex.

Under the heading "During sex in the last year I have experienced" were the following: (9) difficulty getting excited/aroused; (10) feeling distracted; (11) inability to relax; (12) involuntary vaginal spasm so that vaginal entry and/or intercourse was impossible or difficult; (13) inadequate vaginal lubrication; (14) pain during intercourse or other internal stimulation; (15) fantasizing that I am having sex with someone other than my partner; (16) difficulty in reaching orgasm; (17) inability to have an orgasm; (18) reaching orgasm too quickly; (19) my partner seeming distracted; (20) my partner wanting shorter foreplay than I wanted; (21) my partner having difficulty getting aroused. In addition, there were two more items specifically for women with male partners: (22) my partner ejaculating too quickly; and (23) my partner having difficulty getting and/or maintaining an erection. There also was a blank where the respondent could specify "other."

Henceforth, I will refer to these above 23 items as the *overview list.*

The Experiences

The experiences on this overview list are clearly a part of women's lives. Of the 2,295 survey respondents with a previous-year sex partner, 98.6 percent checked at least one as experienced sometimes, often, or all the time. When "sometimes" was omitted, 72 percent had experienced at least one often or all the time.

Problems—or "Just How It Is"?

In 1978, Ellen Frank, Carol Anderson, and Debra Rubinstein, reported the results of their study of 100 predominantly white, college-educated, and happily married couples. They found that although over 80 percent of the couples described their marriages and sexual relationships as happy and satisfying, their sexual lives were far different from those typically portrayed in the media. "Forty percent of the men reported erectile or ejaculatory dysfunction, and 63 percent of the women reported arousal or orgasmic dysfunction. In addition, 50 percent of the men and 77 percent of the women reported difficulty that was not dysfunctional in nature (e.g., lack of interest or inability to relax)" (p. 111).

Influenced by this groundbreaking and often-cited study, we asked respondents to our survey who had experienced any of the items on the overview list to consider which, if any, they thought of as "problems" and which they thought of as "just the way life is." Depending on the item, from 50 percent to virtually 90 percent of those who had a particular experience concluded, "That's the way life is" rather than "this is a problem." No one item was called a problem by more than half of the women who'd had it happen at all, whether sometimes or more frequently.

Our survey demonstrated that, in general, many of us accept the realities and imperfections of our sex lives. There were, however, six circumstances that were more likely than the others to be considered problems, even if experienced only sometimes. I call these "The Big Six;" I will say more about them shortly.

Most Important Sexual Problem or Concern in the Past Year

One survey question asked about the woman's most important sexual problem or concern in the past year. Respondents could indicate an item on the overview list or write in another answer. Table 5.1 categorizes the responses

Table 5.1
Women's Most Important Sexual Concerns and Problems in the Past Year

Problem or Concern Category	Number of Women	Percent of all 1,637 Women
Desire/frequency	555	34
Physical responsiveness	469	29
Lovemaking	261	16
Finding a partner	123	8
Relationship	71	4
Fertility/reproduction	45	3
STIs/safer sex	37	2
Her own body/health	31	2
Miscellaneous—abuse, nonmonogamy, orientation, other	45	3

Source: Adapted from the table on page 258 of C. R. Ellison, *Women's Sexualities: Generations of Women Share Intimate Secrets of Sexual Self-Acceptance* (Oakland, CA: New Harbinger Publications, 2000), 258.

of the 1,637 women who reported a most important concern or problem. There were 547 others who reported having *no* most important sexual problem or concern in the previous year.

Certain issues, particularly those related to fertility, physical responsiveness, and health, tended to vary with age. For example, of the most important problems or concerns related to women's bodies and health, 69 percent were reported by women age 40 or older, while only 45 percent of the respondents were in that age group.

Issues of Desire and Frequency: The American Way of Life

While respondents to the Ellison/Zilbergeld survey all lived in the United States, we suspect that many of our conclusions, particularly with respect to desire and frequency, apply to other Western cultures as well.

Among the factors in Category I of the New View (sexual problems due to sociocultural, political, or economic factors) are "lack of interest, fatigue, or lack of time due to family and work obligations" (p. 6). Category II (sexual problems relating to partner and relationship) includes "discrepancies in desire for sexual activity or in preferences for various sexual activities" (p. 7).

In the Ellison/Zilbergeld survey, the three most marked items on the overview list were being "too tired to have sex," being "too busy," and having "lower sexual desire than I wanted to have." There is no doubt that these are typical experiences of today's American women. The desire and frequency category—these three items plus one not included on the overview list: the woman and her partner having different levels of sexual desire and interest—also led the more specific list of most important sexual concerns and problems. One out of three of the women with a most important concern or problem reported an issue from this category.

Too tired/too busy. Although being too tired to have sex and being too busy to have sex were the items selected most often from the overview list, they were not among the experiences most likely to be considered problems when they occurred; they were among those most likely to be considered as the way life is. Being at least sometimes too tired and/or too busy for sex is a part of the American way of life that many of us take pretty much for granted. Often, both a woman and her partner are affected. A woman in her forties commented: "Lack of sex is due to exhaustion on both our parts. We are coming to terms with the fact we're older, work two full-time jobs, and are actively involved in our three young children's lives." Another woman, who was younger, mentioned "difficulty juggling—balancing—being a parent, a worker, time for myself, my relationship and my sexuality."

In these comments, we see clear examples of role fragmentation: one woman filling many roles. Role fragmentation is a part of the American way of life. Where are the time, energy, and attention to come from for sexual desire?

Lower sexual desire than I wanted to have. Having lower desire than they wanted was reported by women of all ages and was more likely to be considered a problem than being too tired or too busy. Here, too, however, some respondents specifically voiced their acceptance of their low desire for sex. One woman, close to age 50, explained: "I no longer feel my low desire is a 'problem' or 'something wrong with me' but a path to a new way of being sexual. My partner and I are experimenting with sex that is not goal (orgasm) oriented." Some women of reproductive age noted a link between diminished desire and taking birth control pills. Other respondents mentioned links to grief and loss, and to anger and resentment. Some problems and concerns seemed to be more a loss of interest than lack of desire. For example: "I haven't been wanting to be with my primary partner in a sexual way. I am bisexual."

As clinicians we need to consider that we may be pathologizing levels of desire that are normal. Given women's lifestyles and reproductive statuses, low levels of sexual desire are to be expected. Most women with children and stressful lives will rarely, if at all, experience sexual desire fueled by a biological urge for reproduction; nor are they likely to experience often the passionate desires of courtship. Many of these women do, however, frequently experience interest, the idea that they would like to have sex. It is the physical/psychological urgency we call desire that does not often occur. We need to normalize interest, the idea of having sex, as the beginning of the path to sexual activity. We can then help women to create situations in which they can start with interest and let one thing lead to another, including to deeper intimacy, lovemaking, and sex. Although in some cases, rekindling desire is important; it may also at times make sense to bypass desire altogether. I often tell women, "Interest and consent are all you need to start." (See different models of female sexual response in the appendix of this volume.)

Desire discrepancy. Each of us has a personal ebb and flow of sexual interest and desire. Each sexual relationship also has its own ebb and flow that is specific to that partnership. A couple's individual rhythms may more or less synchronize, or there may be a discrepancy in which one partner seems to want noticeably more or less sex than the other. Over 100 survey respondents specifically indicated that their major problem or concern was that they wanted more sex than their partners did. Their partners were avoiding sex or were not as interested as they were. It is noteworthy that many of the comments in this section were from women older than age 40. Heterosexual women ages 40 to 60 described male partners who avoided sex, were less interested in closeness after sex, and had difficulty getting aroused; some men also had delayed ejaculation. Most of these women felt quite strongly about their partners' unavailability for as much sex as they would like. Some younger women also had similar complaints.

While clinically, we typically label these situations as desire discrepancies, we might more realistic think of many of them as discrepancies in interest and willingness to engage in sex.

Problems Related to Physical Responsiveness

Of the reported most important problems and concerns, 28 percent had to do with the physical responsiveness of the woman or her partner. Of the 457 responses in this category, 138 involved a partner's responsiveness, and 329 the survey respondent's. Of these, 186 had something to do with her orgasms, sometimes in combination with another problem or concern.

The Big Six

There are six items on the overview list that I call The Big Six. These were not the experiences of the greatest number of women, but they were the ones most likely to have been called "problems," not just accepted as "the way life is," by those who experienced them. All six have to do with what goes on during sexual activity, something to do with attention or with the physical responsiveness of the woman or her partner. Three have to do with her partner's involvement, and three the woman's own.

Compared to the other items on the overview list, a woman was more likely to experience it as a problem if her partner:

- had difficulty getting and/or maintaining an erection,
- had difficulty getting aroused, or
- seemed distracted during sex.

She also was likely to experience it as a problem if she herself:

- reached orgasm too quickly,
- experienced pain during intercourse or other internal stimulation, or
- experienced involuntary vaginal spasm so that vaginal entry and/or intercourse was impossible or difficult.

There were five other items that were almost as likely to be called problems and not just accepted as the way life is by the women who experienced them. These too have to do with what goes on during sexual activity. They include the woman's own difficulty getting excited/aroused during sex; inability to relax during sex; insufficient vaginal lubrication; inability to orgasm; and one other experience, specifically with male partners, that could well be related to the woman's own difficulties with arousal and orgasm—her partner ejaculating too quickly.

It is clear from the research that many of us can accept being too tired and too busy for sex, or even not desiring very often to do it. We're much less likely to say "that just how it is" when we don't get relaxed and caught up in sex or don't fully enjoy doing it. When we and/or our partners regularly don't seem able physically, mentally, and emotionally to get into the dance of sex, we are likely to experience that as a problem.

A Male Partner's Difficulties with Arousal and Erections

Male partners with erectile difficulties were mentioned by women of all ages. An 18-year-old woman reported: "My partner has difficulty getting aroused and getting erections. He has been taking an orgasm-inhibiting medication (Zoloft, a selective serotonin reuptake inhibitor, SSRI)." Another in her early 20s said: "My partner had what I consider to be erectile dysfunction, and our sexual relationship went nowhere fast. I'd never before had a man I couldn't turn on in a big way." Women whose partners have erectile difficulties often convey this sense of frustration at their powerlessness to elicit a sexual response from their partners. Frequently, however, a man's erectile difficulties have underlying causes that a partner's attractiveness can't overcome. (See chapter 1 in this volume.)

Whenever a man has erectile difficulties, I ask about medications, because these difficulties can be iatrogenic. (See chapter 14 in this volume.) Pharmacological treatment for one aspect of health may be negatively affecting quality of life in another. I ask women about medications, too. Medications for blood pressure, heart conditions, anxiety, depression, allergies—and many others—can affect erections in men and vaginal engorgement and lubrication in women. When a medication is involved, I often recommend that someone having engorgement or erectile difficulties talk to her or his health provider about trying out a different brand, a related drug, or other-than-pharmaceutical interventions to treat the "medical" condition.

Not every woman whose male partner has erectile difficulties finds them a problem. A woman in her 70s told me that her husband of the last four years had difficulty getting strong erections but was "very good with oral. He wasn't at first, but I taught him what I want." A woman in her mid-30s told me, on the other hand, of her frustration with her husband's difficulty with his erections and arousal and added: "When I say I think you should see a doctor, he gets completely upset and refuses, says he just needs time."

This survey was done before the introduction of Viagra (sildenafil). One benefit of the introduction and advertising of Viagra is that men like this woman's husband are much more willing to seek help for their erectile difficulties than previously. In my experience as a therapist, Viagra has been very helpful for some couples, such as those who desire sexual intercourse while the male partner has erectile difficulties due to diabetes. It does concern me, however, when a man is given Viagra without any discussion of the importance of his partner's consent, receptivity, and pleasure. Those who prescribe Viagra often seem to ignore that producing a male's erection should be an enhancement to creating *mutual* erotic pleasure, not an end in itself. I describe my work with couples as intimacy-based sex therapy and sexual choreography. Recommending a drug like Viagra is a very specific intervention I would choose from among many other possibilities. As we are demonstrating, the majority of women's sexual problems and concerns will not be remedied with sexual arousal pills for their partners or themselves. Ironically, one group who might find such pills beneficial are those whose difficulties with sexual responsiveness are caused by other prescribed pills they are taking.

A Male Partner's Difficulties with Ejaculation

Women whose male partners ejaculated too quickly reported difficulties reaching orgasm, anger, frustration, and feeling unsatisfied. Delayed and absent ejaculation were not on our overview list but were among the problems and concerns women noted. Like other aspects of physical responsiveness, delayed or absent ejaculation can be medication- or drug-related as well as indicative of distraction, performance anxiety, physical "armoring," and breathing patterns that inhibit arousal.

Aspects of Women's Physical Responsiveness Other Than Orgasm

We rarely can reduce a problem with physical responsiveness to only one of its aspects. Inability to relax during sex, for example, may lead to and be a part of difficulty getting aroused, which would be reflected as insufficient vaginal lubrication, which could be one of the underlying causes of pain during intercourse or other internal stimulation; pain could lead to involuntary vaginal spasms.

Difficulties with relaxation, distraction, arousal, and vaginal lubrication may be related to a woman's own health, her hormonal status, her female or male partner's difficulties (e.g., her partner's inability to relax or to sustain arousal), to relationship issues, or to numerous other factors. Inability to relax during sex affects women of all ages and may be situational. When a woman is experiencing pain during sex, I refer her for a medical consultation (see volume 2, chapter 11; and chapter 9 in this volume).

Involuntary Vaginal Spasm

While only 6 women marked involuntary vaginal spasm so that vaginal entry and/or intercourse was impossible or difficult as their most important problem or concern in the previous year, 59 women said they had this experience either often or all the time, and that same number considered the experience a "problem" rather than "the way life is." This experience is perhaps more common than many people realize: 10 percent of all respondents to the overview list of sexual circumstances had experienced this kind of vaginal spasming at least sometimes during the previous year (see volume 2, chapter 11; and chapter 9 in this volume).

Partner-Focused Problems and Concerns That May Inhibit Arousal and Orgasms

Category II of the New View addresses "sexual problems relating to partner and relationship." Some partner-related factors that may inhibit a woman's arousal and orgasms involve sexual technique. In my research, women of all ages mentioned partners who wanted shorter foreplay than they wanted; didn't touch or kiss much; didn't like to perform oral sex; didn't make their needs known; weren't aggressive enough; didn't express their excitement more; and who were less interested in performing manual and oral stimulation than the women wanted. One respondent, whose partner was male, noted: "His inhibitions make me more inhibited."

Other issues involved relationship dynamics and the initiation and timing of sex. For example: "My partner chooses inconvenient times. He is a night owl; I am more alert in the morning. He helps little with evening activities of dinner, children's homework, getting kids ready for bed, but expects my sexual receptivity regardless.

THINKING ABOUT INTERVENTIONS

Three hats I wear as therapist include: (1) sexual choreographer, in which I am a coach, facilitator, instructor for creating erotic pleasure; (2) sexual detective/problem solver, in which I try to figure out what is going on and diagnose the sexual problems my clients bring to me; and (3) sexual advisor, in which I assume the role of mentor, knowledgeable teacher, guide, counselor, consultant—and provide solutions and information about, for example, pleasuring techniques, hormones, methods of birth control, or anything else that might be relevant and appropriate.

A Sexual Detective Considers Low Sexual Desire

Attendees at one World Health Organization conference (WHO, 1975) suggested that we define "sexual health" as "the integration of the somatic, emotional, intellectual, and social aspects of sexual being" (*New View*, p. 4). (See volume 1, chapter 1.) In my sex therapist roles of detective and problem solver, I recognize that lower desire for sex than someone wants is not just one simple condition that is the same for all; it can be arrived at by many different paths and often reflects a complex combination of factors. If a woman is currently experiencing less sexual desire than she wants, I consider the following questions:

- When and under what circumstances did she first notice she had lower sexual desire than she wanted?
- Is there anything related to her health that might be affecting her sexual desire?
- Does she eat well and regularly? Does she get enough sleep?
- Does she experience chronic pain? If so, when is it most intense? Least bothersome?
- What birth control pills, medications, and vitamins does she take?
- Does she smoke cigarettes, drink alcohol or coffee, and/or use other recreational drugs? If so, how much? How often? Under what circumstances?
- Does she eat sweets and/or drink soft drinks? If so, how much?
- Is she depressed? If so, how often? Under what circumstances?
- Is she resentful or angry at her partner?
- Does she have sex with her partner when she is not truly consenting?
- Is she trying to get pregnant or concerned that she might become pregnant?
- Is she concerned that she might acquire a sexually transmitted infection?
- Does she get enough time for herself?
- Is she protecting her relationship in some way by not having sex?
- Is her partner a skillful and satisfying lover?
- Are she and her partner effective together at initiating sex?
- Does she have a history of sexual abuse or trauma that is affecting her now?
- What pressures and demands does she have in her life outside of her relationship?

Usually the answers to these questions will deepen our understanding of her sexual desire and suggest changes that might begin to enhance it. Desire is likely to be optimal when a woman is in harmony with her partner and is herself physically, mentally, emotionally, and spiritually in balance.

This method can be applied to any other issues a client might bring to therapy. Many of the same questions apply, for example, to orgasm problems or male erectile difficulties, as well as some others specific to the problem or concern.

Sexual Choreography

The guiding principle of my intimacy-based sex therapy is my definition of "sexual success": a couple is sexually successful when they create erotic pleasure, to whatever level and in whatever form they desire on a particular occasion, if each ends up feeling good about him/herself and the other, and they have a good time. One of the first interventions with practically every couple is to talk about this definition of success. Among the assumptions of this model is the notion that couples can create erotic experience through a process with building blocks in which one thing leads to another.

Transitions

Transitions of two types—personal and interpersonal—are crucial. Most people are most of the time in their not-doing-sex selves. The personal transition is a shift—physically, emotionally, in attention—from one's not-doing-sex self into one's doing-sex self. This shift can be practically instantaneous or occur over an extended period of time. It may be stimulated primarily through something outside of oneself or from hormones, physical changes, feelings, and images within (Ellison, 1984). The interpersonal couple transition is a shift from feeling separate to a sense of connection and togetherness. Many difficulties with physical responsiveness—lubrication, orgasm, erection, ejaculation—are related to or the result of skipping the crucial step of transition into the sexual process.

In recommending activities to facilitate individual and couple transitions, a therapist might recommend, for example, either solo or together, a shower or bath, stretching and breathing deeply, a snack, a glass of wine, playing or listening to music, and so forth. Couple activities that are not specifically sexual, such as a taking a walk or doing a chore together, can be excellent ways to begin feeling close. Such activities provide opportunities to weave in sexual innuendos and play and can give interest and arousal time to build into full desire.

Sexual Invitations

Consent of both partners is a prerequisite for mutuality and intimacy in sex. To consistently create satisfying sexual experiences, couples need to know how to make effective sexual invitations, and each partner needs to know how to successfully accept, reject, and negotiate the invitations the other makes.

One aspect of low sexual desire may be an absence of full consent. A woman might say, "I want to make my partner happy" to explain why she goes along with a partner's requests for sex at times when she doesn't really want to. In some relationships, going along with a partner's wishes makes both partners happier and enhances the relationship. In relationships where it does not do this, however, a partner who is only going along may begin to avoid sex with her partner and to experience diminished sexual desire. In therapy, a couple can learn to more effectively make and respond to sexual invitations so that they can negotiate to mutually consensual, and mutually pleasurable, sexual activity.

Putting a Structure around Spontaneity

While more traditional therapy focuses on getting the genitals ready for action, intimacy-based therapy focuses on facilitating mutual interaction. A therapist might recommend that a couple create rituals for relationship maintenance and enhancement. These are intended to set up their relationship in a way that will increase the likelihood that intimate feelings and sex will regularly occur. While many people believe that sex should be spontaneous, an intimacy-based therapist understands that spontaneity actually is the outcome of a series of incremental steps in which one thing leads to another.

Among interventions in this category are regular dates devoted to creating good feelings together, regular gripe or life-maintenance sessions so that problematic issues don't need to be discussed during the dates, greeting and parting rituals, and rituals that affirm loving and caring the last thing at night before sleep.

Focus of Attention

As an intimacy-based therapist, I encourage individuals to shift attention during sex from "How am I doing?" "Am I going to make it?" or "This is taking too long" to "Am I enjoying what's happening right now?" I also may suggest that they play music to unify their rhythms and attention or that they share their fantasies. And, always, my intentions include facilitating their sexual self-acceptance.

NOTE

This chapter is adapted from C. R. Ellison (2000), *Women's Sexualities: Generations of Women Share Intimate Secrets of Sexual Self-Acceptance* (Oakland, CA: New Harbinger Publications). Much of the material has also appeared in C. R. Ellison (2001), Intimacy-based sex therapy: Sexual choreography,   In Peggy Kleinplatz (Ed.), *New directions in sex therapy,* New York: Brunner-Routledge; and C. R. Ellison (2001), A research inquiry into some American women's sexual concerns and problems, In Ellyn Kaschak, & Leonore Tiefer (Eds.), *A new view of women's sexual problems,* New York: Haworth Press. (Simultaneously published as *Women & Therapy,* vol. 24, nos. 1/2.)

REFERENCES

Barbach, L. (1975). *For yourself: The fulfillment of female sexuality.* New York: New American Library.

Chesser, E. (1957). *Love without fear: A plain guide to sex technique for every married adult.* New York: Rich and Cowan.

Ellison, C. R. (1979). *Beyond the clitoris: Arousal and female sexuality.* Paper presented to the Society for the Scientific Study of Sex, San Diego, CA.

Ellison, C. R. (1980). *A critique of the clitoral model of female sexuality.* Paper presented to the American Psychological Association, Montreal, Canada.

Ellison, C. R. (1981). *Questioning the clitoral model of female sexuality.* Paper presented to the Society for the Scientific Study of Sex, New York, NY.

Ellison, C. R. (1984). Harmful beliefs affecting the practice of sex therapy with women. *Psychotherapy, 21*(3), 327–334.

Ellison, C. R. (2000). *Women's sexualities: Generations of women share intimate secrets of sexual self-acceptance.* Oakland, CA: New Harbinger Publications.

Frank, E., Anderson, C. & Rubinstein, D. (1978). Frequency of sexual dysfunction in "normal" couples. *New England Journal of Medicine, 299,* 111–115.

Freud, S. (1920). *A general introduction to psychoanalysis.* Authorized translation. New York: Boni and Liveright.

Freud, S. (1927). Some psychological consequences of the anatomical distinction between the sexes. *International Journal of Psychoanalysis, 8,* 139.

Greer, G. (1971). *The female eunuch.* New York: McGraw-Hill.

Hite, S. (1976). *The Hite report.* New York: Dell.

Kaschak, E., & Tiefer, L., eds. (2001). *A new view of women's sexual problems.* New York: Haworth Press.

Kinsey, A. C., Pomeroy, W. B., Martin, C. E., & Gebhard, P. H. (1953). *Sexual behavior in the human female.* Philadelphia, PA: W. B. Saunders.

Masters, W. H., & Johnson, V. E. (1966). *Human sexual response.* Boston: Little, Brown & Co.

Masters, W. H., & Johnson, V. E. (1970). *Human sexual inadequacy.* Boston: Little Brown & Co.

Sisley, E. L., & Harris, B. (1977). *The joy of lesbian sex.* New York: Simon and Schuster.

Van de Velde, T. H. (1968). *Ideal marriage, its physiology and technique.* New York: Random House. (First publication 1926.)

Chapter Six

THERAPY UPDATE FOR WOMEN: THE TREATMENT OF LOW LIBIDO IN WOMEN USING AN INTEGRATED BIOPSYCHOSOCIAL APPROACH

Marianne Brandon and Andrew T. Goldstein

Sexual health is a necessary aspect of general health for many adults. Women report feeling more satisfied with various aspects of life when they are comfortable with their sexual functioning (Oberg & Fugl-Meyer, 2005). Several common sexual concerns can leave women feeling sexually dissatisfied, sexually unhealthy, or somehow sexually inadequate, often prompting them to seek help. These issues are addressed in chapters by Ellison, Duplaisse & Daniluk, Graziottin, and Ogden in this book series and can include concerns about orgasm, libido, and sexual pain. In this chapter, we will focus on the treatment of low libido in women.

For men and women alike, libido represents a primary aspect of sexual health. In fact, low libido is the most frequently reported sexual concern among women. A commonly cited study suggests that over a third of women experience decreased libido at some time in their lives (Laumann, Paik, & Rosen, 1999). Patients struggling with low sex drive often report significant emotional discomfort within themselves and in their relationships as a result of their sexual disinterest (Bancroft, Loftus, & Long, 2003; Laumann et al., 1999). Common concerns expressed by women who report prolonged low sex drive include loss of pleasure in feeling feminine, discomfort with their bodies, loss of physical and emotional intimacy with their partners, fear of their partner's infidelity, and even fear of divorce. Women with low libido describe intercourse as unsatisfying, uncomfortable, or even intrusive. They frequently explain that the daily rigors of life take their toll, and that expending even more energy to have sex is often nearly impossible. In addition, they report feelings of guilt and shame about not wanting what they perceive to be a healthy part of life and relationships. How do clinicians best assist such patients in creating fulfilling, rewarding, and gratifying sexual moments for a woman and her partner?

Most practitioners working in the area of women's health are regularly faced with this question. Basson (2006) has summarized the various factors that should be taken into consideration when diagnosing and treating women with desire and arousal disorders. Women of all ages, ethnic backgrounds, and education levels report concerns about low desire. Regardless of whether a woman is actually diagnosed with hypoactive sexual desire disorder (HSDD), if she seeks help for the subjective experience of a decreased libido, practitioners must embrace a theoretical framework for her care. In this chapter, we explore a holistic, integrative, biopsychosocial model for such treatment.

This biopsychosocial treatment model to which we subscribe was the natural outgrowth of our professional collaboration in meeting the needs of our patients. Dr. Goldstein, a board certified gynecologist with a specialized focus in female sexual dysfunction, and Dr. Brandon, a clinical psychologist and diplomat in sex therapy, founded the Sexual Wellness Center in Annapolis, Maryland, after determining that individual private practice care was not addressing women's sexual concerns as effectively as collaborative treatment. In joining forces, treatment for both of us became more productive, efficient, and enjoyable. The treatment benefits to our clients were immediately apparent, as were the advantages to us of a more interesting and satisfying work environment. Like us, many other clinicians have formed similar teams in order to provide optimal treatment options for their clients.

In this chapter we will outline first why we believe the traditional treatment model involving a sole practitioner providing the majority of patient care does not optimally serve patients with low libido. Second, we will review some of the benefits for both patients and clinicians of practicing within a biopsychosocial treatment paradigm. Third, we will describe our particular framework for treating low libido in women. This integrated biopsychosocial treatment model addresses four quadrants of a woman's experience; namely, her physical, emotional, intellectual, and spiritual health, as they relate to her libido. Within each quadrant, issues within her romantic relationship are also explored. The impact of environmental and cultural influences are also considered within each quadrant. This results in an assessment and treatment model that takes into account the full complexity of a woman in the context of her world.

LIMITATIONS OF TRADITIONAL, NONINTEGRATIVE MODELS FOR TREATING LOW LIBIDO

Decreased libido carries a reputation among clinicians as one of the more challenging sexual concerns to treat. There are numerous possible reasons that traditional healing models, which often focus more exclusively on either a woman's emotional or medical health, fail a practitioner. For our purposes in this chapter, we define traditional treatment models as essentially any treatment paradigm that focuses solely on one practitioner's method of healing. Thus any practitioner may be guilty of offering an outdated model in this regard if he or she chooses not to collaborate with complimentary medical and psychological practitioners in patient care. We use the term *outdated* because, for the majority of women, low libido is not one-dimensional. And while the initial etiology of a woman's low sex drive may be understood as either primarily psychological (such as partner difficulties) (Bancroft et al., 2003; Dunn, Croft & Hackett, 1999; Hawton, Gath & Day, 1994) or primarily physiological (such as menopause), over time multiple other aspects of a woman's biology or psychology are apt to be affected. As a result, physicians, sex therapists, marriage and family therapists, and physical therapists can all be guilty of outdated care if they do not function within a conceptualization of treatment that extends beyond their own particular specialty.

NONINTEGRATIVE MODELS DO NOT OPTIMALLY ADDRESS MIND-BODY INTERACTIONS

The mind-body treatment paradigm is becoming increasingly accepted among mental health and medical providers (Weeks, 2005). The length and breadth of this *Sexual Health* series attests to this. One whole volume is devoted to the emotional and psychological aspects of sexual health, one to the physical, and one to the sociocultural aspects of healthy sexuality. Most practitioners acknowledge that physical problems may indeed have an impact on our emotions and, alternately, that emotional conflicts may be expressed through our bodies.

Female libido is a prime example of a mind-body phenomenon. That is, for most women, multiple aspects of the body and mind must be in sync for her libido to thrive. For many women, regardless of how or why her sex drive initially decreases, both mind and body become affected over time. Women readily acknowledge that their thoughts and feelings about themselves, their bodies, their partners, and their relationships impact the willingness and ease with which they express themselves sexually. Likewise, women who feel physically imbalanced, tired, or ill often report less interest in sexual activity. Thus, for most women with low libido, only attention to both realms of mind and body support optimal healing. Traditional treatments that do not embrace a holistic conceptualization of sexuality frequently yield less than adequate outcomes. For example, a sex therapist who primarily spends his time encouraging sensate focus exercises in an effort to help a woman explore herself sensually and sexually will not attend to this woman's emotions and relationship.

A marriage and family therapist who identifies anger between the couple as the primary problem will wonder why improved communication and healthy anger expression between partners does not result in a sexually interested wife. Finally, a gynecologist who prescribes testosterone cream for her patient will be surprised when the cream works well for only several months, but then ultimately the patient is back in the office verbalizing the same libido concerns. These are just a few examples of how traditional healing methods often fail conscientious practitioners and well-meaning patients.

TRADITIONAL MODELS PLACE THE BURDEN OF CURE ON THE PRACTITIONER RATHER THAN ON THE COLLABORATION BETWEEN PRACTITIONER AND PATIENT

Traditional healing models involving one primary practitioner tend to present this practitioner as an all-knowing guide to treatment. Patients in these treatment situations are often encouraged to rely exclusively on their practitioner, adapting a more passive role in the treatment process. Patients are often frustrated with themselves and their bodies by the time they begin treatment. It is not uncommon for a new patient to describe a history of struggling for a year or more with a low sex drive. As a result, these patients seem relieved to "hand over the treatment reins," and wait to be healed.

Such an approach on the part of the patient adapts well to clear-cut medical problems, such as a bone fracture. However, because of the complexity of female sex drive, libido is less responsive to relatively one-sided treatment efforts. This is often the case even when the cause of a patient's decreased libido appears medically straight forward—for example, when it appears that antidepressants or birth control pills have created low desire. Even in these situations, distinct, clear-cut treatment solutions are frequently not enough.

Ultimately, we have found that a practitioner's capacity to treat a woman with low libido is dependent on the cooperation and effort of the patient. For example, it is up to the patient to take the risks involved in deepening her sense of connection to her own body and to her partner. The patient must be willing to experiment with her sensual expression, open to feelings of joy and vulnerability with her partner, and let go of control to her partner. She must get adequate sleep and proper nutrition for her body to respond sexually. In sum, she has the challenging task of taking all that she learns from treatment and manifesting it in her life. She must learn to break old behavior and communication patterns, challenge fears, develop a new sexual identity, and heal old wounds. All this requires tremendous work and effort on her part. She is set up for failure if her role as an active participant in the healing process is not clarified from the beginning of her treatment. Allowing her an expectation that healing depends more on her practitioner, rather than her collaboration with multiple practitioners, opens the door for disappointment when she finds that her treatment is not resulting in a return of her sex drive.

TRADITIONAL MODELS MAY BE LESS ORIENTED TO ADDRESS SECONDARY GAIN

As with most human struggles, sexual or otherwise, symptoms simultaneously serve us, as well as hinder us; protect us, as well as prevent our healing and growth. In this way, most symptoms serve a purpose by offering some kind of benefit to a patient. Secondary gain is common in treatment situations, and it is frequently encountered when treating women with low libido.

Sexual complaints such as decreased desire or sexual pain may serve functions that may not be readily apparent to patients or practitioners. If left unaddressed, the "benefits" of a low sex drive can ultimately appear to practitioners as treatment failure. That is, when a symptom serves a purpose for a patient, whether conscious or unconscious, treatment outcome can be negatively affected. While most of our patients express a desire to change, in fact they are likely to be unconsciously ambivalent about their request for healing. Resistance to change and growth is common for most of us. Treatment models that identify such natural human tendencies may be more likely to guide a patient through fear and resistance, and toward her treatment goals.

We have found that the biopsychosocial treatment model is better positioned than the traditional models to address such issues because of the holistic focus on the patient, including her interaction within her social milieu.

DISTANCE AS A "BENEFIT" OF LOW LIBIDO

Symptoms that are experienced for extended periods of time usually have the effect of maintaining a state of equilibrium. Symptoms become part of a system, whether it is the physical system of the body, or an interpersonal system such as a marriage. When a symptom is resolved, the system it functions within will be thrown into disequilibrium for a period of time. Even when removal of a symptom is desired, patients must gain their footing in the new, healthier environment. An example of this phenomenon is the use of PDE5 inhibitors, such as sildenafil (Viagra), vardenafil (Levitra), and tadalafil (Cialis). A significant number of men who have reported good result with these medications ultimately discontinue their use (Jiamm, Tsai, Wu, & Huang, 2003). Why is that? If a couple is again able to have intercourse after an extended period of physical distance, the marital system is thrown into disequilibrium. Sometimes couples are unable to resolve the emotional conflicts that result from the increased physical intimacy.

Resurrecting a strong libido may have a similar impact on a woman and her intimate relationship. The disequilibrium that can result from the return of a woman's libido can be quite powerful, resulting in a changed relationship with herself and with her partner. For example, low libido may enable a woman to disengage from emotional pain within herself, such as a traumatic sexual history or shame about her body. Low libido may afford a woman the "opportunity" to deny her femininity, or it may allow her to disengage from her physical and emotional needs so that she may never have to feel the vulnerability inherent in exposing them to her partner. In addition, maintaining a low libido may enable a couple to avoid dealing with emotional struggles such as anger, mistrust, or grief. If the couple never becomes close enough to make love, they may never be forced to confront challenging emotional issues. In sum, all of these possibilities ultimately have the potential for increased intimacy when libido is elevated.

Increased intimacy, both physical and emotional, always involves increased risk. Most of us really are ambivalent about how close we want to be with our loved ones, and how close we can tolerate them being with us. This drama can easily be expressed sexually. Thus, for many women, distance feels safe, and this is a benefit of low libido. If a woman allows herself to be truly intimate, enabling her partner access to the most vulnerable aspects of her body, she simultaneously risks being hurt more deeply.

Most women find it helpful to address intimacy concerns in some fashion during treatment for low sex drive. However, they are often unaware of them when seeking help. When expressing a wish to revive her sex drive, a patient's longing for assistance is often clearly evident. Her voice softens, her eyes become wistful—she truthfully wants to desire her partner again. To then wonder how she benefits from her lack of libido probably seems counterproductive at those moments. But for many women, these questions are necessary issues to explore in the treatment process. Offering treatment solutions without taking the time to examine the implications of such change can set up a treatment for failure. But when a patient has the benefit of working with more than one clinician in an integrative capacity, she likely has more opportunity for such complex issues to be identified and explored. Because integrative treatment models tend to take into account the system within which a patient functions, they are more apt to include attention to these necessary but less evident aspects of the healing.

TRADITIONAL TREATMENT MODELS OVERSIMPLIFY THE IMPACT OF ENVIRONMENT

The environment within which our patients heal plays a significant role in their treatment process. This includes the more personal environment of their home, as well as their sociocultural environment. The impact of culture on sexuality is explored extensively in volume 3 of this series. We will thus only mention it here to make the point that female libido is often reactive to cultural influences, and that biopsychosocial treatment models are by design more apt to take such influences into consideration. Traditional treatment models that tend to focus on a woman's biology or inner psychology alone will miss the important impact of a woman's environment on her sexual expression.

Environmental influences can have a tremendous impact on women's comfort with their sensuality and how they express themselves sexually. For example, there is a popular notion in Western cultures that women can "do it all," including being an attentive wife and nurturing mother, work outside the home, have time to care for herself, and still maintain a healthy sex life. Many women cannot compete with these extreme societal ideals. If such unrealistic notions remain unchallenged in a patient's mind, they can leave women feeling sexually inadequate and unworthy. In reality, many women will only feel sexually open and interested if they are not living the intense life of chaos that unfortunately has become the norm for many in Western cultures. Other unspoken messages promoted by Western cultures include such notions as it is alright for sleep and self-care to be a low priority for women with busy lives, or that sexuality should just "flow" if a woman is with the right partner. Again, women endorsing such societal ideals find their libido suffering without understanding why.

When working from a holistic, mind-body model, we are less likely to ignore these potentially destructive societal beliefs. Integrative models take into account not only the emotional and physical aspects of a woman, but also the context within which she lives. When we assist a woman in finding her lost libido, such notions as lack of sleep or not enough time for personal solitude and reflection become as important to her sexuality as a loving sexual partner or scheduling time for making love. We suggest that the more limited traditional models are much less inclined to assist a woman in evaluating her life from a balanced perspective, thus failing to address notions ingrained by society that can leave women feeling unworthy or defective.

THE BENEFITS OF INTEGRATIVE BIOPSYCHOSOCIAL MODELS IN TREATING LOW LIBIDO

Benefits to Women

A biopsychosocial model offers multiple patient benefits. First and most importantly, we find models involving multiple clinicians offer the opportunity for more comprehensive assessments and individualized treatments. Secondly, it is our clinical observation that patients appear more satisfied and confident when they know their concerns are being discussed among several trusted practitioners. Finally, patient's issues are addressed holistically—including interpersonal, intrapersonal, social, and even spiritual. Physically and emotionally, her needs are taken into account on a variety of levels.

Benefits to Practitioners

Patients are not the only benefactors of an integrative framework. A biopsychosocial model places less pressure on the practitioner to offer a single solution. Approaching treatment from such an integrative model enables clinicians to relax in the knowledge that they can hone their skills in their area of expertise, without having to be experts in those aspects falling outside their training. Clinicians may find such integrative care professionally stimulating, and thus more enjoyable, as regular collaboration allows for insights into a variety of healing modalities.

THE HOLISTIC MODEL IN A PRIVATE PRACTICE SETTING

Integrative mind-body models of care may be achieved with relative ease in major medical centers where patients have access to a wide variety of practitioners. Private practice settings may appear to offer fewer opportunities for such collaboration. However, we have found that much can be accomplished via the cooperation of a gynecologist and a clinical psychologist. In addition, we utilize a variety of practitioners in the community to augment our treatment as needed, including chiropractic care, physical therapy, yoga, massage, nutritional counseling, and acupuncture. In this way, patients may be offered the maximum care while minimizing time spent with more costly professional treatments.

At our center, we have formulated our assessment and treatment model to involve the following quadrants of a patient's experience: physical, emotional, intellectual, and spiritual. Each of these quadrants is explained in some detail below. Many new patients are unaware that so many aspects of themselves can influence their sex drive. As a result, it is not unusual for a new patient to request focused attention to only one or two aspects of her symptom experience. For example, a woman with low libido may request only assessment of her hormones, or alternately, only individual therapy. However, we feel that our clients achieve maximum benefit from treatment when all quadrants are addressed.

The Physical Quadrant

The physical quadrant is probably the broadest category in our holistic model, involving both the medical aspects of a woman's body and her emotional relationship to it. Physical issues are often what patients first consider when seeking help for their decreased sex drive. Women will frequently verbalize hope for a quick fix, such as via hormone therapy. However, the ways a woman relates to her physical body are often as important to address in reviving her lost libido. We will now look at each of these aspects in turn.

Medical Issues in the Physical Quadrant

A thorough evaluation of a woman's physical health is an essential component of a biopsychosocial evaluation of decreased libido. At the Sexual Wellness Center we believe that physical wellness cannot be over emphasized as an integral component of a healthy libido. To that end, we encourage our patients to strive for optimal physical health, not just "health" as defined by an absence of disease. Therefore, any evaluation of decreased sexual desire should include a thorough discussion regarding nutrition, smoking cessation, substance abuse, exercise, stress reduction, and sleep habits.

A medical review of systems, history, and physical exam is also part of an evaluation of a woman complaining of decreased sexual desires. A clinician should be able to recognize evidence of general medical conditions such as hypothyroidism, diabetes mellitus, renal dysfunction, or liver disease that may negatively affect sexual desire. A thorough gynecologic history and physical exam should evaluate for symptoms of sexual pain disorders, perimenopause, menopause, and anovulatory conditions such as polycystic ovarian syndrome or hyperprolactinemia.

A complete medical history must include a thorough examination of medications that a woman is currently taking or that she was taking when she began to notice diminished sexual desire. As discussed in chapter 14 of this volume, by Baron-Kuhn & Segraves, many medications can negatively affect libido. As herbal preparations, which patients may not consider medications, can also affect libido, these should be specifically addressed as well.

Evaluation of Urogenital Health

While this chapter's main focus is on sexual desire, libido cannot be divorced from other aspects of female sexual dysfunction including sexual pain disorders and sexual arousal disorders. A woman who experiences sexual pain will very quickly have decreased desire. In addition, a woman who has difficulty becoming sexually aroused or achieving orgasm often will have a corresponding decrease in her libido. Therefore, a thorough gynecologic examination in dorsal lithotomy position (lying on her back with her legs knees and thighs abducted) is an essential part of our biopsychosocial evaluation of decreased sexual desire.

Essential Aspects of Urogenital Exam

A complete, but focused, urogenital exam is used to rule out possible causes of sexual pain disorders or arousal disorders. Specifically, the vulva should be thoroughly examined for atrophy, tenderness, fissures, hyperkeratosis, ulcers, erosions, hypopigmentation, scarring, phimosis of the clitoris, and narrowing of the introitus. These abnormalities may be evidence of a vulvar skin disorder such as lichen sclerosus, erosive lichen planus, lichen simplex chronicus, or vulvar intraepithelial neoplasia. If there is evidence of any of these vulvar skin conditions, a skin punch biopsy should be sent for pathologic evaluation by a dermatopathologist, and the clinician should consider referral to a specialist in vulvar disease.

The vulva and vulvar vestibule should then be carefully palpated with a cotton swab. The swab can help elicit decreased sensitivity of the vulva and clitoris that may be evidence of a sexual arousal disorder. In addition, the swab can elicit areas of tenderness that can be evidence of vulvar vestibulitis syndrome or atrophic vestibulitis (see *Sexual Health: Vol. 2,* chapter 11).

A speculum exam should be performed to look for lesions or ulcerations in the vagina. In addition, the vagina should be examined for a loss of vaginal ruggae, vagina pallor, and petechiae which are evidence of atrophic vaginitis. While the speculum is in the vagina, a sample of the vagina discharge should be obtained for pH, wet mount, and culture. If there is evidence of cervicitis, testing for gonorrhea and chlamydia should be performed. A vaginal pH of 5 or greater can be evidence of atrophic vaginitis or bacterial vaginosis. A wet mount should be evaluated for evidence of atrophy (white blood cells, and parabasal cells), candidiasis (hyphae), bacterial vaginosis (clue cells, white blood cells, positive whiff test), and trichomonas.

A bimanual exam should then be performed to evaluate the bladder, uterus, adnexa, and pelvic floor muscles. Tenderness of the adnexa or uterus can be evidence of chronic pelvic inflammatory disease or endometriosis. Tenderness of the urethra and bladder may be evidence of interstitial cystitis. Hypertonicity, tenderness, and the presence of trigger points in the paravaginal muscles is evidence of pelvic floor dysfunction, which is a key component of dysesthetic vulvodynia and vulvar vestibulitis syndrome.

Evaluation of Hormonal Health

Any evaluation of diminished sexual desire and sexual dysfunction must include an evaluation of the three hormones essential for urogenital health and sexual desire: estrogen, testosterone, and dopamine (Caruso, Agnello, Intelisano, Farina, Di Mari & Cianci, 2004; Chanson & Salenave, 2004; Hull, et al., 1999). However, as previously mentioned, our biopsychosocial model acknowledges that there is a complex mind-body interplay. Therefore, while we believe that decreased levels of these hormones can be responsible for a low libido, we also believe that a low level of sexual desire caused by emotional or relationship issues can lead to lower levels of these hormones. In addition, our

Table 6.1
A Questionnaire That Can Help Identify Relative Testosterone Deficiency

_____ 1. I fantasize or dream about sex less often than I used to.
_____ 2. I masturbate less often than I used to.
_____ 3. During sex, I climax more slowly, and my orgasms feel less intense.
_____ 4. My nipples feel less sensitive.
_____ 5. My pubic hair is thinning.
_____ 6. I have difficulty analyzing problems and thinking clearly.
_____ 7. I seem to be losing muscle mass.
_____ 8. Overall, my energy is low.
_____ 9. One or both of my ovaries have been removed.
_____ 10. I use oral estrogens or birth control pills.

biopsychosocial model acknowledges that the wide range of normal hormone levels in women may be partially responsible for the wide range of libido in women. Therefore, in addition to relying on absolute hormonal blood levels, we also use a series of questions that can suggest if an individual woman has a relative deficiency of these hormones. (See Table 6.1.)

A Biopsychosocial Approach to Estrogen Supplementation

Low estrogen levels can be associated with the natural decrease in estrogen production during perimenopause, menopause, or lactation. In addition, low estrogen levels can be caused iatrogenically with medications (GNRH agonists, oral contraceptive pills, or progestins) or surgically (oophorectomy). Regardless of the cause, decreased estrogen levels are associated with vaginal dryness, decreased sexual arousal, diminished vulvovaginal sensation, and dyspareunia. There is less evidence that decreased estrogen alone is responsible for decreased sexual desire. However, women may have secondary reduction of sexual desire if they experience decreased arousal or dyspareunia associated with low estrogen levels. The symptoms of atrophic vulvovaginitis include vaginal dryness, decreased sensation, and dyspareunia and may be treated by systemic or local (vulvovaginal) estrogen therapy. Systemic estrogen replacement has the advantage of helping to diminish nonurogenital symptoms of decreased estrogen such as hot flashes and night sweats. However, oral systemic estrogen supplementation has the unwanted effect of increasing circulation sex-hormone binding globulin (SHBG) which in turn binds testosterone, thereby lowering bioavailable testosterone. In addition, data from large studies such as Women's Health Initiative has suggested that systemic estrogens increased the risk of stroke, myocardial infarction, and possibly breast cancer. The controversy around this study is further discussed by Dr. Huang in _Sexual Health: Vol. 2,_ chapter 3. We prefer to treat atrophic vulvovaginitis with topical estradiol in the form of tablets, creams, or rings.

A Biopsychosocial Approach to Testosterone Supplementation

It is generally accepted that low levels of testosterone may cause symptoms of fatigue, low energy, a diminished sense of well-being, and decreased sexual desire (Bachmann, Bancroft, & Braunstein, 2002). While there is unresolved academic debate whether there is a "female androgen insufficiency syndrome," there is strong evidence that testosterone supplementation significantly increases both sexual desire and the frequency of satisfying sexual activity. Therefore, testosterone supplementation is an integral part of our treatment. However, as previously mentioned, in our experience, the majority of women have both psychosocial and physical components to their decreased libido. In women who have both low testosterone levels and psychosocial issues, we prefer to initiate treatment for the psychosocial components before starting testosterone supplementation. While we do not have data supporting this approach, it has been our experience that women who just receive testosterone supplementation frequently have a transient increase in libido, but within several months their sexual desire again diminishes. We believe this is because they have not addressed the psychosocial aspects of their decreased libido. In contrast, we have found that women who get counseling to address the psychosocial aspects of their diminished libido and then start testosterone supplementation have a longer lasting increase in their libido. When addressing this philosophy with our patients, we use the analogy of restoring a beautiful, but weathered old house: it would be foolish to repaint the house before assuring that the foundation of the house is sound. We believe that testosterone supplementation without at least a thorough evaluation of the psychosocial health of a woman and her relationship is similarly unwise. A much more satisfying result is achieved by addressing psychosocial issues first and then restoring her natural testosterone levels to reenergize her libido.

An Integrative Approach to Increasing Dopamine Levels

Dopamine is a neurotransmitter partially responsible for motivation, and the "pursuit of pleasure." People who have a relative deficiency in dopamine find it difficult to seek pleasure and don't think about what would be fun or feel good. Obviously, what we call sex drive or libido is, after all, a specific kind of anticipatory drive. As tests are not readily available to measure dopamine levels, we rely on a series of questions that may suggest dopamine deficiency (Table 6.2). If dopamine deficiency is suspected, one of the most effective treatments is high intensity exercise. Regular physical activity stimulates production of dopamine as well as endorphins (Goldfarb, Kamimori, Hegde, Otterstetter, & Brown, 1998; Sutoo & Akiyama, 2003). Obviously, we emphasize this approach in our biopsychosocial treatment plan as exercise has added benefits that improve

Table 6.2
A Questionnaire That Can Help to Identify Dopamine Deficiency

____	1. I always feel tired.
____	2. I sleep more than usual.
____	3. I'm less physically active than I used to be.
____	4. I seem to lack motivation.
____	5. My self-confidence has declined.
____	6. I seldom spend time with friends or make plans for activities that I once enjoyed.
____	7. Generally, I'm not all that happy.
____	8. I am not engaged in life.
____	9. I have given birth or breastfed within the past year.
____	10. I am taking medication for depression or anxiety.

quality of life both inside and outside the bedroom. Exercise can enhance muscle tone and stamina, both of which can improve a woman's sex life. In addition, as exercise can also have the added benefit of weight loss in women who are overweight, it can improve body image. If exercise is not sufficient to raise dopamine levels, bupropion can be used to pharmacologically raise dopamine levels. Bupropion improves libido and orgasmic potential both in depressed and in nondepressed women.

Herbal Supplementation to Improve Libido

For centuries, cultures throughout the world have attached potent sexual powers to an array of natural substances. While many of the prosexual affects of these natural aphrodisiacs are derived from a strong placebo affect, it is likely that some of these compounds do have physiologic properties that may improve sexual response or libido. The desire of a large percentage of women to use "natural" products as opposed to "synthetic" pharmaceuticals should not be underestimated or discounted. In addition, we recognize in our biopsychosocial model that the patient must be an active participant in choosing a personalized treatment approach. We have found that when a woman is given a "cookbook" treatment regimen she is less likely to make the necessary lifestyle changes that are essential to improving her libido. Therefore, if a woman so desires, we will include herbal supplementation as part of a biopsychosocial treatment regimen after we have discussed with her that there is little scientific data supporting the efficacy, safety, and quality control of these products. In addition, we also discuss that supplements are not required to follow the strict controls that the FDA requires of prescription medications. Therefore, there can be inconsistency in dosage and contamination that does not occur with prescription medication. Some of the herbs that we have recommended are discussed below.

Yohimbe

A traditional herbal remedy in West Africa, yohimbe has a centuries-old reputation for its libido-enhancing properties. The herb, which comes from the bark of the corynanthe yohimbe tree, plays a role in tribal fertility celebrations, marriage ceremonies, and mating rituals. Spurred by yohimbe's effects, some of these ceremonies involve sexual activity that may go on for days, or even weeks.

Since the late 1930s, researchers have been studying yohimbe to substantiate the prosexual claims for the herb. No less than 30 scientific articles have shown that the active ingredient in yohimbe, the alkaloid yohimbine, increases urogenital blood flow, and stimulates the central and peripheral nervous systems (Meston & Worcel, 2002; Tam, Worcel, & Wyllie, 2001; Vogt, et al., 1997). Further studies have shown that yohimbine can counteract the negative sexual side effects of SSRI antidepressants. However, yohimbine can cause hypertension (increased blood pressure), tachycardia (rapid heart beat), palpitations (abnormal heart beat), restlessness, and insomnia (inability to sleep). For these reasons, we do not recommend yohimbe or yohimbine for anyone with a history of coronary artery disease, stroke, heart arrhythmias, high blood pressure, migraines, panic attacks, schizophrenia, or bipolar disorder.

Damiana

Damiana is a wild shrub that grows in parts of Mexico, Central and South America, and the West Indies. Recently, it has been cultivated in Texas and California. Its botanical name, *Turnera diffusa aphrodisiaca*, hints at its reputation as a libido-enhancing plant. The ancient Mayans used damiana for its prosexual properties. And for centuries, Mexican women have been brewing tea from the plant's leaves to improve their sexual satisfaction. Damiana has been the subject of some research. In a double-blind placebo controlled trial, an herbal preparation called ArginMax for Women—which combines damiana with other reputed sex-enhancing herbs—boosted sexual desire, reduced vaginal dryness, increased the frequency of sexual intercourse and the frequency and intensity of orgasm, and improved clitoral sensation in women who took it (Ito, Trant, & Polan, 2001). In fact, almost three-quarters of the women in the study showed positive changes in these sexual variables, compared with only slightly more than one-third of the women who took a placebo.

Gingko and Ginseng

Chinese culture is rich in the study and use of aphrodisiacs and sex-enhancing herbs. For centuries, Chinese people have relied on the nuts and leaves of the ginkgo tree to help improve their sexual vigor, as well as their mental acuity. Though limited, recent scientific research suggests that ginkgo may benefit sexual function by increasing blood flow (Hong, Ji, Hong, Nam, & Ahn, 2002). Two separate studies involving men with erectile dysfunction found that the herb helps to restore erections without side effects. In a study involving women, a preparation of ginkgo mixed with other herbs improved orgasms and overall sexual satisfaction (Ito et al., 2001).

Perhaps the best known of the Chinese herbs is ginseng. It has been used in Asia for more than 5,000 years to boost energy and alertness. It also is known for improving sexual response, increasing sexual energy, and reviving libido. There are three different types of ginseng: Asian, or "red," ginseng (*Panax ginseng*); American, or "white," ginseng (*Panax quinquefolius*); and Siberian ginseng (*Eleutherococcus senticosus*). Ginseng contains ginsenosides, compounds that have been shown to stimulate the hypothalamus. It is purported that ginseng acts locally on the vagina and clitoris to increase genital blood flow which enhances lubrication, sensation, and arousal. In randomized placebo-controlled trials, Asian ginseng has improved sexual response in men with erectile dysfunction (Hong et al., 2002). And in combination with ginkgo and damiana, ginseng appears to boost sexual arousal and overall sexual satisfaction in women (Ito et al., 2001).

Psychological Issues in the Physical Quadrant

A woman's relationship to her body has a profound impact on how she thinks and feels about herself. Obviously, her sexual identity has much to do with how she understands herself as a sensual woman. As a result, for a woman to feel open and engaged with her partner sexually, she must first be aware of, and comfortable with, her body and her sensuality. Otherwise, it is unlikely that she will allow a sexual partner to intimately explore her body.

To enjoy her sex drive, a woman must not only know her body, but she must have experience and comfort with feeling pleasure through it. Otherwise, it is unlikely that she will allow herself the more intimate experience of sensual or sexual pleasure. This goal of comfort in feeling nonsexual, physical pleasure is not as easy as it may initially seem. It is here that many women begin their work in finding their libido.

Women in Western cultures are often disconnected from their bodies. This is evident when listening to women speak about themselves. For example, it is common for women to describe being unable to physically relax, even when on vacation or during a long weekend, let alone at the end of a day. Many women struggle to decipher their body's natural cues, such as knowing the difference between hunger pains versus an emotional desire to "fill up" with food. Some women refuse to look at themselves naked in a full length mirror, feeling shame in relation to their body size or shape. Other women abuse caffeine rather than allow their body's natural needs for sleep. Many women are "addicted" to substances such as alcohol or food, which can have a numbing effect not only emotionally, but physically as well. Women are often not tuned into their body's natural rhythms.

Many women are not just cut off from their bodies; they also spend little time enjoying them. Most low libido patients will report little if any time spent in daily activities that feel sensually pleasurable, such as a soak in the tub, a yoga class, or a walk outside. Instead, women spend long hours in front of desks and computer screens, behind the wheel of a car, or sitting in front of a TV. For many women, and especially for women with low libido, sensual pleasure occurs rarely and often only with the help of a glass of wine or a piece of chocolate.

In our fast-paced and often chaotic society, women eat when they tell their body it is time, they expect to sleep when they lay down to rest, and they intend to want sex when their partners initiate it. Female libido, however, is just not that simple. When women are not used to feeling their bodies, let alone feeling pleasure in them, it is hard to imagine that they will immediately be able to feel sexual pleasure when their partner suddenly expresses an interest in making love. Women innately feel the truth of this concept when it is presented to them. If a woman is more used to inhabiting her thoughts than her body, she will likely struggle to enjoy her partner's physical touch, foreplay, or even orgasms. Instead, she will engage in sex as she does in life more generally—reacting with logical thought rather than feeling: "Do I really want to make love right now?" "He's touching me that way again." "Is the phone ringing?" "What are the children doing?" She will find herself unable to turn off her thoughts, the possibility of physical pleasure becoming more and more remote.

How do practitioners assist women in reinhabiting their bodies, learning again how to feel relaxation, physical pleasure, and sexual enjoyment? Experiential homework, including journaling and exercises designed to heighten a woman's awareness of her body and her sensual and sexual relationship to it, are often quite helpful in this regard. Sex therapists know well the process of guiding women to focus on their senses and physical sensation. Approaching sexual concerns with body techniques does tend to take women closer to their treatments goals. For most women, this process takes time, commitment, and a significant amount of motivation. Unlike book learning, reconnecting with one's body occurs at the body's pace—often slowly and deliberately, over an extended period of time. Much of this work is thus physical and experiential, and actually happens outside a typical therapy room. Usually this translates into a regular practice, such as yoga, dance, massage, meditation, or almost any experience in which a woman is focused and aware of her body, and her emotions. It is in this fashion that a woman becomes reacquainted with the deepest aspects of herself, her feelings, and her sex drive. In fact, we suggest that, for many if not most women, maintaining a regular body practice of some sort is a lifelong requirement to staying connected to her libido. Libido is not controlled like a light switch, turned on and off at will. It is more like a flower, requiring regular care and attention to thrive. It should be noted that many of our patients initially find our recommendations about "body work" to be taxing or burdensome. They will resist following through with such a program, claiming that they have no time or interest in such activity. Interestingly, it is often the women most resistant to these experiential types of treatment who ultimately benefit the most from them.

We find it imperative to support patients in finding a body discipline that they are comfortable with and assist them in finding sound practitioners of these particular healing methods. Patients are often new to such techniques and have little experience evaluating quality care. Simply suggesting to a patient that she do body work will probably not provide her with enough support to obtain effective help. We encourage practitioners to educate themselves about the resources available in their community so that they may assist patients by making sound referrals in this arena.

EMOTIONAL QUADRANT

For many women, therapeutic work in the emotional quadrant is a key element in igniting their desire. Most women's experiences of sensuality and sexuality are rich and replete with emotional meaning and depth. As such, it is almost impossible to quantify the myriad of ways emotional issues can interfere with a woman's desire for sex. In exploring the emotional components of low libido, most women are best served by addressing this quadrant from both individual and couples' perspectives.

Probably the most obvious emotional saboteur of libido is *depression* Research demonstrates that depression affects approximately 12 percent of women each year (National Institute for Mental Health, 2000). And since libido loss is actually one diagnostic criterion for this disorder, many women experience a mood-related libido loss in their lifetimes. However, we find at our center that a woman does not have to suffer from a full-blown diagnostic depression for her libido to be negatively impacted by her mood. Simply feeling depleted, overburdened, or overwhelmed by life for a period of time can be enough. Attention to a woman's mood is thus frequently a necessary first step in addressing issues of libido

Similarly, *anxiety disorders* are the most commonly occurring class of psychiatric disorder, affecting 19 million people each year in the United States; women almost twice as often as men (Centers for Disease Control, 1994). Women who struggle with anxiety describe a sense of being unable to relax or focus their thoughts away from their worries. Anxious women report that they feel jittery and uncomfortable in their bodies. Sex is less pleasurable, and as a result, women are less inclined to feel sexual desire. Obviously, as with depression, anxiety issues must usually be treated first before a woman experiences increased libido.

We cannot review the common emotional issues relating to low libido without addressing *sexual shame* and *guilt*. Practitioners working in sexual health know that women commonly report shame and guilt about being sexual. Many of these women logically acknowledge that healthy sexuality is a real and appropriate part of feminine life. However, at the same time, women frequently report histories of negative sexual experiences. But women need not have a sexual trauma history to feel sexual shame or guilt. One unfortunate outgrowth of a patriarchal society is that women may develop a belief that femininity is of less value than masculinity. Believing her femininity to be substandard, she may hide from it, resist it, and venture far from this core in an effort to protect herself from shame. Thus, for some women, low sex drive is the cost of the shame she carries for simply being female.

It is not only the abundance of uncomfortable emotions, such as depression or shame, that can result in a lowered sex drive. The opposite effect, that of *emotional disengagement,* can have a similar negative impact on a woman's desire for sex. If a woman copes via emotional disconnection, it is likely that her libido will be impacted. It is difficult to explore this concept without at least making a cursory comment about addictions. For the purpose of this chapter, we use the term *addiction* loosely, and not necessarily in a diagnostic sense. Instead, addictions for our purpose here represent any excessive activity or focus which takes a woman's attention away from her deepest self, her emotions, and thus, her sex drive. Addictions serve the function of emotional numbing. Whether they are to alcohol, food, shopping, work, or her child's homework assignments, women who cope by repeatedly tuning out of their emotional life will likely find themselves less tuned into their libido. That is, any method she may use of "tuning out" will probably have the effect of dulling all sensation, including sex drive. As a result, reconnecting with sexual interest for some women includes a process of letting go of addictive behaviors so that she may experience herself on a deeper emotional, and sexual, level. For many women, this process can be time consuming and emotionally painful.

Interpersonal Issues

The emotional quadrant consists not only of internal emotional issues but also relationship issues. Regardless of what seems to cause low libido initially, couples' issues usually require therapeutic attention over time. Often, what masquerades as low libido in a woman is actually her healthy reaction to unhealthy couple's dynamics. Many relationship issues can play a causal role in a woman's low sex drive. (Bancroft et al., 2003; Dunn et al., 1999; Hawton et al., 1994). Issues including communication, sexual style, and unexpressed emotions such as anger or grief must be explored in the treatment room. A woman who has difficulty trusting or opening to her partner will obviously feel less interested in making love. The possible relationship dynamics that may interfere with a woman's desire for sex are too numerous to list here. Astute practitioners must be observant to all such possibilities.

Loss of sexual "tension" is another common emotional issue that leads women to loose interest in sex. Over time in intimate relationships, couples may become better friends than lovers. The result may be a lack of sexual passion, resulting in "boring sex." For many women, an unimaginative or invariable sexual script leads to a loss of libido. Couples can learn to re-create sexual passion by becoming more present emotionally with each other, allowing their relationship to grow in depth and adventure. This therapeutic work takes much effort on the part of both partners.

No discussion of couple's issues common to women with low libido would be complete without addressing the likely impact of her partner's emotional issues on a woman's sex drive. That is, any emotional issue her partner may be struggling with is likely to affect a woman's experience of making love to him/her and thus affect her sex drive. In this way, a woman's failed libido may actually be a healthy response to an unhealthy dynamic in her partner. Such issues can be blatant, such as alcoholism or major depression, or less obvious, such as emotional disengagement from his/her partner. Women may or may not be aware of these issues when they present for treatment. Again, a clinician must be astute and thorough to comprehend the complex dynamics contributing to a woman's lack of sexual interest.

Ultimately, couples' therapeutic needs vary depending on the issues at hand and the personalities of the particular partners. Some couples benefit from regular weekly couples therapy for periods of time; others require a less intensive focus. Sometimes, simple discussions about the effect a woman's low sex drive has had on the marriage will suffice. More commonly, however, deeper emotional work is necessary to create an emotional environment where both partners feel heard, understood, and supported. This necessary aspect of treatment can be quite challenging for couples. Women with partners unwilling to participate often feel rejected and angry, and ultimately less interested in improving their low libido.

INTELLECTUAL QUADRANT

"I hope he doesn't want to make love again tonight." "I wish he'd just hurry up and get it over with, I can't stand foreplay." "I hate how my body looks naked." "I don't know why we even bother to try making love, I know how it's going to feel." These types of thoughts are not unusual for women with low sex drive. Obviously, the way a woman thinks about sex can have a powerful impact on her actual sexual experience, and on her sex drive. The old adage that the brain is our largest sex organ cannot be overstated.

Many women with low libido report difficulty "turning off" their thoughts during sex. Instead, they find themselves obsessing about "to do lists," the way their body appears naked, or how their partner is touching them. All this takes the focus away from experiencing physical pleasure, emotional connection, and sexual gratification. Her libido will suffer as she struggles to focus on pleasure rather than her thoughts.

The intellectual quadrant encompasses the ways a woman thinks about sex: her perceptions, expectations, as well as the meanings she places on her sexual experiences. It also relates to her general sense of feeling intellectually stimulated in her life. If she's not interested and intellectually engaged in her life in a broad sense, she's unlikely to be interested more specifically in sex. Women who report feeling underutilized, bored, or understimulated in their lives generally appear less likely to find sex stimulating or exciting. And of course, if sex isn't stimulating and exciting, she's unlikely to want to participate in it.

The intellectual quadrant is impacted by cultural, social, religious, and family held beliefs about sex. Many of these issues are thoroughly explored in other chapters of this volume. To address these issues, a woman must explore the origins of her thoughts about sex. Girls develop concepts about sex from a very young age. They watch their mothers model adult female sexuality, and they develop expectations for themselves based on these observations. Children are also exposed to sexual information through their environment outside their family. They interpret this material based on what those of authority are saying—be it in the media, religious institutions, or peers. These early conceptualizations often linger throughout her lifetime, sometimes whether or not she acknowledges them, or even agrees with them, as an adult. For example, a girl may learn that "good girls don't," and even after she grows and becomes married, that mantra may still affect her sexual expression.

A woman's expectations about sex, how it will feel, and what will happen are likely to affect the outcome of any particular sexual experience. Most women with low libido expect sex to feel emotionally or physically uncomfortable. If she determines that sex won't feel good, it is likely that she will act in ways that will encourage this outcome. She will begin the sexual interaction with a frustrated tone, perhaps avoiding eye contact with her partner, keeping her muscles stiff and unyielding. This approach will obviously result in a different experience than if she were physically open and relaxed, curious about what will happen and how it will feel to her. Thus, when working with a woman in this quadrant, we encourage her to explore the ways her thoughts, expectations, and resultant behavior impacts what she creates with her partner. In anticipating the possibility of a positive encounter, she will increase the chances that sex will feel good, and over time, her libido may very likely respond in kind. In addition, techniques that assist a woman in being present with her body and her partner are often useful at these times, such as making eye contact, deep breathing, or engaging in sexual banter with her partner.

Our biopsychosocial model teaches women to use their thoughts as a sexual asset. Many women find it helpful to begin by generating enjoyable sexual thoughts and images throughout the day. Essentially, she will be creating a kind of thinking foreplay for herself. Eventually some women find it helpful to cultivate these thoughts into sexual fantasies about herself and her partner. Writing positive affirmations of a sexual nature may also be helpful. The repetitive phrases can help guide her toward positive thinking patterns rather than hurtful ones. Giving herself permission to explore sexually, enabling her sense of sexual creativity and adventurousness, can assist women in breaking free from outdated thinking patterns that no longer serve her sexual self. Finally, we find eye movement desensitization and reprocessing (EMDR) to be a helpful therapeutic tool in these circumstances. EMDR utilizes repetitive eye movements to assist patients in exploring and processing difficult emotional material. It can be utilized for women with low libido in a variety of ways, including the exploration and redefinition of negative thinking patterns.

SPIRITUAL QUADRANT

Women whose sexual relationship(s) lacks a spiritual essence tend to describe sex as "boring," "dry," or "unemotional." Alternately, a woman who has developed a spiritual flavor in her sexual expression uses terms like "deep," "rich," and "gratifying" to describe her sexual experiences. This woman feels rejuvenated from sex rather than experiencing it as an energy drain. She enjoys and looks forward to making love. Sexual expression becomes much more than simple physical release. It becomes a way for her to experience herself, her partner, and perhaps her world in a more meaningful way.

For our purposes, spirituality is a broad concept, taking into account an individual woman's needs and personality. It may be defined as a woman understanding herself and her place within her relationships and society. It allows a woman to reach deeper into herself and/or her sexual partner, and to explore the meanings, emotions, and richness she finds there. Rather than experiencing sex as a purely physical act, making love becomes much more—a channel to levels of experience and emotion that take sex out of the realm of the mundane and into the extraordinary. When we speak of spirituality we are not necessarily referring to religiosity, although they are synonymous for some women. In fact, spirituality cannot be quantified in any particular way for all women. What opens one woman spiritually will close another. As a result, adding a spiritual dimension to a woman's sexual experience is a personal, intimate, and individual process.

The realm of spiritual sexual expression can easily become complicated. That is, while "extraordinary sex" may sound enticing, in actuality it is a difficult place for many people to explore. Experiencing sex from this perspective often means letting go, opening one's heart and body in deep and profound ways. This level of vulnerability is often avoided and feels frightening to those unfamiliar to connecting deeply to themselves or others. Instead, men and women tend to value self-control, safety, and thinking versus feeling in the daily activities of life. Both sexes also tend toward limiting their exposure to others. In most cases, the people we encourage our patients to open to (their sexual partners) are the people whose faults they are most acutely acquainted with. As a result, the initially exciting concept of bringing sacredness and spirituality to sexuality can quickly devolve into an uncomfortable situation to be avoided. Patients often require much guidance and support at these times in treatment.

How then, can clients be led into such territories? We are delighted to note that an entire following chapter (by Ogden) in this volume is devoted to the bridging of spirituality and sexuality. Much useful information is available there. Some practitioners find it useful to educate themselves about the Eastern sexual traditions such as Tantra or Tao. Many books and workshops are available on the subject, thus the interested reader is encouraged to pursue such educational opportunities. In our clinic, we begin by supporting those couples who express an interest in deepening their spiritual sexual experience through basic homework exercises described below. Synchronized breathing and heart meditations offer a safe place for couples to gently cultivate a more sacred feeling to their sexual experience. Over time, those couples may wish to explore other levels of spirituality both in their lives more generally and in their sexual experiences together.

Synchronized breathing is just that—a focused breathing technique in which both partners adjust their breathing so that they inhale and exhale at the same rate. In this exercise the couple may choose to lay together, either facing each other or "spooning." In order to synchronize the breath, individuals must focus on their own body as well as their partner's body. If practiced over time, this type of exercise trains people to leave their minds and develop both an intensive body focus, as well as an intimate awareness of their partner's physical experience. A woman without a partner may practice by focusing on her breath and body, maintaining a deep, steady breathing rhythm over time.

Heart meditations are basically meditations focused on opening one's heart, thus facilitating loving feelings toward oneself and one's partner. For this exercise, couples are encouraged to sit cross-legged in front of each other, with eyes open and soft, gazing at the other. It may be helpful to instruct a participant to put her hand over her heart so that she may support her mental focus with a physical one. Alternately, couples may enjoy placing a hand on their partner's heart for the same purpose. Couples then breathe together, tuning in to the loving feelings that this exercise generates. Women working alone may do this exercise focusing on her own heart, or perhaps looking at herself in a mirror. Breathing slowly and deeply encourages a deepening of the meditation and the emotional experience. These meditations encourage loving feelings, which is, for many women, the most powerful form of foreplay.

These exercises are particularly useful for women with low libido, although many of them will report emotional discomfort as they practice. That is in part because women with low libido often report difficulty letting go and leaving their minds behind during sex. They are used to focusing on their thoughts and their bodies, usually in negative, frustrated terms such as "I wish he'd not touch me that way" or "That doesn't feel good." Synchronized breathing and heart meditations encourage women to disengage from such a focus, supporting instead an intimate and open emotional and physical experience with a partner. Patients will often resist such homework, calling it silly or boring. It is usually these women, who are living the paradox of resisting intimacy yet longing for exciting sex, who can most benefit from this exercise.

CONCLUSION

Working with women reporting low libido can be a hugely gratifying experience for practitioners. Libido issues are frequently complex, requiring a treatment model that encompasses a vast array of possible etiologies. Traditional treatment models involving a solo practitioner; thus they rarely provide adequate insight into these challenging cases. We find a biopsychosocial treatment model, which addresses the physical, emotional, intellectual, and spiritual quadrants of sexual health, to be extremely valuable in this regard. We believe that such a holistic, mind-body treatment focus offers a woman the richest opportunities to create gratifying sexual experiences, leaving her feeling interested and desirous of intercourse.

REFERENCES

Bachmann, G., Bancroft, J., Braunstein, Burger, H., Davis, S., Dennerstein, L., Goldstein, I., Guay, A., Leiblum, S., Lobo, R., Notelovitz, M., Rosen, R., Sarrel, P., Sherwin, B., Simon, J., Simpson, E., Shifren, J., Spark, R., & Traish, A. (2002). Female androgen insufficiency: The Princeton consensus statement on definition, classification, and assessment. *Fertility and Sterility, 77*(4), 660–665.

Bancroft, J., Loftus, J., & Long, J. S. (2003). Distress about sex: A national survey of women in heterosexual relationships. *Archives of Sexual Behavior, 32*(3), 193–208.

Basson, R. (2006). Sexual desire and arousal disorders in women. *New England Journal of Medicine, 354,* 1497–1506.

Caruso, S., Agnello, C., Intelisano, G., Farina, M., Di Mari, L., & Cianci, A. (2004). Placebo-controlled study on efficacy and safety of daily apomorphine SL intake in premenopausal women affected by hypoactive sexual desire disorder and sexual arousal disorder. *Urology, 63*(5), 955–959.

Chanson, P., & Salenave, S. (2004). Diagnosis and treatment of pituitary adenomas. *Minerva Endocrinol, 29*(4), 241–275.

Dunn, K., Croft, P., & Hackett, G. (1999). Association of sexual problems with social, psychological, and physical problems in men and women: A cross sectional population survey. *Journal of Epidemiological Community Health, 53*, 144–148.

Goldfarb, A. H., Jamurtas, A. Z., Kamimori, G. H., Hegde, S., Otterstetter, R., & Brown, D. A. (1998). Gender effect on beta-endorphin response to exercise. *Medicine and Science in Sports and Exercise, 30*(12), 1672–1676.

Hawton, K., Gath, D., & Day, A. (1994). Sexual function in a community sample of middle-aged women with partners: Effects of age, marital, socioeconomic, psychiatric, gynecological, and menopausal factors. *Archives of Sexual Behavior, 23*(4), 375–395.

Hong, B., Ji, Y. H., Hong, J. H., Nam, K. Y., Ahn, T. Y. (2002). A double-blind crossover study evaluating the efficacy of Korean red ginseng in patients with erectile dysfunction: A preliminary report. *Journal of Urology, 168*(5), 2070–2073.

Hull, E. M., Lorrain, D. S., Du, J., et al. (1999). Hormone-neurotransmitter interactions in the control of sexual behavior. *Behavioural Brain Research, 105*(1), 105–116.

Ito, T. Y., Trant, A. S., & Polan, M. L. (2001). A double-blind placebo-controlled study of ArginMax, a nutritional supplement for enhancement of female sexual function. *Journal of Sex & Marital Therapy, 27*(5), 541–549.

Jiamm, B. P., Tsai, J. Y., Wu, T. T., and Huang, J. K. (2003). What to learn about cildenafil in the treatment of erectile dysfunction from 3-year clinical experience. *International Journal of Impotence Research, 15*(6), 412–417.

Laumann, E. O., Paik, A., & Rosen, R. C. (1999). Sexual dysfunction in the United States. *Journal of the American Medical Association, 281* (6), 537–544.

Meston, C. M., & Worcel, M. (2002). The effects of yohimbine plus L-arginine glutamate on sexual arousal in postmenopausal women with sexual arousal disorder. *Archives of Sexual Behavior, 31*(4), 323–332.

National Center for Health Statistics, Centers for Disease Control and Prevention. (1994). *Health, United States, 1995.* Hyattsville, MD: U.S. Public Health Service.

National Institute of Mental Health. (2002). *Depression.* Bethesda, MD: National Institute of Mental Health, National Institutes of Health, U.S. Department of Health and Human Services [reprinted 2002; cited January 26, 2004]. (NIH Publication Number: NIH 02–3561). 23 pages.

Oberg, K., & Fugl-Meyer, K. S. (2005). On Swedish women's distressing sexual dysfunctions: Some concomitant conditions and life satisfaction. *Journal of Sexual Medicine, 2*(2), 169–173.

Sutoo, D., & Akiyama, K. (2003). Regulation of brain function by exercise. *Neurobiology of Disease, 13*(1), 1–14.

Tam, S. W., Worcel, M., & Wyllie, M. (2001). Yohimbine: A clinical review. *Pharmacology and Therapeutics, 91*(3), 215–243.

Vogt, H. J., Brandl, P., Kockott, G., Schmitz, J. R., Wiegand, M. H., Schadrack, J., Gierend, M. 1997). Double-blind, placebo-controlled safety and efficacy trial with yohimbine hydrochloride in the treatment of nonorganic erectile dysfunction. *International Journal of Impotence Research, 9*(3), 155–161.

Weeks, G. R. (2005). The emergence of a new paradigm in sex therapy: Integration. *Sexual and Relationship Therapy, 20*(1), 89–103.

Chapter Seven

SPIRITUAL DIMENSIONS OF SEXUAL HEALTH: BROADENING CLINICAL PERSPECTIVES OF WOMEN'S DESIRE

Gina Ogden

In this age of Viagra and other media messages about sexual function and dysfunction, the dominant discourse about sexual health centers on performance—that is, a goal of physical orgasm generated by intercourse and/or genital stimulation. Definitions of sexual health and performance are so thoroughly conflated that from the perspective of clinician, client, and consumer these concepts often seem interchangeable. But my research shows that goal-oriented norms represent only a fraction of human sexual experience and play only a bit part in creating sexual desire for women (Ogden, 1999, 2002, 2006). After more than half a century of focusing on the quantifiable aspects of performance (e.g., Kaplan, 1979; Kinsey et al., 1948, 1953; Laumann et al., 1994; Masters & Johnson, 1966), sex researchers have yet to find a definitive answer to the question famously posed by Sigmund Freud: "What do women want?" (Freud, 1938).

In my practice of sex therapy since the mid-1970s, I have found that equating sexual health with performance is not only inaccurate, but can also be harmful, especially to women. By reifying the performance aspects of sex, generations of sex researchers and therapists have unwittingly reinforced that women are the "second sex" (DeBeauvoir, 1952), historically less sexually interested and less functional than men. From the clinical point of view, performance norms are basic to *DSM-IV-R* definitions (2000, pp. 23–24; also see the appendix in this volume) and they constitute a distorted standard of sexual health that predicts how clinicians are likely to diagnose and treat women who present with complaints about low sexual desire (e.g., Tiefer, 1995; Tiefer & Kaschak, 2001). It is no wonder that sex research has consistently found that a high percentage of American women lack desire for performance oriented sex—43 percent is the number most recently and most broadly cited (Laumann, Paik, & Rosen, 1999).

Performance definitions of sexual health leave out the emotions and meanings that are arguably crucial for desire, satisfaction, and healthy sexual relationship. (Daniluk, 1998; Ellison, 2000; Espin, 1987; Foley, Kope, & Sugrue, 2002; Kitzinger, 1983; Kleinplatz, 2001; Savage, 1999; Sugrue & Whipple, 2001). Women in my clinical practice have routinely linked their positive sexual experiences with qualitative issues such as self-esteem, love, passion, compassion, altruism, empathy, acceptance, release, beauty, reverence, and grace, and the sense of ongoing personal power when all of these are present. Although such emotions and meanings cannot be objectively quantified, they are nonetheless real, part of what visionary psychiatrist Carl Jung has called the "irrational facts of experience" (Jung, 1959). When applying them to issues of human sexuality, I have referred to them as the spiritual dimensions of sexual health (Ogden, 2002, 2006).

The purpose of this chapter is to broaden the clinical base for understanding the emotions and meanings that are implicit in women's sexual desire, and to broaden the scope of questions clinicians might ask women who present with sexual desire problems. Information in this chapter is based on results of an independent exploratory survey I conducted on integrating sexuality and spirituality (ISIS) (Ogden, 2002, 2006). The ISIS methodology has been detailed elsewhere (Ogden, 2002, 2006); a brief description follows here, to give context. Excerpts from the ISIS questionnaire are listed in Table 7.1.

Table 7.1
Excerpts from the ISIS Survey

The survey begins with demographic inquiries and is then followed by specific questions:

Here are some comments people have made about sex and spirituality. (check all that reflect your experience)

1. "Sex usually means intercourse."
2. "For me, sex is much more than intercourse; it involves all of me—body, mind, heart, and soul."
3. "I associate spirituality mainly with going to church."
4. "When I open myself to warmth, desire, depth, expansion, and trust, there is no separation between sex and spirit."
5. "Sex is for conceiving babies and has little to do with spirituality."
6. "It's through my senses that I often experience God."
7. "All my life I've been told that people who love sex too much will go to hell."
8. "Mainly, sex means connection with my partner."
9. "Sex is physical, but it also involves love, romance, even mystical union."
10. "For people who have been sexually disappointed or hurt, consciously giving and receiving sexual pleasure can be healing."

Table 7.1
(Continued)

Sexual romance and religious worship have many kinds of symbols and rituals in common.

(check all that you associate with both your sexuality and your spirituality)

1. Candles
2. Incense
3. Flowers
4. Wine
5. Music
6. Dancing
7. Special foods
8. Words of comfort
9. Words of love
10. Laying on of hands
11. None of the above
12. Other (please specify)_____

When I use the word "spirituality" in the context of my sexuality, I mean: (check one)

Spirituality but not religion
Religion but not spirituality
Spirituality and religion combined
Other (please specify)_____

To me, it seems sacrilegious to talk about sex and spirituality together.

1 Yes   2 No

Sex needs to have a spiritual element to be really satisfying. (check one)

1. Always true for me
2. Sometimes true for me
3. Neither true nor untrue for me
4. Seldom true for me
5. Never true for me

With which of the following has sex been a spiritual experience for you? (check all that apply)

1. Husband
2. Wife
3. Committed partner
4. Casual encounter
5. Affair while committed to someone else
6. Self
7. None of the above
8. Other (please specify)_____

(Continued)

Table 7.1
(Continued)

Which of the following have contributed to sex being a spiritual experience for you?
(check all that apply)

1. Being in love
2. Conceiving a baby
3. Being pregnant
4. Having no fear of getting pregnant
5. Feeling committed to my partner
6. Feeling free of responsibility to my partner
7. Feeling safe
8. Experiencing a personal crisis
9. Feeling in control
10. Feeling controlled
11. Being in the mood
12. Aggressive thrusting
13. Danger
14. Drinking or drugs
15. None of the above
16. Other (please specify)_____

Which of the following have you done to help bring a spiritual dimension to your sexual experiences? (check all that apply)

1. Made eye contact with my partner
2. Lit candles or incense
3. Bathed
4. Enjoyed special foods
5. Meditated before getting physical
6. Made love in a special place
7. Touched reverently
8. Kissed soulfully
9. Played music
10. Danced
11. Fantasized or daydreamed
12. Laughed together
13. Let go of control
14. Did nothing special
15. Other (please specify)_____

How have your spiritual beliefs led you to express your sexuality more fully? (check all that apply)

1. By affirming that love is good in all its forms and expressions
2. By teaching that making love is holy
3. By opening me to risk deeper intimacy

**Table 7.1
(Continued)**

4. By giving me faith when I've felt like running away from pleasure
5. By sanctioning my feelings of longing and passion
6. By making the physical part of relationship into a sacrament
7. Other (please specify)_____

How have your spiritual beliefs prevented you from expressing your sexuality as fully as you might? (check all that apply)

1. By giving me the message "good girls don't"
2. By making sexual desire a source of guilt
3. By making the body a source of shame
4. By teaching that sex is not for pleasure, but for procreation (conceiving babies)
5. By teaching that pleasure is more important for a man than for a woman
6. By keeping me from exploring sexual taboos
7. Other (please specify)_____

Has anything else in your life prevented you from experiencing a sex-spirit connection? (check all that apply)

1. Childhood abuse
2. Abuse as an adult
3. Drinking and/or drug use
4. Depression and/or anxiety
5. Physical disabilities
6. Worry about how I look
7. Getting older
8. Not having a partner
9. Pregnancy
10. Parenthood
11. My partner only thinking about physical kicks
12. Not loving my partner
13. My partner not loving m
14. Sex isn't that interesting to me
15. Spirituality isn't that interesting to me
16. I've never thought of spirituality as a part of sex before now
17. Other (please specify)_____

Have you ever experienced sexual ecstasy?	1 Yes	2 No
Have you ever experienced spiritual ecstasy?	1 Yes	2 No

The ISIS survey questionnaire can be adapted for expanded sex history–taking, for assessment and evaluation of clients, and for educating students and clients. Countless ISIS respondents have written that the questions themselves were both thought-provoking and therapeutic for them. The entire survey questionnaire can be found at http://www.GinaOgden.com.

THE ISIS SURVEY—BROADENING DEFINITIONS OF SEXUAL EXPERIENCE

The ISIS survey is the first large scale survey to explore elements of sexual response beyond the performance criteria commonly used to evaluate sexual function and treat sexual dysfunction. Questions on the ISIS survey all derived from my clinical practice since the mid 1970s.

The survey was conducted between 1997 and 1999. There were 3,810 respondents (82% were women). About a third of these respondents were contacted personally by me, or by sexologist colleagues. Printed questionnaires were handed to individuals from "known groups"—in this case, cohorts of people generally considered to hold widely diverse views about both sexuality and spirituality. These groups included clergy (Catholics, Methodists, Mormons, and Unitarian Universalists), health providers (doctors, nurses, psychologists, social workers, and sex therapists), and students (of sexology, family therapy, and theology). They also included sexual abuse survivors, incarcerated male and female sex offenders, lesbian, gay, bisexual, and transgendered individuals, sex industry workers, and homemakers. The remaining two-thirds of the ISIS responses came as a result of the questionnaire being published in *New Age* magazine (January–February 1998), whose readership consisted primarily of men and women interested in holistic and spiritual health, and *New Woman* magazine (July 1998), whose readership consisted primarily of women interested in self improvement.

The ISIS sample is clearly not representative of all women, or all American women. It is nonetheless diverse and inclusive, even beyond the diversity of the groups mentioned above. Ages of women respondents ranged from 18 to 86. Their geographical locations included every state in the United States and two Canadian provinces (Ontario and British Columbia). Most of the women were Caucasian, but 18 percent were racially diverse. Seventy-one percent of the women said their religion of origin was Catholic or Protestant, but by adulthood the overall sample of women was practicing twenty-two religious faiths and about a quarter of the sample reported no formal religious practices at all. Almost two-thirds of the women had college degrees, but their overall socio-economic range was broad, including students, manual laborers, white-collar workers, and professionals. Eighty-nine percent of the women were heterosexual, 11 percent were bisexual or lesbian, fewer than one percent were transgendered.

The ISIS questionnaire required no narrative replies, but 1,465 respondents sent narratives describing how they connected sexuality and spirituality. These narrative documents vary in length and detail, but together they add an unprecedented body of qualitative information to the literature on sexual response and sexual health.

Major Finding

The foundational finding of the ISIS survey is that for most of these respondents sexual experience was intrinsically multidimensional. ISIS descriptions broaden sexual experience beyond the phases of physiological desire, arousal, and orgasm (Masters & Johnson, 1966; Kaplan, 1979; volume 1, chapter 11). For ISIS women, sexual response consisted of much more than the discrete sequence of immediate physical events. Not only did it include a wide range of feelings and meanings, such as those mentioned above by my clients, it tended to take place over a period of time. That is, their sexual responses were informed by a spectrum of factors that ranged from the physical, emotional, and mental impact of day-to-day interactions to early memories of pleasure and pain. Many women wrote that old feelings and memories greatly influenced their present experiences of sexual pleasure, both positively and negatively. This finding corroborated my long-term clinical observation that when we are appropriately loved and touched in our early years we are likely to feel enthusiastically sexual as adults, if the circumstances are right (see volume 1, chapter 5). The body remembers those early experiences and positive messages are fed directly into our adult responses to pleasurable sexual stimulation. By the same token, memories of neglect and abuse can feed fear and even loathing to our here-and-now sexual response (see volume 1, chapter 13).

ISIS women also reported a concomitant observation about sexual response and time: that the effects of their sexual experiences sometimes lasted long beyond the bedroom, to alter the course of their lives. When the effects were positive, these women felt energized and sometimes their entire outlooks on life expanded. When the effects were negative, the women felt lingering anger, fear, and a diminished sense of self. Because most of the ISIS questions were focused on sexual health, many respondents reported an ongoing sense of creative energy: "alive, present, and in oneness," "tuned in to life." Some ISIS women asserted that sexual experience literally transported them to other times and spaces. "It was not just sensual, sexual, or even conceptual; it was an experiential reality of Oneness, an opening unto Wholeness, into which I had somehow found a doorway," wrote a 56-year-old artist from Waialua, Hawaii. She went on to explain that this sense of sexual wholeness involved:

> a deeper understanding of the multi-faceted nature of the relentless Creative Spirit of the Vital Life Force ... all woven together, and still evolving, as I endeavor to move beyond my conditioning, various cultural illusions of mind/body/spirit separation, and live within the sacred circle of Life and Sexuality with an open heart, a more conscious mind, compassionate awareness, and practical feet.

Thus, the ISIS finding that sexual response is multidimensional not only corroborated my own clinical observations about the spiritual possibilities of pleasure, orgasm, and ecstasy, it is consistent with findings of contemporary brain research. What I had not known before I began the ISIS study is that human beings are actually hard-wired for the kinds of emotional and spiritual sexual experiences described by my clients and by ISIS women. In a landmark study conducted at Rutgers and Wake Forest Universities beginning in 1999, sex researchers Beverly Whipple and Barry Komisaruk were able to run brain scans on ten women during vaginal and cervical self-stimulation and orgasm. They found that multiple regions of the brain were simultaneously activated during sexual response—including the amygdala, which controls emotional response, and the temporal lobe, which controls religious ecstasy (Komisaruk, Beyer, & Whipple, 2006).

EXPERIENCING SEXUAL AND SPIRITUAL ECSTASY

Many ISIS women used the term "ecstasy" to describe the union of sex and spirit. For some women, ecstasy meant love and nurturing—a soul-mate, an empathic partner, a sense of deep connection with their partners, and also with themselves. Others expressed a sense of being on an emotional journey or in a delicious limbo outside of clock time. For still others the ecstasy connection was part of creating new human life—conception, childbirth, or breastfeeding a baby—occurrences that literally embody the spirit of sexual union. These women often waxed lyrical in their descriptions: Sexual ecstasy was "holy," "transcendent," "a path to God and Goddess," "an entry into the primordial waters, the ocean of universal love" (Table 7.2).

What stands out for me in these figures is that so many ISIS women affirmed that a significant part of their sexual satisfaction lay outside the performance definitions of sex. The numbers indicate that most ISIS women had experienced positive sexual outcomes beyond the usual goal of orgasm. Nearly half of these women said they found physical sex to be a direct path to God—and that spirituality can be a path to physical pleasure.

How do these ISIS women compare with the rest of the world's women? There is no way of knowing. The ISIS responses are unique because questions

Table 7.2
ISIS Women by the Numbers: Ecstatic Experiences

85 percent said they had experienced sexual ecstasy

67 percent said they had experienced spiritual ecstasy

47 percent said they had experienced God in a moment of sexual ecstasy

45 percent said they had experienced sexual feelings in a moment of spiritual ecstasy

about sex and spirit have never been systematically researched on a large scale before. What is important is how these women's perceptions may help us broaden our clinical perceptions of sexual health for women so that we can more effectively guide our clients.

The scope of sexual desire changes when the voices of these ISIS women are factored in. Their stories of sexual ecstasy include themes that range from a sense of personal purpose to a profound awareness of communion with the divine. The list below offers an overview of these themes. The list is not arranged in hierarchical order because ISIS women indicated no hierarchy. Nor did ISIS women necessarily associate all of these elements with each ecstatic experience. Rather, the themes were woven into reports of their ecstatic experiences. These themes are far larger and more complex than the wish for "sexual activity" and "function" that the *DSM* lists as representative of healthy sexual desire (see the appendix in this volume).

What ISIS Women Said Sexual Ecstasy Includes

- Suddenness and/or synchronicity
- A sense of oneness, unity
- A sense of understanding and purpose
- A paradoxical and simultaneous ego-loss, a sense of *not*-knowing
- Love and altruism toward the world
- Religious awe
- Heightened meaning for the event
- A sense of moving or being on a journey
- A sense of timelessness
- Awesome beauty
- Letting go of control
- Surrender to a larger reality—physical, mental, emotional, spiritual

Many ISIS women spoke of heart-and-soul connections that went beyond performance definitions. A 40-year-old musician from Bellingham, Washington wrote that her most ecstatic experiences included what she called "orgasms of the heart."

> I clearly entered an altered state. I cannot even remember if we had intercourse or physical orgasms. All I remember is him pressing gently with his hand at different points on my chest and abdomen. I experienced waves of ecstasy emanating from my heart. The waves would pulsate rhythmically, then subside, then a new wave would come along.

Some ISIS women said they discovered sexual ecstasy through their spiritual practices, which included meditation, breath work, dance, chanting, singing in the church choir, journeying to shamanic drumming, worship in earth-based religions such as Wicca, and astral travel—shifting the consciousness to realms beyond the body. A 39-year-old physical therapist from Chico, California, offered a musical metaphor for how her spiritual practice changed her experience of sexual ecstasy: "My body hums with different music—more of an orchestra as opposed to a solo. Or maybe a soloist backed by a really fine orchestra."

Despite her sensitivity to energy, this woman wrote that she had not always been open to the subtleties of sexual energy. An "uptight Protestant" upbringing had instilled in her a high degree of sexual guilt and shame. Not until her mid-thirties, after two husbands and an unmarried partner, had she been able to allow herself full permission to enjoy sexual pleasure.

> I had gone through a profound spiritual transformation around the time of splitting up with partner number three. The depth this has given and continues to give to my life is the reason I know the difference between "spiritual sex" and just plain "fucking." (A roll in the hay, just "plain old sex", etc.)

She wrote that she had gained increasing confidence as a healer—helping others reconnect with what she called "life-force energy." By the time she responded to the ISIS survey, however, she said she was ready for a spectacular relationship of her own.

> My explorations and experiences as an energy worker have brought me into contact with others who are as sensitive as I am. However, I have yet to experience a LOVER with my abilities. When I do have the pleasure of sharing on this level with my partner, well . . . planet Earth will get the ride of her life.

THE RELIGIOUS LANGUAGE OF SEXUAL ECSTASY

The performance language of sexual experience expresses only a small part of the whole picture. Many ISIS women described the flush of sexual ecstasy as if it were a religious experience: "holy," "sacred," "a revelation," "a sacrament." They felt a merging of body and soul. At the height of passion they cried out "Oh, God!"

That ISIS women's descriptions of sexual ecstasy often reflected the language of religion harks back to ancient customs where sexual union was built in to worship—sometimes to wild excess, as in Bacchanalian orgies and Celtic May Day ceremonies, replete with bonfires and gluttonous mating. Lustiness was next to godliness, along with feasting, drinking, and dancing. Pleasure, orgasm, and ecstasy were not sins. They were routes to the deity.

Some religions are still predicated on the notion that sex can be a path to spirit. These include Tantric Buddhism, Chinese Taoism, Wicca, and countless indigenous practices. Even some of the major world religions carry vestiges of the early sexual rituals. Candles and incense, wine, flowers, music, anointing with oil, laying on of hands—all these come from those early rites (Eisler, 1995; Gadon, 1989). We have adapted them into ceremonies such as the Catholic mass and protestant Eucharist without acknowledging their pagan sexual roots. We have also adapted them into our courtship and mating rituals without acknowledging their spiritual connections.

I have found that understanding these connections can help some clients release the physical and emotional tension that keeps them from opening to their deepest sexual desires. Such understanding offers them historical context for what they feel and intuit in their sexual interactions, imagery through which they can identify what they want and do not want, and occasionally language to help them translate their wishes to their partners. In addition (and sometimes most importantly), it provides context for their lack of desire. They can understand that separating sex and spirit has been built into the culture over the centuries, and represents a kind of social control that is beyond their power to change. This has allowed some clients to stop blaming themselves for sexual pathology and focus on the aspects of sexual pleasure to which they are most drawn.

TANTRA: "WINDOWS TO THE UNIVERSE"

Tantra is a sexual practice that originated in both Buddhist and Hindu scripture some 4,000 years ago as a ritual bridge between the physical realm of sex and the subtle realm of spirit. Tantric practices were popularized in the Western world in the 1970s by Bagwan Shri Rashneesh ("Osho") and later by the books and workshops of Margo Anand and others (e.g., Anand, 1989, 1996; Stubbs, 1999). At this writing there are almost two thousand Tantra books listed on Amazon.com and close to half a million Tantra websites appearing on a Google search. Tantra is not all there is to spiritual sex, but has become so synonymous with sacred or spiritual sex that it may provide an entry for clinicians to open a discussion about a sexual philosophy that goes beyond performance goals.

For some ISIS women, Tantra was their primary path to sexual ecstasy. A woman from Tucson, Arizona described herself as a Tantra teacher and a "spirit in a 50-year-old body." She wrote of finding "windows to the universe" through the Tantric practice of gazing. Her description offers insight into how it is possible to shift one's belief systems by aligning one's personal intentions with practices that already exist.

> My first conscious response to Tantric practices was to know that this would expand my capacity for pleasure—in all ways. It helped open all my senses to pure enjoyment of the physical universe, then steadily increased my awareness of my sexual response to life. My involvement has created bigger windows to the universes beyond the

physical and has led me to now teach it to an appreciative group of exquisite souls who are curious about how to integrate sexuality and spirituality. We are learning together.

As usually practiced in the West today, Tantra, or Tantric yoga, involves intention, breath, eye-contact, sound, movement, touch, and ritual to help practitioners reach a higher consciousness during sexual interaction. Sexual excitement is framed as the rising of kundalini energies coiled in the pelvis. The word *kundalini* comes from the Sanskrit *kunda,* literally "a lock of the beloved's hair." In energetic terms, *kundalini* means "creative potential, which uncoils upward to activate the sacred, loving, universal mind." "High sex," as in *The Art of Sexual Ecstasy,* "helps bring heightened awareness to the body, heart, and mind and to tune these three aspects . . . into a harmony that allows higher, more intense levels of pleasurable experience" (p. 45)

The ancient texts outlined elaborate rules for courting, kissing, aphrodisiacs, sexual play, and intercourse. (Anand, 1989; Bishop, 1996; Khalsa, 2000.) Some of these can be adapted into lovemaking rituals that add an element of attention and mystery for Western lovers. Tantric techniques include:

- Meditation with a partner
- Gazing into a partner's eyes and heart
- Invocation of spirits and deities, especially of Shakti and Shiva, the Hindu female and male principles
- Visualization of *yantras:* diagrams of energy fields depicting the sexual play of Shakti and Shiva
- *Mantras:* chanting ritual syllables such as *om mani padme hum*—"the (male) jewel in the (female) lotus"
- *Mudras:* ritualized hand gestures that represent transition from body to spirit
- *Yoni puja:* worship of the vagina through attention and touch
- *Lingam puja:* worship of the penis through attention and touch
- Yogic postures that create circuits for sexual energy to progress from body to spirit
- Ritualized intercourse that includes delayed ejaculation.
- Physical orgasm extended for long periods: "gateway to bliss." Heart orgasms or energy orgasms, centered in the heart and breath, require no physical touch.

COSMIC, MYSTICAL, MAGICAL, AND OTHERWORLDLY EXPERIENCES OF SEX AND SPIRIT

If ecstasy means entering fully into the center of one's sexual experience, sexual magic means stepping all the way through the center and entering an entirely new territory, a dimension that opens minds and transforms lives. One of the great surprises of the ISIS narratives was the extent to which women described cosmic, mystical, magical, and otherworldly experiences of sex and spirit—the "irrational facts" that lie beyond the goals of sexual performance. I have found that acknowledging these irrational facts can help "low libido" clients vividly visualize sexual desires they may not have been aware they had—desires beyond lubrication and orgasm on-demand, and also beyond the good-girl just-say-no messages that are built into the culture.

When ISIS women found sexual experience shifting beyond orgasm and ecstasy and into magical experience they reported entering a consciousness that was well beyond performance definitions of sex. Entrenched beliefs about the material world tended to fade, and with them expectations of specific sexual outcomes—the desire-arousal-orgasm model of sexual completion and success. The landscape sometimes grew ethereal or fantastical. Colors brightened. Time and space tended to ebb and flow like ocean tides. Symbolic shapes and gestures held potent meaning. What was often judged as "unbelievable" or "incredible" when respondents returned to ordinary reality was experienced as utterly authentic in the realms where sexual and spiritual experience merged. In some instances, even the concept of sexual partnership shifted and changed. Partners morphed into luminescent beings, sometimes from another time and place.

What ISIS Women Said Their Cosmic, Mystical, and Magical Experiences Included

- Spontaneous healing
- Extraordinary luminescence
- Existing beyond clock time, where past and future merge
- Ability to perceive auras, energy fields, and other extrasensory phenomena
- Raised vibrations—opening to higher dimensions of reality
- Reexperiencing prior lifetimes
- Intimate communication with spirit guides and teachers, guardian spirits, power animals, and divine beings
- Merging with universal energy—direct experiences of God and the cosmos
- Transformation and change—personal, relational, emotional, spiritual, physical

It was most often in their love relationships that women found the essence of sexual magic. But ISIS women also affirmed that the mystical qualities of sex could be found "everywhere"—in breathing and moving the body, in nature, in substances that altered the mind and shifted the spirit. Some women experienced the magic as primarily spiritual, mystical, and creative; some located it primarily within the body. Some women sensed that they were connected with the natural forces of the cosmos—earth, wind, rain, the divine light of heaven.

Others said this sense of magic was palpable. One said she felt as if she were making love with the universe.

The ISIS survey did not ask direct questions about cosmic, mystical, and magical experiences. It is therefore noteworthy that many women chose to describe such experiences in detail. Table 7.3 lists responses to the few questions from the ISIS survey that might have related to these phenomena.

A number of ISIS women described spontaneous sexual encounters with energy bodies and divine beings that were beyond direct physical, sensuous, and rational experience. Some identified these beings as angels, trees, sun, moon, or star-born beings. Others identified them as Christ, Shiva, God, Goddess, the hand of God, the eye of God, or the voice of God. Others wrote that they recognized beings from what they intuited were prior lifetimes—a lover from ancient Greece or a Wild West saloon. Some of these cosmic encounters were initiated by genital stimulation, others by meditation and prayer. Still others were initiated by love, passion, and other energy created within the relationship.

Encounters like these may stretch the bounds of credibility when taken out of context. Clearly they fall outside the boundaries of performance definitions, and yet they appear in the sexological literature (Ogden, 1999; Savage, 1999; Wade, 2004). There is also wide documentation of similar experiences in other disciplines. The psychological literature cites instances of trauma resolution through patients suddenly "seeing the light" and following the call of spirit. Such stories also abound in the self-help literature from addiction recovery to near-death experiences. Stories like these also appear in academic works, such as Maslow's exploration of peak experiences (1952) and Jung's exploration of archetypes (1959). They exist even in the medical literature, which cites instances of "miraculous" recoveries and faith healings, after ordinary therapeutic interventions have failed. (Chopra, 1998; Northrup, 1995; Siegel, 1986; Simonton, Simonton, & Creighton, 1978; Weill, 2000).

The most definitive validation for ISIS stories of cosmic and magical sex resides in the religious literature. Rita Brock (1988), Carter Heyward (1989), Thomas Moore (1998), James Nelson (1992), and Joan Timmerman (1992) are among the theologians who legitimize erotic energy as a form of prayer

Table 7.3
ISIS Women by the Numbers: Cosmic, Mystical, and Magical Experiences

85 percent said sex involved love and mystical union

63 percent said they connected sex and spirit by letting go of control

54 percent said sexuality involved oneness with a Higher Power

45 percent said it was through their senses that they often experienced God

39 percent said sexual satisfaction involved oneness with nature

and worship that communicates directly with God. From a mystical point of view, one has only to read the biblical *Song of Songs,* where sexual desire is inseparable from the holy bounties of nature: "thy breasts shall be as clusters of the vine" (chapter 7, verse 8). Or the diaries of St. Teresa of Avila, the sixteenth-century Carmelite nun who enumerated her sensual "raptures" with Christ and his flame-bearing angels (Peers, 1991). Or accounts of ceremonial invocations from shamans of the Amazon rain forests and the Siberian steppes; researchers like Mircea Eliade (1972) and Michael Harner (1990) have compiled a rich lode of information about sexual encounters with animal, angelic, and mythical beings. Swiss chemist Jeremy Narby (1998, 2005) has corroborated their "reality" by comparing such accounts to images from the chemistry laboratory. In analyzing the ladders and spirals repeatedly used by indigenous artists to connect human beings with animal and heavenly bodies, he found marked parallels to the ladders and spirals we now identify as our DNA.

Several ISIS women observed that sexual magic can arise from the most "ordinary," or "routine," experiences rather than from exotic practices. A sweet kiss, a tender conversation, or just holding each other on a Saturday afternoon when the rest of the family is out playing touch football.

A 38-year-old elementary teacher expressed a sense of merging with the universe that altered her awareness of herself and her relationship to the world. She described entering this magical space through the portal of the body—her own and her partner's. It was the opening of hearts that transported her to a realm where she could connect with a supernatural presence. Note that she took care to state that her experience did not include orgasm.

> When I was 22, I experienced a union with all things while making love with my former husband. He became my body and I his—our hearts opened, our bodies merged and I felt the rushing wind of an angelic presence, music played in my head and I laughed out loud. The room seemed to explode into light. There was another presence, the two became three and one all at once (I had no genital orgasm).

The level of union she described here is well beyond the usual performance standards, and my students have found it instructional to understand how using different standards of judgment may affect how they assess treatment plans for their clients. By *DSM* definitions this woman's story could point to severe pathology. Her merging with her husband could be seen as dysfunctionally codependent. Her experience of angelic presence, light explosion, head music, and spontaneous laughter could suggest that she suffers from dissociative disorder and/or delusional ideation. Perhaps these warrant an exploration of repressed childhood abuse and a prescription for psychotropic drugs. Yet from an ISIS point of view, this woman's ability to love wholeheartedly is highly valued. Her communication with sacred beings is a manifestation of cosmic grace. Finally, her ability to let go of control is an attribute many sex therapy clients strive for.

For many ISIS women, nonordinary sexual experience was signaled by light and a kind of extrasensory "knowing," qualities usually associated with spiritual experience. A 41-year-old woman wrote of an "inner explosion of energy" that she called "sublime" and "almost holy." Most interestingly, in terms of the woman quoted above, she addressed the issue of control, a crucial sexual and spiritual issue for many women even beyond the ISIS sample. She said that letting go of control—including the illusion of control—was for her the key to connecting with a larger reality of all-encompassing universal understanding in love: "Frequently it leaves me feeling a sort of awe mixed with tenderness for all of humanity. Like I get it all—why we're here—why I'm here. It all makes sense. I see my purpose."

A homemaker from Sarasota, Florida, described a different kind of "magical connection." She framed it within what she called the "completely spiritual" and ever-deepening relationship with her husband.

> From the first time we had sex, [15 years ago] it wasn't sex. It first was like a normal thermometer and when I had a climax the mercury broke. I ended up floating up in outer space and I could see my utter essence, my soul, transcend as reaching out onward, onward until there was utter darkness then a bursting of light.

She went on to parse this experience of light in terms of "auras," the energy fields around the body that some people are able to see. Although our energy fields are not always visible, they are nonetheless there and it is possible to work with them to change our physical, emotional, and mental reality (Brennan, 1987). This homemaker went on:

> Now when we're making love, different colors escape from our auras—pink, blue, white, then when it gets really passionate the color turns deep purple. It is as if the auras from our souls join in spiritual union. The complete colors, the oneness is so complete, that now I don't know where one leaves off and the other begins. There is also a oneness with nature and with an outside great spirit. It is all-encompassing. It is physical, sexual, spiritual—everything.

To my ISIS consciousness, it could be no coincidence that the colors of the energy fields this woman described matched the colors usually ascribed to various chakras, vital energy centers in the body (see below). Note that the "cool" colors—white, purple, blue, and green—belong to the four higher (or more spiritual) chakras and that the "hot" colors—red, orange, and yellow—belong to the three lower (or more physical) chakras.

If we allow ourselves to venture beyond performance standards of sexual health, it is possible to use these chakra colors as part of our diagnostic and therapeutic tool kit. If working with colors seems too far-fetched for either client or clinician, it may help simply to acknowledge that there is such a tradition as the chakra system, and that it is a venerable part of Eastern medical practice. There may be instances, even for allopathically trained clinicians, where such acknowledgement can offer clues to imbalances of sexual energy and desire and help restore their balance.

The Chakra System

The chakra system is an ancient *schema* to chart energy flow (*chakra* is the Sanskrit word for "wheel"). Although this *schema* differs somewhat from culture to culture, in its basic form it is most often diagrammed as seven energy centers in the body. These energy centers or wheels move in circular patterns, beginning with the root chakra at the base of the spine and culminating with the crown chakra at the top of the head. The meanings and other attributes associated with the chakras may also vary from culture to culture, but they are most often presented as outlined below (Brennan, 1988; Bruyere, 1994; Judith, 1999). These are offered here not as a substitute for a medical diagnosis, but as suggestions for expanding clinical options for assessing and discussing sexual desire problems (Table 7.4).

The narrative from the ISIS homemaker above suggests that lovemaking triggered intense activity in her upper, or more "spiritual," chakras, as distinct from her lower, or more "physical," chakras. Note that her experience of these energy centers also corresponds to the earlier-cited brain research that shows activation of the temporal lobe, or "spiritual" center of the brain, during physical stimulation (Komisaruk, Beyer, & Whipple, 2006). In this sense, the ISIS homemaker's description spans two belief systems at once: the scientific and the mystical. In her words, the experience was "all-encompassing."

Some ISIS women said that during sexual experience they sensed activity in both their lower and upper chakras. A 50-year-old massage therapist from Bozeman, Montana used a striking image: "It feels as if the clitoris must be related to the third eye."

> When I have a strong orgasm, my body dissolves into light and I sense an opening in the third eye area—an opening into unconditional love and/or a feeling of oneness with all. All fears and worries are forgotten. In fact, it seems as if when I am having frequent and full love-making that I rarely experience stress and overwhelming worries and fears. It has the strength of prayer—it is a body prayer to love.

Table 7.4
Diagram of the Chakra System

Meanings and Colors Usually Associated with Chakras

Chakra Level	Meaning	Color
7—Top of head, crown	Bliss, connection with universal energy "I know"	Violet, white
6—Brow, third eye	Imagination, intuition psychic "second sight" connection with archetypal patterns "I see"	Indigo, amethyst
5—Throat	Communication, creativity expressiveness "I reach out"	Blue
4—Heart	Love, self-acceptance empathy, peace, community "I love"	Pink, green
3—Solar plexus	Power, will, ego, focus on self rational thinking "I deserve"	Yellow
2—Sacrum	Emotional feelings sexuality, desire "I want"	Orange
1—Base of spine, perineum	Support, grounding physical sensations "I am	Red

Source: This table is based on information drawn from Barbara Brennan's *Hands of Light* (Bantam, 1988), Rosalyn Bruyere's *Wheels of Light* (Fireside, 1994), and Anodea Judith's *Wheels of Life* (Llewellyn, 1999).

THE HEALING CONNECTION

It is important for clinicians to understand the parameters of pleasure so that they can better inform and assess their clients. It is also important to understand that pleasure can induce spontaneous healing in some women. An author and producer, from Ontario, Canada, wrote of this healing aspect of sexual pleasure and its power to transform a deep emotional shadow that had settled over her personal life. She described living in a "soul-destroying" marriage to a man who had refused to stand up for her in the face of his abusive grown children. This had devolved into a connubial hell, in which she said communication had finally "crumbled into belittling snubs and angry retorts." The healing experience came for her in the form of a sudden energetic, orgasmic merging at what she called the "soul level."

One night as we lay in bed, gloomy in the blackness, I listened as he finally settled into sleep. I was lying there, hurting and questioning, when what I'm convinced is his soul, a blue light lifted itself from his body, moved over to mine and somehow melted into my body. Every single inch of me was stroked by a body-length cellular orgasm. I will never forget this moment. I hold it as the hope for reconciliation. No matter what he says, some part of him knows better.

Again, note the color this woman cites in her letter: "a blue light" that moved from her husband's body to hers. From correspondences on the chakra chart, this suggests an activation of throat chakra energy, and a spontaneous clearing of communication on a spiritual plane. It served to give hope and meaning to a situation that she wrote had been systematically killing her "cell by cell." It also serves here to provide a graphic—and even colorful—example of spiritual orgasm, or as she phrased it, "orgasm without sex."

Is this woman describing potential relationship health or ingrained personal pathology? Again, it depends on where one bases one's judgment. In ISIS terms this woman's sense of a unified and loving universe might well signify a journey to infinite wisdom, a most auspicious mating and merging with the universal mind. In the predominantly one-dimensional yet dualistic culture of today's medical model, such an interpretation requires an expanded belief system, or at least a suspension of ordinary disbelief. Whatever the eventual answer, I believe it is crucial for health practitioners to be familiar with more than one modality so that they can ask such fundamental questions of themselves and their clients.

CONCLUSION: CLINICAL AFFIRMATION AND CLINICAL CHALLENGE

ISIS narratives that inform this chapter were sent from every part of the United States and also from Canada and Israel. They were written by women whose ages and occupations varied widely. Their sexual experiences also varied, along with their relationship choices, which included cohabitation, affairs, chance encounters, and celibacy as well as marriage. Their sexual orientations included lesbian and bisexual as well as heterosexual. Yet along with the intensely individual stories expressed in these narratives there also run common strands that impact on women's experience of sexual desire.

There is commonality of content in recurring references to light, love, intimacy, healing, and general abundance. There is another commonality, too. Many of these narratives seem to have been written in isolation, as if each women's thoughts and feelings were being expressed for the first time, perhaps born separately out of some cultural black hole where little or no language had existed before. Some of these ISIS women seem to have been inventing their own new language and with it a new persona. "It is difficult to find the words to explain this experience, and to fit it into a questionnaire is utterly impossible," wrote a 51-year-old antique dealer from San Jose, California. "My spirituality exploded and enveloped everything. I have begun to see everything with new eyes—nothing is the same. I am like a baby, fresh and new, knowing nothing and having to start all over again."

The cumulative effect of 1,465 such narratives suggests that women's sexual experience is far broader than the performance limits indicated by *DSM* definitions. It also suggests that we need a broader clinical perspective for understanding the full range of women's sexual experience—the parameters of sexual health as well as the parameters of sexual pathology. Such a perspective is based on the premise that sexual experience is multifaceted and multidimensional rather than only physical. Broadening the notion of sexuality in this way allows for sexual experience to encompass an ecstasy connection as well as a goal of physical orgasm. This is a sexual perspective characterized by chaos, flux, and flow rather than neat definitions formed by activities that can be counted and measured.

Many women can benefit from clinical affirmation for their ecstatic experiences. It is therefore important to frame these experiences as part of a continuum of normal (if unique) response to sexual stimulation—to place them within an acknowledged universe of sexual health. At the same time, it is important to provide positive language for these experiences, which are so often stated in negative terms ("indescribable," "I can't explain it") because there is not yet a fully developed vocabulary to describe them. Finally, it is important for clinicians to legitimize these experiences as more than isolated sexological theory or anecdotal clinical observation.

In short, we need to broaden our definitions of sexual health, and ask more mindful questions of our women clients. With an enlarged and more complex picture in mind, there can be more comprehensive discussion of relationship, religion and culture, sexual desire, and sexual healing. Moreover, there can be more comprehensive discussion of the roles these play in women's lives. Further, it can be possible to envision new potentialities for sexual partnership, including the radical notion that many men may feel the same way these women do. But that is the subject of another chapter.

REFERENCES

American Psychiatric Association. (2000). *Diagnostic and statistical manual of mental disorders.* Fourth Edition, Text Revision. (DSM-IV-TR.) Washington, D.C.: American Psychiatric Association.

Anand, Margo. (1989). *The art of sexual ecstasy: The path of sacred sexuality for western lovers.* Los Angeles: Jeremy Tarcher.

Anand, Margo. (1996). *The art of sexual magic.* Los Angeles: Jeremy Tarcher.

Beattie-Jung, Patricia, Mary E. Hunt, & Radhika Balakrishnan. (2001). *Good sex: Feminist perspectives from the world's religions.* New Brunswick, N.J.: Rutgers University Press.

Beauvior, Simone de. (1952). *The second sex.* New York: Knopf.

Bishop, Clifford. (1996). *Sex and spirit.* Boston: Little, Brown & Co.

Bonheim, Jalaja. (1997). *Aphrodite's daughters: Women's sexual stories and the journey of the soul.* New York: Fireside.

Brennan, Barbara. (1987). *Hands of light: A guide to healing through the human energy field.* New York: Bantam Books.

Brock, Rita N. (1988). *Journeys by heart: A Christology of erotic power.* New York: Crossroad.

Bruyere, Rosalyn. (1994). *Wheels of light: Chakras, auras and the healing energy of the body.* New York: Fireside.

Chopra, Deepak. (1998). *Ageless body, timeless mind: The quantum alternative to growing old.* New York: Three Rivers Press.

Daniluk, Judith C. (1998). *Women's sexuality across the life span.* Binghamton, NY: Guilford Press.

Eisler, Riane. (1995). *Sacred pleasure: Sex, myth, and the politics of the body.* San Francisco: Harper Collins.

Eliade, Mircea. (1972). *Shamanism: Archaic techniques of ecstasy.* New York: Princeton University Press.

Ellison, Carol. (2000). *Women's sexualities: Generations of women speak about sexual self acceptance.* Oakland, Calif.: New Harbinger.

Espin, Oliva M. (1987). Issues of identity in the psychology of Latina lesbians. In Boston Lesbian Psychologies Collective, *Lesbian psychologies.* Urbana: University of Illinois Press.

Foley Sallie, Sally Kope, & Dennis Sugrue. (2002). *Sex matters for women: A complete guide to taking care of your sexual self.* Binghamton. New York: Guilford Press.

Freud, Sigmund. (1938). Three contributions to the theory of sex. *The basic writings of Sigmund Freud.* A. A. Brill (Trans. and Ed.). New York: Random House.

Gadon, Elinor W. (1989). *The once and future goddess.* New York: Harper & Row.

Gimbutas, Marija. (1989). *The language of the goddess.* San Francisco: Harper & Row.

Harner, Michael. (1990). *The Way of the Shaman.* San Francisco: Harper San Francisco

Heyward, Carter. (1989). *Touching our strength: The erotic as power and the love of God.* New York: Harper Collins.

Hunt, Valerie V. (2000). *The infinite mind: Science of human vibrations of consciousness* (3rd ed.). Los Angeles, CA: Malibu Publications.

Judith, Anodea. (1999). *Wheels of life: A user's guide to the chakra system.* St Paul, MN: Llewellyn Publications.

Jung, Carl G. (1959). *The archetypes and the collective unconscious.* R.F.C. Hall (Trans.). New York: Pantheon Books.

Kaplan, Helen Singer. (1979). *Disorders of sexual desire.* New York: Brunner/Mazel.

Khalsa, Shakta Kaur. (2000). *Kundalini yoga.* Toronto: Whole Way Library.

Kinsey, Alfred C., Wardell B. Pomeroy, & Clyde E. Martin. (1948). *Sexual behavior in the human male.* Philadelphia, PA: W.B. Saunders Co.

Kinsey, Alfred C., Wardell B. Pomeroy, Clyde E. Martin, & Paul H. Gebhard. (1953). *Sexual behavior in the human female.* Philadelphia, PA: W.B. Saunders Co.

Kitzinger, Sheila. (1983). *Woman's experience of sex: The facts and feelings of female sexuality at every stage of life.* New York: Putnam.

Kleinplatz, Peggy J. (Ed.). (2001) *New directions in sex therapy: Innovations and alternatives.* Philadelphia: Brunner-Routledge.

Komisaruk, B.R., Beyer-Flores, C., & Whipple, B. (2006). *The Science of Orgasm.* Baltimore: The Johns Hopkins University Press.

Laumann, Edward O., John H. Gagnon, Robert T. Michael, & Stuart Michaels. (1994). *The social organization of sexuality: Sexual practices in the United States.* Chicago: University of Chicago Press.

Laumann, Edward O., Anthony Paik, & Raymond Rosen. (1999, February 10). Sexual dysfunction in the United States: Prevalence and predictors. *Journal of the American Medical Association, 281,* 537–544.

Maslow, Abraham. (1952). *Toward a psychology of being.* Princeton, N.J.: Van Nostrand.

Masters, William H., & Virginia E. Johnson (1966). *Human sexual response.* Boston: Little, Brown & Co.

Moore, Thomas. (1998). *The soul of sex: Cultivating life as an act of love.* New York: Harper Collins.

Narby, Jeremy. (1998). *The cosmic serpent: DNA and the origins of knowledge.* New York: Tarcher.

Narby, Jeremy. (2005). *Intelligence in Nature.* New York: Tarcher.

Nelson, James B. (1992). *Body theology.* Louisville: Westminster/John Knox Press.

Northrup, Christiane. (1995). *Women's bodies, women's wisdom: Creating physical and emotional health and healing.* New York: Bantam.

Ogden, Gina. (1999). *Women who love sex: An inquiry into the expanding spirit of women's erotic experience.* (Rev. Ed.). Cambridge, MA: Womanspirit Press.

Ogden, Gina. (2002). Sexuality and spirituality in women's relationships: Preliminary results of an exploratory survey. *Working Paper 405.* Wellesley College Center for Research on Women, Wellesley, MA.

Ogden, Gina. (2006). *The Heart and Soul of Sex: Making the ISIS connection.* Boston: Shambhala.

Peers, E. Allison. (Trans. and Ed.). (1991). From the critical edition of Teresa of Avila (c. 1575). *The life of Teresa of Jesus: The autobiography of Teresa of Avila.* Silverio de Santa Teresa. New York: Doubleday.

Savage, Linda E. (1999). *Reclaiming goddess sexuality: The power of the feminine way.* Carlsbad, CA: Hay House.

Shaw, Miranda. (1994). *Passionate enlightenment: Women in tantric Buddhism.* Princeton, N.J.: Princeton University Press.

Siegel, Bernie. (1986). *Love, medicine and miracles.* New York: Harper and Row.

Simonton, O. Carl, Stephanie M. Simonton, & J. L. Creighton (1978). *Getting well again.* New York: Bantam.

Stubbs, Kenneth Ray. (1999). *The essential tantra: A modern guide to sacred sexuality.* New York: Jeremy Tarcher.

Sugrue, D.P., & Whipple, B. (2001). The consensus-based classification of female sexual dysfunction: barriers to universal acceptance. *Journal of Sex and Marital Therapy, 27,* 221–226.

Tiefer, Leonore. (1995). *Sex is not a natural act and other essays.* Boulder, Colo.: Westview Press.

Tiefer, Leonore, & Ellyn Kaschak (Eds.). (2001). *A new view of women's sexual problems.* Binghamton, NY: Haworth Press.

Timmerman, Joan H. (1992). *Sexuality and spiritual growth.* New York: Crossroad.

Wade, Jenny. (2004). *Transcendent sex: When lovemaking opens the veil.* New York: Paraview Pocket Books.

Weill, Andrew. (2000). *Spontaneous healing: How to discover and embrace your body's natural ability to maintain and heal itself.* New York: Ballantine Books.

Whipple, Beverly, John D. Perry, & Alice K. Ladas. (Rev. Ed.). (2005). *The G spot: And other discoveries about human sexuality.* New York: Owl.

Chapter Eight

GENDER VARIABILITY: TRANSSEXUALS, CROSSDRESSERS, AND OTHERS

Dallas Denny, Jamison Green, and Sandra Cole

In the Western world, gender variance has long been associated and confused with sexual orientation. Gender variance occurs in human beings when a male-bodied individual expresses or displays, consciously or unconsciously, a preponderance of characteristics that are typically associated with femaleness or femininity, and the reverse for a female-bodied individual. Feminine-appearing men have long been thought to be homosexual, and it has been a common misperception that masculine women are "trying" or generally "wanting" to be men so they might legitimately demonstrate their erotic attraction to women. These stereotypes have long plagued homosexual, lesbian, bisexual, transsexual and transgendered people.

Gender identity is a person's concept of herself as masculine or feminine; gender expression is the gender-based characteristics that a person displays as part of his outward social interactions. There is no direct correlation between gender identity and sexual orientation. There are gay men who are very masculine, lesbians who are very feminine, bisexual people who are not confused about who they are or to whom they are attracted, and transgendered people who are heterosexual (and bisexual, and homosexual).

The classic notion of a transsexual is "a man in a dress," and there seems to be a general sense that transgender is the new, politically correct word for transsexual. This is a narrow, oversimplified view. There is so much more to gender variance. If we are to understand gender variance and how it differs from and compliments human sexuality, we must clarify what transgender means, and particularly what it means to be transsexual or transgendered in the modern world.

UNDERSTANDING GENDER VARIANCE

In the early 1990s, *transgender* arose from the grassroots as an umbrella term to refer to all types of individuals whose gender identities or presentations differed from binary male/female norms (Green & Brinkin, 1994). The term quickly gained popularity, appearing in both the gay and mainstream press. Today, the term has become ubiquitous and many people who might once have called themselves transsexuals, crossdressers, or drag queens proclaim themselves "transgenders" (Lev, 2004, pp. 6–7; Taylor & Rupp, 2004).[1]

Bornstein (1994, p. 141) considers transgender shorthand for "transgressively gendered." In fact, many, and perhaps most human beings find themselves in conflict with gender rules at some times in their life. When Shannon Faulkner enrolled at Charleston, South Carolina's all-male Citadel academy in 1993, she made history (Bennett-Haigney, 1995). So did Los Angeles Rams defensive lineman Rosie Greer, when he took up needlepoint in the 1970s (Beller, 2006). The very definitions of what is "right and appropriate" for men and women to wear, how they groom themselves, and their roles in society have changed dramatically over the past several centuries (and even before that) as a result of individuals who, like Faulkner and Grier, have refused to abide by and have rebelled against society's rules of gender. Trousers, which are now everyday attire for most North American women, were illegal women's wear in some states less than 100 years ago (cf. *Atlanta Constitution,* February 26, 1911, February 2, 1913).

As with any other class of people, gender-variant individuals are as a group quite diverse. Transsexual people are those who either have a psychological sense of themselves, or simply desire to live, as members of the non-natal sex (see Benjamin, 1966). Many, and perhaps most, transsexuals lack the finances, social support, or sheer nerve to live publicly as members of the other sex, and they remain in their natal sex throughout their lives. Others seek professional help, with a goal of altering their bodies with hormones, surgeries, and, often for those vectoring toward female, electrolysis, so they may publicly live in the non-natal gender role; this is called "sex reassignment" (Green & Money, 1969), or, in the vernacular, a "sex change." Yet others manage this obstacle course without any help from, and often in spite of, mental health professionals (see Richards & Ames, 1983, for an example of an obstructive psychoanalyst).

Most transgendered people do not in fact identify as transsexual. They may dress in a gender-neutral manner, blend elements of male and female clothing styles, or dress wholly or partially, full- or part-time in clothing ordinarily worn by members of the non-natal gender. Some modify their bodies in the same ways as do transsexuals, but don't necessarily seek genital surgery or consider themselves to be members of the non-natal sex (Boswell, 1991; Feinberg, 1992).[2] Some individuals (often heterosexual) identify as crossdressers, and yet others as drag queens or drag kings. Increasingly, nontranssexual transgendered people have come to describe themselves as having characteristics of both sexes, as blending genders, or as inhabiting "third-gender," "transgenderist," or "genderqueer" space (see Bolin, 1994; Bornstein, 1994; Boyd, 2003; Devor, 1989; Nataf, 1996; Nestle, Wilchins, & Howell, 2002; Norbury & Richardson, 1994; Rothblatt, 1994).

The reasons for bending or breaking society's laws of gender display and identity are many and varied. Many men and some women crossdress for erotic reasons; they find it sexually stimulating (Prince, 1978). Some of these men and women may crossdress only once or twice; for others, it is a lifetime interest or, in come cases, obsession (Docter, 1988, pp. 10–19).

Many heterosexual male crossdressers report that over the years, the erotic component of wearing the clothing of the non-natal sex fades away as a feeling of comfort and belongingness grows (Prince, 1978). Many crossdressers give considerable thought to sex reassignment, and more than a few will eventually describe themselves as transsexual (Docter, 1988).

Transsexuals crossdress in order to make manifest their internal views of themselves; to them, wearing the clothing of the non-natal sex is congruent—normal and ordinary. Many transsexuals report having never felt comfortable in the clothing they were "supposed" to wear (see Green & Brinkin,1994, pp. 1–25).

Most transsexuals report no or minimal history of erotic crossdressing, but a minority of male-to-female transsexuals have recently claimed eroticism as a primary motivator of their sex reassignment (see Allison, 1999, and Lawrence, 1998, for opposing points of view). One sensationalistic writer has denied that male-to-female transsexuals change genders because they identify as members of the non-natal sex; he has claimed on the basis of interviews with transsexuals in night clubs that all male-to-female transsexuals are sexually motivated (Bailey, 2002).[3]

There are many other motivations for crossdressing. Some are external. Many natal males and an increasing number of natal females use drag personas in order to provide entertainment, often as a livelihood (cf. Norbury & Richardson, 1994; Troka, Lebesco, & Noble, 2003). Cross-dressing can also help to attract sexual partners: drag queens get lots of attention; and oftentimes, transgendered prostitutes find they can make more money when dressed as a woman than as a man (cf. Denny, 2006; Rodriguez-Madera & Toro Alfonso, 2005, p. 117). Bisexual or homosexual male crossdressers tend to prefer being in the female role when having sex with men (cf. Morgan, 1973; Novic, 2005). Yet another external reason for crossdressing is rehearsal: as an eligibility requirement for genital sex reassignment surgery, transsexuals must dress and live 24 hours a day as a member of the non-natal sex (Meyer et al., 2001).

By far, however, most reasons for crossdressing are internal, having to do with expressing an inner sense of masculinity or femininity. Crossdressing—even temporarily—can reduce stress by providing an escape from the financial and social pressures of the natal gender role, or, for transsexuals, reduce the dissonance of living in a nonpreferred gender role, providing relief and increasing self-confidence (see Brown & Rounsley, 1996, pp. 61–62).

Most transgendered people report developing feelings of differentness and a conscious realization of transgender feelings or identity from early childhood (Brown & Rounsley, 1996, chapter 2). A significant percentage describe an awakening or intensifying of transgender feelings or crossdressing at puberty. Some individuals repress their feelings for most of their lives, often waiting until middle age to begin experimenting with crossdressing or looking into the possibility of sex reassignment. There may a number of reasons for this delay: internal shame and guilt about being transgendered, fear of rejection by their families, fear of loss of employment or social standing, religious convictions, or a concern that they may not "pass" convincingly as a member of the non-natal sex.

The past decade has seen larger numbers of young people coming out as transgendered. This may be an effect of increased visibility of not only transgendered persons, but gay men and lesbians in the media and in real life settings. When transgendered people recognize that they are not isolated and alone, they often feel encouraged to reveal themselves earlier than they might have if they never had seen another person who seemed to feel the same way.

HISTORICAL AND CROSS-CULTURAL MANIFESTATIONS OF GENDER VARIANCE

Examination of the anthropological and medical literature shows that historically, gender-variant people have been common (though frequently repressed by political or religious powers) throughout recorded history, and are present in tribal societies on six continents and many inhabited islands (see Bullough & Bullough, 1993; Feinberg, 1996; Taylor, 1996).

Most non-Western societies have traditionally viewed their transgendered and transsexual members as normal variants of the human condition. Hundreds of tribal societies have socially sanctioned roles for their gender-variant members; indeed, some tribes view those who fit and fill these roles with a combination of awe, respect, and apprehension, often considering them to have special insight, wisdom, and powers, including the ability to view life from "both sides" (Herdt, 1994; Roscoe, 1988, 1990; Williams, 1986). Indeed, cross-cultural research has shown that gender-variant people tend to fill important social roles as educators, shamans, healers, storytellers, and entertainers (Whitam, 1997).

When tribal customs and worldviews are influenced by and diminished by the customs and mores of North American and European societies with their rigid binary constructions of gender, traditional tribal roles for gender-variant people tend to be diluted or supplanted with modern Western sexual identity constructions like homosexuality (Jackson & Sullivan, 1999; Roscoe, 1998, Chapter 8, Williams, 1986, p. 210); it should be noted, however, that in Native North American tribes, the belief by the white scientific community that transgender traditions have disappeared in some tribes may have been largely an effect of tribal members learning not to talk to anthropologists (see Williams, 1986, chapter 9). Nonetheless, mainstream cultural influences can result in shame of or contempt for gender-variant people who were once accepted and acceptable in their native cultures. Today, there is a movement afoot to reclaim traditional gender-variant identities in Native American communities (cf. Jacobs, et al., 1997; Roscoe, 1998; Williams, 1986, chapter 10).

The patriarchal religious belief systems that attempted to rigidly control sexual behavior tended to confuse gender variance with sexual degeneracy (see volume 3, chapter 4). These regimes cast transgendered people from their previous incarnations as valuable tribal members and religious leaders, proclaiming them sinners and driving them largely underground. Nonetheless, there have been a variety of high-profile gender-variant people in Western history, including kings, queens, authors of note, and, arguably, one pope whose femaleness was not discovered until she gave birth during a Papal procession (cf. Ackroyd, 1979; Bullough & Bullough, 1993; Dekker & Van de Pol, 1989; and Feinberg, 1996; for biographies and autobiographies of representative individuals, see such works as Bullough & Bullough, 1993; Cromwell, 1999; De Eraso, 1996; Durova, 1988; Feinberg, 1996; and Kates, 1995).

Deriving perspective from Judeo-Christian social beliefs, early sexologists turned their attention to gender variance and issues of sexual orientation in the late 1800s (see Irvine, 1990, for a history). Sexual orientation and gender variance were at first conflated by these early social scientists; for instance, Karl Uhlrichs believed homosexuality to be the result of a blend of male and female emotions and feelings, a "hermaphroditism of the mind" (Ulrichs, 1994). Patients we would today consider transgendered or homosexual were called "urnings" or "sexual inverts" (Ellis & Symonds, 1897; Ulrichs, 1994).

Sexologists Havelock Ellis and Magnus Hirschfeld differentiated gender identity from sexual orientation in the early twentieth century, but as Vern Bullough has pointed out, Hirschfeld's work was unfortunately not translated into English until 1991, and so had minimal impact in the United States (Bullough, 1991, pp. 11–14; Ellis, 1906; Hirschfeld, 1910; Meyerowitz, 2002, pp. 14–15). Hirschfeld's Berlin Institute for Sexual Research and magnificent sexological library, which contained many case studies of people we might today call crossdressers or transsexuals, was destroyed by Nazis on May 6, 1933 (Rudacille, 2005, p. 49).

In the United States, homosexuality and gender variance have been historically confused and conflated. Early and mid-twentieth century stereotypes of gay men and lesbians tended to be of, respectively, effeminate males and masculine women (Van, Maupin, & Stryker, 1996, pp. 16–17); in fact, Radclyffe Hall's prototypical "lesbian" novel of 1928, *The Well of Loneliness,* is a classic description of a female-to-male transgendered person. Hall's protagonist even uses the name Stephen.

Social beliefs about homosexuality have changed in recent decades, not because of new scientific knowledge, but as a result of the gay rights movement that coalesced after the Stonewall Riots in 1969 (Clendinen & Nagourney, 1999; Duberman 1993). Post-Stonewall, many gay men and women have come to reject, respectively, stereotypes of effeminacy and mannishness in favor of more-or-less conventional models of masculinity and femininity (Dahir, 2006; for a portrayal of contemporary homosexual masculinity, see director Ang Lee's Oscar-winning 2005 film *Brokeback Mountain*; for a portrayal of contemporary lesbian femininity, see *The L Word* on Showtime cable television). Of course, feminine males and masculine females continue to be found in gay and lesbian communities, but most gay men are conventionally masculine in dress and demeanor, and seek "straight-acting, straight-looking" men as sexual partners (see the personal ads in almost any major metropolitan alternative newspaper, such as the *San Francisco Bay Times*). With the rise of feminist consciousness, "butchness" fell out of favor in the lesbian community, until "rediscovered" in the early 1990s (cf. Burana, Roxxie, & Due, 1994; Feinberg, 1993; Munt, 1998; Nestle, 1992).

Before the early sexologists began to pay attention to gender and sexual minorities, gender-variant individuals tended to be viewed by the general public, when they were thought of at all, as sinful or wicked or degenerate. As a result of the writings of sexologists like Krafft-Ebing (1894), gender-variant people began to be seen as mentally ill, as "patients" with "conditions" which could hopefully—at least someday—be cured by medical treatments. This set the stage for an unfortunate dynamic when transsexualism came dramatically to the attention of the press, the general public, and the scientific world.

THE MENTAL ILLNESS MODEL OF TRANSSEXUALISM

In December 1952, news media around the world trumpeted the news that George Jorgensen, an American ex-G.I. from the Bronx, had undergone medical treatments in Denmark which had changed his secondary sex characteristics and genitals from male toward female; George had become Christine

Harry Benjamin International Gender Dysphoria Association (HBIGDA).[11] In 1979, HBIGDA published Standards of Care for Hormonal and Surgical Sex Reassignment, which are updated periodically (see Meyer et al., 2001, for the latest revision). The Standards are minimal consensual guidelines developed by HBIGDA members for the hormonal and surgical treatment of transsexual and other transgendered people. The Standards recommend repeated sessions with mental health professionals; resulting letters of authorization recommend clients' access to hormonal therapy and surgical sex reassignment procedures. These letters are presented by the clients to their physicians and surgeons. The Standards further recommend the completion of a one-year real-life experience before genital surgery is performed.

Ongoing revisions of the Standards of Care reflect changes in philosophy and new knowledge about gender identity issues. The Standards serve a valuable purpose in that they are designed to protect both those seeking medical procedures and those who provide them. However, they are unique in that they impose restrictions on therapies for gender-variant people that other classes of people do not have. Nontransgendered people can often obtain the same technologies (hormonal therapy and plastic and cosmetic surgical procedures) with no special restrictions imposed upon them.

While most helping professionals, and for that matter most transsexuals see some value in placing restrictions on access to medical treatment, in their twenty-five years of existence, the HBIGDA Standards of Care have generated no data to either support or question their effectiveness.[12] They are supported only by the clinical judgment of the members of HBIGDA—and the organization's members are not of a single mind about the Standards. After more than 25 years, transsexual and other transgendered people are placed in the unique and unenviable position of being required to follow guidelines which restrict their access to medical care, despite the lack of objective and conclusive evidence that the guidelines are effective.

The DSM

The American Psychiatric Association's *Diagnostic and Statistical Manual of Mental Disorders (DSM)*, now in its text-revised fourth edition, is the primary nosological sourcebook of the mental health field. In 1980 *DSM* introduced gender variance into the third edition—coincidentally, the edition in which homosexuality was removed as a mental disorder.[13] Transsexualism and Gender Identity Disorder of Adolescence or Adulthood, Nontranssexual Type (the latter added in the 1987 revision), were listed under the heading "Disorders Usually First Evident in Infancy, Childhood, or Adolescence," as was Gender Identity Disorder of Childhood. Transvestic Fetishism was included under the heading "Sexual Disorders as a Paraphilia."

This changed with 1994's *DSM-IV*. Transvestic Fetishism was moved to the category "Paraphilias," and Transsexualism was dropped. Gender Identity Disorder was subsumed under the category "Sexual and Gender Identity Disorders." Gender Identity Disorder of Childhood was moved to the "Sexual and Gender Identity Disorders" category.

There has been a great deal of debate about the inclusion of gender identity disorders in the *DSM*, and there have been calls for removal or reform (cf. Wilson, 1998, 2000; Wilson & Hammond, 1996). Criticisms have included the sexism that permeates the *DSM*, the *DSM*'s rigid delineation of sex roles, and the use of prejudicial language. Critics have noted that while *DSM* diagnosis saddles the gender-variant diagnosee with the stigma of mental illness, the corresponding social and financial benefits of mental illness are often denied. For instance, although insurance companies require a diagnostic code before they will pay for treatment, most insurers specifically deny reimbursement for expenses related to sex reassignment. Also, transgendered people are specifically excluded from the Americans with Disabilities Act of 1990.

Without a doubt, the most problematic *DSM* category is Gender Identity Disorder of Childhood. Activists have long considered this category a backdoor reintroduction of homosexuality, as its diagnostic criteria fit many prehomosexual men and women (Vasey, 2000). GID of Childhood has provided a means of forcing involuntary incarceration of children and adolescents for the purpose of "converting" them into heterosexuals; for a graphic description of this, see Scholinski, 1997.

Transgendered people are themselves divided about the issue of inclusion in the *DSM*. Some seek reform, some seek removal, and some hope that more insurance companies will one day reimburse transgender-related expenditures, for which they expect a diagnosis of some kind will be required.[14]

Mental Health Issues

The simple fact of being gender-variant can impose tremendous stress on an individual; this can come both from within and from external sources.

Most transgendered and transsexual people report having experienced intense negative emotions related to their feelings and behaviors; these include fear, shame, guilt, and anxiety. Their gender-variant behaviors and desires may be ego dystonic, causing them to hide and deny them and become overcome with shame and guilt. Many gender-variant people eventually overcome these negative feelings by a coming out process analogous to that of gay men and lesbians, but many more struggle with negative or ego-dystonic emotions all of their lives; Lev (2004) calls the process of growth and acceptance "Transgender Emergence."

Hiding or denying transgender feelings can result in a constellation of self-destructive behaviors. These can include withdrawal from daily activities or attempts to self-medicate with tobacco, alcohol, and other drugs (Tayleur, 1994). Sometimes the individual will compensate by engaging in hypermasculine or hyperfeminine behavior. Natal females may marry, bear children, find jobs which have been historically considered the province of females, and do their best to fulfill societal stereotypes of femininity (cf. Kailey, 2005). Males may marry and father children, build up their bodies with exercise, join street gangs, tattoo themselves, enlist in the military, or seek hypermasculine careers (see Brown, 1988). Many seek and fulfill leadership roles in their communities. Both males and females may engage in extreme sports and other high-risk behaviors. Suicide attempts, body cutting, genital self-mutilation, and sexual acting out, including promiscuity and unprotected sex, are common (cf. Beatty, 1993; Farmer, 1994).

Those who have come to terms with their inner natures are much less likely to engage in such behaviors. Even after such balance is reached, however, individuals who have struggled for years in inner turmoil may bear psychic scars which manifest as residual chronic depression, dissociative disorders, or other diagnosable mental conditions. Additionally, they must live with histories which may include poor or nonexistent work history, poor coping skills, substance abuse, criminal records, and the burden of a long history of secrets, unpleasant memories, and fear of discovery.

It should be noted that while most gender-variant people struggle with these issues, many are mentally healthy (Lev, 2004). The transgender community abounds with individuals who have excelled in all aspects of their lives.

Discrimination

Most gender-variant people report having been bullied, and many report having survived physical attacks (Wilchins, et al., 1997). Rejection by parents, siblings, extended family members, friends, and sexual partners is common, and teachers, church and government officials, law enforcement, and medical personnel are often nonsupportive or actively hostile (cf. Green, 1969). Many gender-variant youth are turned out of their homes and must support themselves on the street (see *Our trans children*, 2004, Parents and Friends of Lesbians and Gays). Transgendered adults are often shunned or bullied on the street, harassed in their jobs and neighborhoods, and expelled from churches and social organizations.

Social ostracism and ridicule is not limited to those who transition gender roles. The very differentness of gender-variant people often provokes ridicule, harassment, or attack. This reactive negative behavior is often imposed on family members and friends of gender-variant people as well. Even being perceived as gender-variant can be fatal. On July 29, 2001, Willie Houston, a nontransgendered heterosexual man, was shot to death at Opryland Park in Nashville, Tennessee. The reason: he was carrying his girlfriend's purse and escorting a blind friend to the men's room (see *Crimes against transgender individuals,* National Gay and Lesbian Task Force.)

Many gender-variant people report histories of extended sexual or physical abuse; this can lead to dissociative disorders, post-traumatic stress syndrome, and other disorders (see Cole, Denny, Eyler, & Samons, 2000, pp. 170–171). Under the pathology-based medical model, it was assumed that any co-existing mental condition was part and parcel of the "syndrome" of transsexualism. While mental illnesses can certainly co-occur with gender-variant behavior, it should be noted that such disorders are frequently sequelae of abuse related to the stigma and disenfranchisement of being transgendered rather than part of the gender identity issue per se (Lev, 2004, p. 203).

Sexuality

All human beings manifest sexual behavior, and transgendered and transsexual people are no exception. Unfortunately, observers frequently make unwarranted assumptions about the sexual orientation and behavior of gender-variant people. Perhaps because of a history of mutual struggle for rights, respect, and identity shared by gay men and lesbians and the transgendered, many people presume that gender-variant people are homosexual (as determined by their natal gender role). In fact, some people, despite overwhelming evidence to the contrary, cannot be dissuaded from this opinion (cf. Varnell, 1996). One of the most frequent criticisms of transsexualism is that those who seek or undergo sex reassignment are attempting to escape from internalized feelings of homophobia—that is, that they are dealing with their homosexuality by seeking to reconstruct it, by changing sex, as heterosexual. This theory ignores the fact that it makes no sense to "escape" from a stigmatized minority (homosexuality) into a minority that is much more heavily stigmatized (transsexualism). About half of both pre- and non-operative male-to-female transsexuals are sexually attracted exclusively to females (Green, 2004). Many female-to-male transsexuals identity as gay men and live as such after gender-role transition; many others are exclusively sexually oriented towards females.

The issue of sexual orientation of gender-variant individuals is a complex one. Terms such as heterosexuality and homosexuality lose their meaning when cast loose from the moorings on which they are based—femaleness and maleness:

> Should homosexuality be considered in relation to the individual's natal sex, or their new role? Is a transsexual woman who is still fulfilling the role of husband in a marriage in a lesbian relationship? Certainly, it does not seem so to the world, which

sees a heterosexual relationship. And yet five years later, when the individual has transitioned into the woman's role, the same couple, if publicly affectionate, will be perceived as lesbian. What of a post-transition nonoperative transsexual woman in a sexual relationship with a male? The public sees a heterosexual couple, and yet, in the bedroom, their genitals match. Should their sexual act be considered heterosexual or homosexual? Does it matter if the feminized partner does or does not take the active role in intercourse? And what if the same individual then has surgery and finds a female partner? Is this relationship homosexual or heterosexual? Finally, what if a nonoperative transsexual man has as a partner a post-operative transsexual man? Is this a gay relationship? A straight one? Are any of these people bisexual? And most significantly, can the term bisexuality have any meaning at all when gender is deconstructed? (Denny & Green, 1996, pp. 88–89)

Gender-variant people are nonetheless sexual beings who must interpret their own sexual attractions and desires. They may partner with natal males, natal females, or both, or with other transgendered people. They may be abstinent or promiscuous, kinky or "plain vanilla." They are perhaps the best arbiters of whether their relationships are "heterosexual" or "homosexual" or something else altogether.

Relationships

Gender-variant individuals do not live in vacuums. They are connected to other human beings through family relationships, marriages, parenting, community, church, school, the workplace, and through their citizenship in cities, states, and nations. When the individual changes gender role, not only the individual, but every individual with whom he or she has a relationship is in some way, great or small, affected.

Those most impacted are family members. It can be devastating to learn that a loved father or mother, sister or brother, or son or daughter, cross-dresses or is considering sex reassignment. How does one relate to a co-worker, employer, or employee who will be coming to work with a different gender presentation? What is the church's position on this? How will you remember to call your bowling partner by his or her new name?

Many gender-variant people are visibly "different" from an early age. They are simply unable or unwilling to suppress or hide their feelings and identity. This can result in hostility to the child by the family (Burke, 1997). Other individuals successfully hide their gender variance from their loved ones.

A decision to change sex later in life may strike others as sudden, capricious, or ill-considered, although it almost never is. The prior secrecy and closeted behavior regarding the transgender identity can reinforce this perception. When a transgendered person's gender variance becomes known, the family often reacts as if the lack of previous disclosure was intentional and purposefully deceitful. The withholding of information is in truth best recognized as a reflection of the transgendered person's fear of being abandoned by loved ones. For many families, the discovery of truth can predictably be experienced as a major emotional trauma which may have been triggered by the discovery of a secret cache of clothing, the accidental opening of a letter, or a spontaneous confession. Reaction can be profound, ranging from tearful acceptance to permanent rejection. Under such traumatic emotional conditions, it is essential that the family seek counseling or therapy (see Rosenfeld & Emerson, 1998, for a systems approach to family counseling; see also Lev, 2004).

Clearly, issues of how, when, and from whom the disclosure was made can have a huge impact on the way the revelation or discovery of gender variance is initially received. For example, a wife who has returned home unexpectedly early to find her husband wearing her clothing and makeup can understandably feel traumatized, and can easily be catapulted into extreme feelings of betrayal, fear, and anger (Cole, 1997, 1998; Cole et al., 2000).

It is perhaps in the area of family and loving relationships that therapists can be most effective. Reaching out to the family as a whole, each member of which may react to such sudden information and change with shock, fear, or rejection, is undoubtedly therapeutically valuable. Uninformed people presume that because the mother or father in such a family is changing gender roles, it is inevitable that the marriage will dissolve, with custody of minor children going to the nontransgendered parent. However, it is more likely that, with thoughtful clinical intervention and education, the family has a solid opportunity to remain intact (Cole, et al., 2000).

Many marriages endure with the presence of occasional crossdressing. The social and medical life changes imposed upon the family by a member's sex reassignment, however, can be profound. External supports such as peer support and especially counseling may be essential in helping the family remain intact as they work through gender-role transition. Partners and families can ultimately stay together with love and respect.

Transgender Health Issues

Gender-variant people experience the same constellation of aches, pains, illnesses, and malignancies as do the nontransgendered. Maintaining wellness can be problematic for the transgendered—but there are real health risks which are specific to transgendered people, and they are at increased risk for other health hazards.

Transgendered and transsexual individuals often fear discovery and rejection from health professionals from whom they seek medical assistance; consequently, some tend to avoid visits to healthcare practitioners. Male crossdressers may avoid routine medical checkups because they are self-conscious about shaved legs and chests. Both male-to-female and female-to-male transsexuals may avoid checkups or delay or fail to seek treatment because they are self-conscious about or ashamed of their bodies and the reactions of caregivers. If the individual has transitioned gender roles but has not had genital surgical sex reassignment, he or she may be realistically concerned about a negative reaction from health care providers if and when their genital status is discovered (see Green, 1960). If the individual has not transitioned gender roles and presents for treatment in the natal gender role, he may still be concerned that the physician will somehow be able to determine his transgender status. Those with such fears include not only those who have altered their bodies with hormones, electrolysis, or surgery, but those whose body shape and physical characteristics naturally fall outside the traditional male and female norms.

This avoidance can translate into undiagnosed illnesses. Beyond avoidance, there may be so much dissonance about the body that the individual neglects to properly care for it. Natal females may avoid gynecological examinations and breast exams; natal males may avoid prostate exams. Both may avoid dental care and tests for HIV and other sexually transmitted infections (STIs), and neglect chronic conditions like diabetes, high blood pressure, and heart disease. They may fail to seek treatment to stop smoking or reduce alcohol or drug use (Sperber, Landers, & Lawrence, 2005).

Gender-variant people face a number of health risks specifically associated with being transgendered.[15] Female-to-male transsexuals have a higher than usual risk of polycystic ovarian syndrome, an endocrine disorder (Balin, et al., 1993). Gender-variant individuals may have undiagnosed intersex conditions like Klinefelter Syndrome (an XYY chromosomal pattern; cf. Davidson, 1966) or congenital adrenal hyperplasia (a virilizing endocrine syndrome; see Ehrhardt, Evers, & Money, 1968).

Ingestion or injection of opposite-sex hormones can produce not only the usual risks associated with their use, but pose additional risks such as embolism, especially in the absence of medical monitoring (Cole et al., 2000).[16] Female-to-male transsexuals may develop acne following initiation of testosterone therapy and may develop abnormal lipids that can lead to coronary artery disease (Prior & Elliott, 1998). Clearly, it is advisable to have frequent medical monitoring for hormonal tolerance and equilibrium following a laboratory test of blood levels and organ function to create a baseline (Basson & Prior, 1998; Cole, et al., 2000; Prior & Elliott, 1998).

Transsexuals often avail themselves of non-genital plastic surgeries to enhance their internal image of themselves. In male-to-female people, these can include rhinoplasty (nose surgery), laryngioplasty (tracheal shave or reshaping of the Adam's apple), surgery to increase vocal pitch, face lifts, brow lifts, hair transplant or relocation, chin and cheek implants, injections of fat cells or collagen, breast implants, liposuction, and shaving of the facial bones to reduce strong male characteristics and cause the individual to more closely resemble the desired female form (see Lynn Conway's Facial Feminization Surgery Page at http://ai.eecs.umich.edu/~mirror/FFS/LynnsFFS.html). Genital surgeries include orchiectomy (castration) and can include penectomy (removal of the penis); these can occur as separate operations, although more frequently they are part of vaginoplasty (surgical creation of a neovagina). Male-to-female transsexuals usually have various forms of electrolysis and laser treatment to remove facial hair. Female-to-male transsexuals often have surgery to remove breast tissue and create a more masculine chest contour, and may have metaoid-ioplasty (a procedure which modifies the testosterone-enlarged clitoris into a more penis-like erectile organ), phalloplasty (surgical creation of a phallus), fusion of the labia and testicular implants, and (rarely) surgery to masculinize the face. Additionally, FTMs may undergo hysterectomy and oophorectomy (removal of the ovaries) to avoid medical complications. (See Green, 1995, 2004, for a discussion of FTM surgeries; Hage, 1992, and Schrang, 1998, for discussion of vaginoplasty.)

Even when performed by accomplished surgeons, surgical procedures can pose risks to health. When they are performed by inadequately-trained physicians, the results can be devastating. Unfortunately, in their desperation, transgendered people can fall victim to charlatans. After plastic surgeon John Ronald Brown lost his medical license, he continued to do vaginoplasties, often in non-sterile conditions, with usually poor results. Brown continued his "practice" for years, operating out of Tijuana, Mexico, before finally being arrested and sentenced in San Diego for fatally removing a healthy leg from an aged man (Williams, 1999). Lately, authorities have become aware of and have begun prosecuting unlicensed "practitioners" who engage in the widespread, occasionally fatal practice of injecting non-medical grade liquid silicone into cheekbones, breasts, hips, and just about every other part of the body; this is done in an attempt to gain "instant curves" (cf. Curtis, 2005; see also *Silicone use: Illicit, disfiguring, dangerous*, Gender Education & Advocacy, July 2, 2003). Health problems resulting from silicone injection can include disfigurement, respiratory and systemic illnesses, and death. Once injected, silicone cannot be completely removed, and even incomplete removal can lead to further disfigurement.

Gender-variant people are at risk for hepatitis and HIV/AIDS if they share needles for injection of estrogen, testosterone, silicone, or illegal drugs. Many male-to-female gender-variant people make their living as sex workers, often performing (at the request of their clients) sex acts without protective devices like condoms. Studies have shown astonishingly high seropositivity rates among such populations (see Elifson, et al., 1993; see Bockting & Avery, 2005, for recent needs assessments).

Male-to-female transsexuals have been unfairly accused of having a pathological need for multiple surgeries (cf. Raymond, 1980). Multiple surgeries are necessary for some MTF individuals in order to achieve a viable presentation in the non-natal gender, which can enhance employability and decrease the risk of discrimination, harassment, and physical attack. Cranial reshaping and facial plastic surgery procedures can make a considerable difference in a person's appearance and result in a dramatic improvement in way she is treated in public (Allison, 2001). It should be noted, however, that a few transgendered people share with some nontransgendered people an unhealthy need for repetitive surgeries. Similarly, some transgendered people will dress and groom themselves in a conspicuously excessive manner. This is usually an effect of rehearsal, and will disappear with time, but fetishistic individuals may prefer an outrageous or outlandish appearance and some genderqueer-identified people will deliberately dress to give a gender-ambiguous appearance.

Transgender-Caregiver Interactions

In the course of their careers, both mental and physical health professionals are likely to encounter a number of clients with gender identity issues. Although most practitioners understandably choose not to specialize in issues of gender and sexuality, it is nevertheless important that all caregivers be sensitive to the needs of the client and responsible for learning and understanding enough information about the transgender population to provide minimal or palliative care until referral to a more experienced caregiver can be made. It is certainly not appropriate to blindly turn away the transgendered client simply because she is transgendered.

It's important for caregivers to realize that many of the issues which confront transgendered people are only peripherally related to their gender identity issues, that many of their medical and psychological needs are essentially the same as those of other clients, and that they can almost always be helped by almost any practitioner. The client with gender identity issues should be considered as a whole person, with needs in areas which often don't require a sex or gender specialist, and should be offered services if the caregiver specializes in the areas of need. Caregivers inexperienced with gender identity issues should be aware of their prejudices and biases, continue to educate themselves about transgender issues, and seek advice and supervision from peers.

The actual gender issue is best handled by a professional with special training and experience in gender identity issues. Unfortunately, practitioners with such training and experience are relatively rare, and nonexistent in some parts of North America.

Some professionals—usually those working within certain religious frameworks—believe that gender variance is a mental illness and that God intended human beings to live in the bodies into which they were born.[17] They take it as their duty to "protect" such people from themselves by doing whatever they can to dissuade them from accepting their transgender natures and convince them to embrace rigidly heteronormative gender norms. This is usually ineffective, and it is unethical to impose personal values on a client. The responsible professional will, after making certain the client is aware of available treatment options, assist that client to realize his goals.

Even today, few caregivers receive training to work with gender-variant individuals. Many of the most experienced professionals in the field are considered pioneers, as they began their work in a time when there was little available literature and no opportunities for professional training. They typically began their work with transgendered clients with no sources for referral, and no knowledge or supervision, learning from their clients. Learning from clients without identifying and consulting external sources continues today, often needlessly, as much literature, clinical guidelines, and case history treatment protocols are available and realistically helpful. Many gender-variant people complain that they have paid to educate their therapists about gender identity issues; that is, any number of therapy sessions are taken up by helping the therapist understand about transgender issues. While it once may have been necessary and effective for the therapist to learn specifics of the transgender process at the client's expense, it is no longer so. Therapists now can consult with peers who already have specialized knowledge about gender variance, subscribe to journals like HBIGDA's *International Journal of Transgenderism*, join organizations like HBIGDA, The Society for the Scientific Study of Sexuality, the American Association for Sexuality Educators, Counselors, and Therapists, and can attend training institutes and national and international conferences on transgender issues.

Therapy

Transgendered people seek therapists for a variety of reasons. First, they have the same needs for therapy as the general population. Secondly, there are unique stresses related to being transgendered. The financial, marital, and social disruption and the loss and discrimination that accompany gender-role transition place additional pressures on the individual, increasing the usefulness of therapy. And finally, there is the issue of the letters that are needed for initiation of hormonal therapy and genital sex reassignment surgery.

Therapy can center on assisting the transgendered individual to cope with his feelings about choosing to or having to remain in their natal gender role, or, if she is exploring transition, assist her to guide herself through the difficult process of changing her gender role.

A prime responsibility of the therapist is to assist the client in developing a realistic life plan to accommodate the many challenges that lie along the transgender journey. Many gender-variant people don't fully understand their options. Therapists can and should assist them to understand that they can make a myriad of choices about the ways they will live their lives.

Therapy should be nondirective; the object is not to convince the client to accept a particular outcome, but to enable the client to make a wise choice after considering all of the available options. Unfortunately, there is a long history of abusive relationships between therapists and their transgendered clients (see Bolin, 1988; Kessler & McKenna, 1978). This frequently takes the form of promising and then withholding the necessary authorization letters for hormones and surgery. This dynamic is perhaps unsurprising, considering the power imbalance inherent in the therapy setting and general societal prejudices about transgendered people, but it unfortunately continues.

The therapist should come to an agreement with the client about the goals of therapy, and, if authorization letters are to be written, should reach a negotiated understanding with the client about just what will need to be done by both therapist and client in order for the therapist to write the letters. It is often helpful to formalize this via a written contract.

Regardless of whether the individual is considering transition, it may be necessary to assist him in identifying and negotiating boundaries for expressing his transgender nature that will respect and maintain his marriage, relationships with his family and communities, and employment.

The transgendered client can benefit from referral to peer support organizations. We strongly recommend this, as support groups can provide the individual with model coping strategies and help to build a network of supportive friends. The caregiver can direct the client to literature and make appropriate referrals to other professionals as indicated by the client's needs. It is of primary importance to include and engage the spouse and other family members in the counseling process.

The time may come when the therapist is asked to write a letter of recommendation to a family doctor, endocrinologist, or plastic surgeon as part of the HBIGDA Standards of Care, for initiation of hormonal therapy or for genital surgery. If, in the judgment of the therapist, the individual has met the guidelines for eligibility and readiness spelled out in the HBIGDA Standards of Care, and if the therapist does not have reality-based concerns about the individual's welfare if he undergoes such treatment, it is appropriate to write the letter of recommendation.

Wellness-Based Medical Treatment Models

New models of transgender medical treatment are developing which have as an underlying basis the presumptions that transgendered and transsexual people are mentally healthy individuals, and that their gender variance is integral to the healthy people they are. These models provide the same medical treatments as did the earlier pathology-based medical treatment model, but benefit from improved caregiver-client interactions and a lack of the limiting beliefs of the earlier model. Moreover, they are providing new and nonpathologizing language to gender-variant people (Cromwell, Green, & Denny, 2001) and helping to develop a literature that does not unfairly characterize or blame transgendered people for deficiencies in the treatment process.[18] The new models have caused a profound difference in the professional literature, which now squarely addresses the patient-caregiver dynamics of the treatment process.

These new models take a number of forms. One example is the walk-in clinic. Since 1993, San Francisco's transgender residents have known that on any Tuesday, they can attend the Tom Waddell Clinic to address acute or chronic mental or physical health problems. They can get prescriptions for hormones and have their blood levels monitored, receive treatment of HIV and STIs, or attend a peer-support group (Sondegaard, 1994; see also www.dph.sf.ca.us/chn/HlthCtrs/transgender.htm).

Another model treatment program, the Gender Identity Project at the Gay and Lesbian Community Service Center of New York, is peer-based. The Project offers one-on-one peer counseling and professionally and peer-facilitated groups for women and men of transsexual experience and parents, family and friends of transgendered people, focused on "[assisting] individuals to overcome the shame and guilt associated with gender-based oppression so that each of them can build a life which will promote growth, development, and freedom" (Blumenstein, Warren, & Walker, 1998, p. 429). GIP participants have access to the Center's other activities and services, including HIV/AIDS services and groups focused on bereavement and grief, "coming out," and recovery. A liaison with the Community Health Project, which has offices in the Center, resulted in the Transgender Health and Education Clinic, which opened in 1995, providing medical care.

The past decades have seen the reinvention of gender identity clinics in North America.[19] Following the collapse of the gender clinics in the late 1970s, the Program in Human Sexuality eventually took on the administrative responsibility of the University of Minnesota's gender program. PHS, which offers a full range of services to transgendered and transsexual people,[20] took an early lead in exploring nonsurgical options and HIV in the transgender population and has been active in HBIGDA and publishing research papers and books on transgender issues.

Since 1993, the University of Michigan Health System Comprehensive Gender Services Program has provided a full range of services to transgendered people and their families. This academic, multidisciplinary program, which includes medical and mental health care, a variety of surgeries, including genital sex reassignment, and allied health services including speech/language therapy and dentistry, focuses on issues of wellness and whole-person health care. The transgendered client/patient is centrally involved as a participant in the decision-making process at all stages of the health care experience (Cole, 1997, 1998). This includes identifying and developing realistic life goals, reviewing self-progress, and being fully educated to his own unique health needs. CGSP interacts with campus student health and with the program offerings of the office of Gay, Lesbian, Bisexual, and Transgender Affairs. Transgender community affiliates and organizations comprise the extended services of CGSP; this includes bookstores, welcoming restaurants and entertainment, specialty clothing boutiques, and legal services. The University houses the National Transgender Library & Archive, a large collection which was donated by Gender Education & Advocacy, Inc., a nonprofit with which all three authors are affiliated.

These and other programs provide services in settings which allay many of the fears of their transgendered clients and continue to develop new models of transgender health care which respectfully include the active participation of transgendered people and their families.

Transgender Politics

Before about 1995, transgender organizations were primarily educational in nature. This is hardly surprising, considering that it was almost impossible to find information about crossdressing and transsexualism, and the scant information that could be found tended to sensationalize gender variance or emphasize its negative aspects. This has changed dramatically over the past decade. The formation of an active and vital community, and especially the development of the Internet has resulted in an explosion of information which has focused activism, reached spouses, families, and transgender youth, and enabled transgendered people in rural areas to find support. Now there are transgender political organizations working on local, state and national levels to advocate for the civil rights and social safety of all transgendered people.[21] In many metropolitan areas, public health advocates have taken on transgender access to health care as both a social and political cause. Working in tandem with gay, lesbian, bisexual, and intersex activists, social progress has been significant. In 1995, only one state (Minnesota) and four cities (Minneapolis; Seattle; Santa Cruz, CA; and San Francisco) had limited antidiscrimination protection for transgendered and transsexual people. Today, nearly one-third of all Americans are protected by their cities, counties, or states against hate crimes or discrimination, or both (Currah, et al., 2000; for an up-to-date listing, see http://www.nctequality.org/aprilnews06.asp). Many colleges now have courses and even programs in gender studies, and new scholars abound. Hundreds of texts have appeared, and gender-variant characters make frequent appearances in books and on the silver and television screens. Movies about transgendered characters have won awards at film festivals like Cannes and Sundance, and even at the Golden Globe and Oscar ceremonies.

In spite of this new visibility, the battle for the legal rights of gender-variant people is hardly over. Opposition—primarily from the radical religious right and conservative activists—is ongoing, highly coordinated, and often venomous. Battles are being conducted daily in every level of the courts, in city halls and in state and federal legislatures, where the civil rights of both gender-variant and gay and lesbian individuals are highly contested: Don't Ask, Don't Tell; the right to marriage and domestic partnership; adoption; and antidiscrimination and hate crimes bills and ordinances are at issue in jurisdictions across the country. Can a person change her sex? Should a person be able to have a legally sanctioned relationship with another person of the same sex, even if one of the parties has changed her appearance to that of the opposite sex? Should transgendered people be able to be parents, retain parental rights after a divorce, or adopt children? Should a transsexual person be eligible to serve in the military? Should a military veteran who is also transsexual or otherwise transgendered be eligible for medical treatments through the Veteran's Administration? What happens to transgendered people if they enter the prison system: are they housed according to the shape of their genitals or according to their gender presentation? All of these questions and more are at issue in the early twenty-first century. But when we understand that transgendered and transsexual people, through their gender variance, are simply experiencing a different relationship to their bodies and genders than nontransgendered people do, it becomes easier to see that they deserve the same rights and accommodations as any other person receives, and they can go on about their lives as do other human beings, with self-esteem, dignity and respect.

NOTES

The authors are founding directors of Gender Education & Advocacy, Inc. (see note 21).

1. It should be noted that some transsexuals dislike and disidentify with the term *transgender.* This is because, having permanently transitioned gender roles, they consider that they have little in common with those who cross gender lines only partially or temporarily (Lev, 2004, p. 6).

2. Virginia Prince used the term *transgenderist* to describe those who, like herself, lived permanently in the non-natal role without having or wanting genital sex reassignment surgery (Ekins & King, 2005).

3. Many in the transgender community perceive Bailey's book as an insult. Certainly, Bailey makes broad negative claims without substantiating them. He was investigated by his university (Northwestern) after several of his "research" subjects lodged complaints against him, claiming they were unaware that he was using them as subjects (Wilson, 2004).

4. The first reported "modern" sex reassignment surgery was Abraham (1931); see Cowell, 1954; Dillon, 1946; Hoyer, 1933; and Meyerowitz, 2002, for other examples.

5. Perhaps the single most important characteristic of transsexuals, as noted by the medical personnel to whom they turned for treatment, was discomfort—often acute—experienced at being forced to live in bodies that did not correspond to their gender identities. Today's transsexuals feel the same anguish, but, thanks to the Internet and the wide availability of printed material, have more opportunities to share their feelings with others and develop effective coping strategies than was true in the second half of the twentieth century.

6. Indeed, complete reassignment of sex, with plastic surgery to transform the genitals, was the only treatment—aside from remaining in the natal gender—that either medical professionals or the transsexuals of the day seem to have even considered. Only one person—Virginia Prince (1997)—argued for an intermediate path (living in the non-natal gender role without genital surgery). It was nearly twenty years before others echoed Prince's call (Boswell, 1991; Feinberg, 1992). For a short autobiography, see Prince (1997).

7. One transsexual woman has reported being required to engage in homosexual behavior:

"'I'm not homosexual. Nor do I want to be. I want to be a woman.'

"He banged his fist on the table. 'We're not here to negotiate! You've heard our terms. Take them or leave them.'"

—"Margaux," in Denny, 1992, p. 15

8. Some post-transition transsexuals choose to construct their new lives in such a way that nobody "knows" they are living in the non-natal gender role; see Duncan Tucker's film *TransAmerica* for an example of this).

9. One (Meyer) was the clinic's director, the other (Reter) a secretary.

10. Ekins and King (2005) place Prince's concept of transgenderism, or nonsurgical crossliving, as early as 1968.

11. After this chapter was submitted, HBIGDA changed its name to the World Professional Association for Transgender Health.

12. Most social science research is generated in corporate or university environments. Most private practitioners lack the funding, personnel, and equipment necessary to design, conduct, evaluate, and publish research. The scarcity of university-affiliated gender identity programs in North America has resulted in a decrease in research and publication on transgender and transsexual issues.

13. Homosexuality was removed as a mental disorder from 1973's *DSM-II* as the result of considerable discussion and politicking; see Bayer, 1980. The diagnostic category Ego-Dystonic Homosexuality remained in the *DSM* until 1980.

14. See Lev, 2004, chapter 5, for an excellent discussion of issues of diagnosis.

15. See Cole et al., 2000, for a discussion of health risks facing transgendered people.

16. In a misguided effort to hasten masculinization or feminization, some transgendered people take dangerously high dosages of hormones. This can result in severe medical complications or even death. The first author has anecdotally known of several cases in which the medically monitored initiation of estrogen therapy in natal males was immediately followed by gall bladder disease necessitating surgery. Bolin (1988) reported the death of one individual who was self-administering high dosages of estrogen (chapter 9).

17. Often conveniently forgetting or ignoring the myriad other ways in which we modify our bodies or have them modified.

18.   See Gorton, Buth, & Spade, 2005; Israel & Tarver, 1998; & Lev, 2004 for excellent examples of this emerging literature.

19.   Gender clinics survive in many places in the world. Progressive university-affiliated clinics in Netherlands have generated dozens and perhaps hundreds of research studies and developed a treatment model for adolescent transsexuals (Gooren & Delemarre-van Wall, 1996). There are clinics in most other European countries and in many other nations throughout the world.

20.   The exception is genital sex reassignment surgery, which is not provided on-site, but through referrals, when appropriate.

21.   Cf. www.gender.org (Gender Education & Advocacy); *www.ifge.org* (The International Foundation for Gender Education); and *www.nctequality.org* (National Center for Transgender Equality).

REFERENCES

Abraham, F. (1931). Genitalumwandlungen an zwei männlichen Transvestiten [Genital transformation in two male transvestites]. *Zeitschrift für Sexualwissenschaft und Sexualpolitik, 18,* 223–226.

Ackroyd, P. (1979). *Dressing up. Transvestism and drag: The history of an obsession.* New York: Simon & Schuster.

Allison, R. A. (1999, Summer). Autogynephilia: Reply to Dr. Anne Lawrence. *Transgender Tapestry, 1*(87), 50–52.

Allison, R. A. (2001, Winter). Passing: Points of view. *Transgender Tapestry, 1*(96), 49–50.

American Psychiatric Association. (1980). *Diagnostic and statistical manual of mental disorders* (3rd. ed.). Washington, D.C.: American Psychiatric Association.

American Psychiatric Association. (1987). Diagnostic and statistical manual of mental disorders (3rd. ed., revised). Washington, D.C.: American Psychiatric Association.

American Psychiatric Association. (1994). *Diagnostic and statistical manual of mental disorders* (4th. ed.) Washington, D.C.: American Psychiatric Association.

Americans with Disabilities Act. (1990). http://www.usdoj.gov/crt/ada/adahom1.htm.

Americans with Disabilities Act. (1969). Press release: Statement on the establishment of a clinic for transsexuals at the Johns Hopkins Medical Institutions [Appendix to chapter 17]. In R. Green & J. Money (Eds.), *Transsexualism and sex reassignment,* 267–269. Baltimore: Johns Hopkins University Press.

Bailey, J. M. (2002). *The man who would be queen: The science and psychology of gender-bending and transsexualism.* Washington, D.C.: Joseph Henry Press.

Balen, A. H., Schachter, M. E., Montgomery, D., Reid, R. W., & Jacobs, H. S. (1993). Polycystic ovaries are a common finding in untreated female-to-male transsexuals. *Clinical Endocrinology, 38*(3), 325–329.

Basson, R., & Prior, J. C. (1998). Hormonal therapy of gender dysphoria: The male-to-female transsexual. In D. Denny (Ed.), *Current concepts in transgender identity,* pp. 277–296. New York: Garland Publishing.

Beatty, C. (1993). *Misery loves company.* San Francisco, CA: Glamazon Press.

Beller, Thomas. (2001). Gotta knit. Retrieved February 23, 2006. from http://www. mrbellersneighborhood.com/story.php?storyid=292.

Benjamin, H. (1966). *The transsexual phenomenon: A scientific report on transsexualism and sex conversion in the human male and female.* New York: Julian Press.

Bennett-Haigney, L. (1995). Faulkner makes history at the citadel. Retrieved on February, 23, 2006, from http://www.now.org/nnt/08–95/citadel.html.

Blanchard, R., & Sheridan, P. M. (1990). Gender reorientation and psychosocial adjustment. In R. Blanchard & B. W. Steiner (Eds.), *Clinical management of gender identity disorders in children and adults,* 159–189. Washington, D.C.: American Psychiatric Press.

Blumenstein, R., Warren, B. E., & Walker, L. (1998). Appendix: The empowerment of a community. In D. Denny (Ed.), *Current concepts in transgender identity,* pp. 427–430. New York: Garland Publishing.

Bockting, W., & Avery, E. (2005). *Transgender health and HIV prevention: Needs assessment studies from transgender communities across the United States.* Binghamton, NY: Haworth Press.

Bolin, A. (1988). *In search of Eve: Transsexual rites of passage.* South Hadley, MA: Bergin & Garvey Publishers, Inc.

Bolin, A. E. (1994). Transcending and transgendering: Male-to-female transsexuals, dichotomy, and diversity. In G. Herdt (Ed.), *Third sex, third gender: Essays from anthropology and social history,* pp. 447–485. New York: Zone Publishing.

Bornstein, K. (1994). *Gender outlaw: On men, women, and the rest of us.* New York: Routledge.

Boswell, H. (1991). The transgender alternative. *Chrysalis Quarterly, 1*(2), 29–31. Reprinted in *Transgender Tapestry, 1*(98), Summer, 2002, 15–17).

Boswell, H. (1997). The transgender paradigm shift toward free expression. In B. Bullough, V. Bullough, & J. Elias (Eds.), *Gender blending,* pp 53–57. Amherst, NY: Prometheus Press.

Boyd, H. (2003). *My husband Betty: Everything you always wanted to know about crossdressing but were afraid to ask.* New York: Thunder's Mouth Press.

Brown, G. R. (1988). Transsexuals in the military: Flight into hypermasculinity. *Archives of Sexual Behavior, 17*(6), 527–537.

Brown, M., & Rounsley, C. (1996). *True selves: Understanding transsexualism for family, friends, coworkers, and helping professionals.* San Francisco: Jossey-Bass Publishers.

Bullough, V. (1991). Introduction. In M. Hirschfeld (Michael A. Lombardi-Nash, translator), *Transvestites: The erotic drive to cross dress,* pp. 11–14. Buffalo, NY: Prometheus Books.

Bullough, V. L., & Bullough, B. (1993). *Cross-dressing, sex, and gender.* Philadelphia: University of Pennsylvania Press.

Burana, L., Roxxie, & Due, L. (Eds.). (1994). *Dagger: On butch women.* New York: Cleis Press.

Burke, P. (1997). Gender shock. New York: Anchor.

Clemmensen, L. H. (1990). The "real-life test" for surgical candidates. In R. Blanchard & B. W. Steiner (Eds.), *Clinical management of gender identity disorders in children and adults,* 119–135. Washington, D.C.: American Psychiatric Press.

Clendinen, D., & Nagourney, A. (1999). *Out for good: The struggle to build a gay rights movement in America.* New York: Simon & Schuster.

Cole, S. S. (1997). *The Michigan model: University of Michigan Medical Center Comprehensive Gender Services Program.* Paper presented at the XV Harry Benjamin International Gender Dysphoria Association Symposium: The State of Our Art and the State of Our Science, Vancouver, British Columbia, Canada, September 10–13, 1997.

Cole, S. S. (1998). The female experience of the femme: A transgender challenge. In D. Denny (Ed.), *Current concepts in transgender identity,* pp. 373–390. New York: Garland Publishing.

Cole, S. S., Denny, D., Eyler, A. E., & Samons, S. (2000). Diversity in gender identity: Issues of transgender. In L. Szuchman & F. Muscarella (Eds.), *The psychological science of sexuality,* pp. 149–195. New York: John Wiley & Sons, Inc.

Cowell, R. (1954). Roberta Cowell's story. London: William Heinemann, Ltd. Reprinted (1955), New York: Lion Library.

Cromwell, J. (1999). *Transmen & FTMs: Identities, bodies, genders, and sexualities.* Urbana: University of Illinois Press.

Cromwell, J., Green, J., & Denny, D. (2001). *The language of gender variance.* Paper presented at the XXIV Harry Benjamin International Symposium on Gender Dysphoria, Galveston, TX, October 31–3 November 3, 2001.

Currah, P., Minter, S., & Green, J. (2000). *Transgender equality: A handbook for activists and policymakers.* Washington, DC: National Gay and Lesbian Task Force.

Curtis, C. (2005, February 4). Woman gets 5 years for silicone death. *PlanetOut.* Retrieved September 9, 2006, from http://www.gay.com/news/article.html?2005/02/04/2

Dahir, M. (2006, March 17). No one likes a nelly homo: Why are gay men so obsessed with butch and machismo? *Washington Blade.* Retrieved May 17, 2006, http://www.washblade.com/2006/3–17/view/editorial/nellyhomo.cfm.Davidson, P. W. (1966). Transsexualism in Klinefelter's syndrome. *Psychosomatics, 7*(2), 94–98.

De Eraso, C. (S. & G. Stepto, Trans.). (1996). *Lieutenant nun: Memoir of a Basque transvestite in the New World.* Boston: Beacon Press.

Dekker, R. J., & van de Pol, L. C. (1989). *The tradition of female transvestism in early modern Europe.* New York: St. Martin's Press.

Denny, D. (1992). The politics of diagnosis and a diagnosis of politics: The university-affiliated gender clinics, and how they failed to meet the needs of transsexual people. *Chrysalis Quarterly, 1*(3), 9–20. Reprinted in *Transgender Tapestry, 1*(98), 17–27.

Denny, D. (1994, Fall). Behavioral treatment in gender dysphoria: A review of the literature and a call for reform. *TV-TS Tapestry, 1* (69), 54–56.

Denny, D. (1995, Spring). Writing ourselves. *TransSisters: The Journal of Transsexual Feminism,* 38–39.

Denny, D. (1998). Black telephones, white refrigerators: Rethinking Christine Jorgensen. In D. Denny (Ed.), *Current concepts in transgender identity,* pp. 35–44. New York: Garland Publishing.

Denny, D. (2004). *A critique of the medical and psychological literature of transsexualism.* Presented as part of the Trans-Progressing Symposium, Fantasia Fair, Provincetown, MA, October, 2004.

Denny, D. (2006). Down and coming out at the Ross Fireproof Hotel: An essay on class in the transgender community. In G. Teague (Ed.), *The new goddess: Transgender women in the twenty-first century,* pp. 106–111.

Denny, D., & Green, J. (1996). Gender identity and bisexuality. In Firestein, B. (Ed.), *Bisexuality: The psychology and politics of an invisible minority,* pp. 84–102. New York: Sage.

Devor, H. (1989). *Gender blending: Confronting the limits of duality.* Bloomington: Indiana University Press.

Devor, H. (1996). Female gender dysphoria in context: Social problem or personal problem? In R. C. Rosen, C. M. Davis, & H. J. Ruppel (Eds.), *Annual review of sex research, 7,* pp. 44–89. Mason City, IA: Society for the Scientific Study of Sexuality.

Devor, H. (1997). *FTM: Female-to-male transsexuals in society.* Bloomington: Indiana University Press.

Dillon, M. (1946). *Self: A study in ethics and endocrinology.* London: Heinemann.

Docter, R. F. (1988). *Transvestites and transsexuals: Toward a theory of cross-gender behavior.* London: Plenum Press.

Dressed in men's clothes, chorus speeders arrested. (1911, February 26). *Atlanta Constitution*, p. C7.

Dr. Walker arrested because of male garb. (1913, February 2). *Atlanta Constitution*, p. 10B.

Duberman, M. B. (1993). *Stonewall.* New York: Dutton.

Durova, N. (M.F. Zirin, Trans.). (1988). *The cavalry maiden: Journals of a female Russian officer in the Napoleonic Wars.* London: Paladin Grafton Books.

Ekins, R., & King, D. (2005). Introduction to special issue: "Virginia Prince: Pioneer of transgenderism." *International Journal of Transgenderism, 8*(4), 1–4.

Ellis, H. H. (1906). *Studies in the psychology of sex: Erotic symbolism, mechanism of detumescence, the psychic state in pregnancy.* Philadelphia. PA: F. A. Davis Co.

Ellis, H. H., & Symonds, J. A. (1897). *Sexual inversion.* London: Wilson & MacMillan.

Ehrhardt, A. A., Evers, K., & Money, J. (1968). Influence of androgen and some aspects of sexually dimorphic behavior in women with the late-treated adrenogenital syndrome. *Johns Hopkins Medical Journal, 123,* 115–122.

Elifson, K. W., Boles, J., Posey, E., Sweat, M., Darrow, W., & Elsea, W. (1993). Male transvestite prostitutes and HIV risk. *American Journal of Public Health, 83,* 260–262.

Farmer, D. (1994). Propelled to self-mutilation. *Chrysalis Quarterly, 1*(7), 9–10.

Feinberg, L. (1992). Transgender liberation: A movement whose time has come. New York: World View Forum.

Feinberg, L. (1993). *Stone butch blues.* New York: Firebrand Books.

Feinberg, L. (1996). *Transgender warriors: Making a history from Joan of Arc to Ru Paul.* Boston: Beacon Press.

Fisk, N. (1974). Gender dysphoria syndrome: The conceptualization that liberalizes indications for total gender reorientation and implies a broadly based multi-dimensional treatment regimen. *Western Medical Journal, 120,* 386–391.

Fleming, M., Steinman, C., & Bocknek, G. (1980). Methodological problems in assessing sex-reassignment: A reply to Meyer and Reter. *Archives of Sexual Behavior, 9*(5), 451–456.

Gooren, L., & Delemarre-van Wall, H. (1996). The feasibility of endocrine interventions to juvenile transsexuals. *Journal of Psychology and Human Sexuality, 8* (4), 69–74.

Gorton R., Buth J., & Spade D. (2005). *Medical therapy and health maintenance for transgender men: A guide for health care providers.* San Francisco, CA: Lyon-Martin Women's Health Services. Green, J. (1995). Getting real about female-to-male surgery. *Chrysalis: The Journal of Transgressive Gender Identities, 2*(2), 27–33.

Green, J. (2004). Becoming a visible man. Nashville: Vanderbilt University Press.

Green, J., & Brinkin, L. (1994). Investigation into discrimination against transgendered people. Human Rights Commission, City and County of San Francisco, 25 Van Ness Avenue, Ste. 800, San Francisco, CA 94102–6033.

Green, R. (1960). Attitudes toward transsexualism and sex-reassignment procedures. In R. Green & J. Money (Eds.), *Transsexualism and sex reassignment,* pp. 235–242. Baltimore, MD: The Johns Hopkins University Press.

Green, R. (1969). Conclusion. In R. Green & John Money (Eds.), *Transsexualism and sex reassignment,* pp. 467–473. Baltimore, MD: The Johns Hopkins University Press.

Green, R., & Money, J. (Eds.). (1969). *Transsexualism and sex reassignment.* Baltimore, MD: The Johns Hopkins University Press.

Hage, J. J. (1992). *From peniplastica totalis to reassignment surgery of the external genitalia in female-to-male transsexuals.* Amsterdam: Vrieji Universiteit Press.

Hall, R. (1928). *The well of loneliness.* New York: Avon.

Hamburger, C., Stürup, G.K., & Dahl-Iversen, E. (1953). Transvestism: Hormonal, psychiatric, and surgical treatment. *Journal of the American Medical Association, 12*(6), 391–396.

Hamburger, C. (1953). The desire for change of sex as shown by personal letters from 465 men and women. *Acta Endocrinologica, 14,* 361–375.

Herdt, G. (Ed.). (1994). *Third sex, third gender: Essays from anthropology and social history.* New York: Zone Books.

Hirschfeld, M. (1910). *Die transvestiten: Eine untersuchung uber den erotischen verkleidungstrieh.* Berlin: Medicinisher Verlag Alfred Pulvermacher & Co.

Hoyer, N. (1933). *Man into woman: An authentic record of a change of sex. The true story of the miraculous transformation of the Danish painter, Einar Wegener (Andreas Sparrer).* New York: E.P. Dutton & Co. Reprinted in 1953 in New York by Popular Library.

Irvine, J. M. (1990). *Disorders of desire: Sex and gender in modern American sexology.* Philadelphia, PA: Temple University Press.

Israel, G., & Tarver, D. (1998). *Transgender care: Recommended guidelines, practical information, and personal accounts.* Philadelphia, PA: Temple University Press.

Jackson, P. A., & Sullivan, G. (Eds.). (1999). *Lady boys, tom boys, rent boys: Male and female homosexualities in contemporary Thailand.* Binghamton, NY: Harrington Park Press.

Jacobs, S-E., Thomas, W., & Lang, S. (Eds.). (1997). *Two-Spirit people: Native American gender identity, sexuality, and spirituality.* Chicago: University of Illinois Press.

Jorgensen, C. (1967). *Christine Jorgensen: A personal autobiography.* New York: Paul S. Ericksson, Inc. Reprinted in 1968 by Bantam Books; in 2000 by Cleis Press.

Kailey, M. (2005). *Just add hormones: An insider's guide to the transsexual experience.* Boston: Beacon Press.

Kates, G. (1995). *Monsieur D'Eon is a woman: A tale of political intrigue and sexual masquerade.* New York: Basic Books.

Kessler, S. (1998). *Lessons from the intersexed.* Brunswick, NJ: Rutgers University Press.

Kessler, S. J., & McKenna, W. (1978). *Gender: An ethnomethodological approach.* New York: John Wiley & Sons. Reprinted in 1985 by The University of Chicago Press.

Krafft-Ebing, R. von. (1894). *Psychopathia sexualis* (C.G. Chaddock, Translator). Philadelphia: F.A. Davis. Reprinted in 1931 in Brooklyn by Physicians & Surgeons Book Co.

Lawrence, A. (1998, Winter). "Men trapped in men's bodies": An introduction to the concept of autogynephilia. *Transgender Tapestry, 1*(85), 65–68.

Lee, Ang (Director). *Brokeback mountain* [Motion Picture]. (2005). United States: Focus Features.

Lev, A. I. (2004). *Transgender emergence: Therapeutic guidelines for working with gender-variant people and their families.* Binghamton, NY: Haworth Clinical Practice Press.

Lothstein, L. M. (1982). Sex reassignment surgery: Historical, bioethical, and theoretical issues. *American Journal of Psychiatry, 139*(4), 417–426.

McHugh, P. R. (1992). Psychiatric misadventures. *American Scholar, 61* (4), 497–510.

Meerloo, J.A.M. (1967). Letter to the editor: Change of sex and collaboration with the psychosis. *American Journal of Psychiatry, 124*(2), 263–264.

Meyer, J. K., & Reter, D. (1979). Sex reassignment: Follow-up. *Archives of General Psychiatry, 36*(9), 1010–1015.

Meyer, W., Cohen-Kettenis, P., Coleman, E., DiCeglie, D., Devor, H., Gooren, L., Hage, J.J., Kirk, S., Kuiper, B., Laub, D., Lawrence, A., Menard, Y, Patton, J., Schaefer, L., Webb, A., & Wheeler, C. (2001). Harry Benjamin International Gender Dysphoria

Association's The Standards of Care for Gender Identity Disorders, Sixth Version. Dusseldorf: Symposon Publishing. See also http://www.hbigda.org/soc.htm.

Meyerowitz, J. (2002). *How sex changed: A history of transsexuality in the United States.* Cambridge, MA: Harvard University Press.

Money, J. (1968). *Sex errors of the body: Dilemmas, education, and counseling.* Baltimore: The Johns Hopkins University Press. (Reprinted in 1994 by Paul H. Brookes Publishing Co.).

Money, J., & Primrose, C. (1968). Sexual dimorphism and dissociation in the psychology of male transsexuals. *Journal of Nervous and Mental Disease, 147*(5), 472–486.

Morgan, P., as told to Hoffman, P. (1973). *The man-maid doll.* Secaucus, NJ: Lyle Stuart, Inc.

Munt, S. R. (1998). *Butch/femme: Inside lesbian gender.* London: Cassell.

Nataf, Z. I. (1996). *Lesbians talk transgender.* London: Scarlet Press (Available in the United States from Inco, Inc., Chicago).

National Gay and Lesbian Task Force. Crimes against transgender individuals. Press release. National Gay and Lesbian Task Force, Washington, D.C. Retrieved on February 28, 2006, from http://www.thetaskforce.org/downloads/hatecrimevictims.pdf.

Nestle, J. (1992). *The persistence of desire: A femme/butch reader.* Boston, MA: Alyson Publications, Inc.

Nestle, J., Wilchins, R., & Howell, C. (2002). *Genderqueer: Voices from beyond the sexual binary.* Boston: Alyson Press.

Norbury, R., & Richardson, B. (1994). *Guy to goddess: An intimate look at drag queens.* Berkeley, CA: Ten Speed Press.

Novic, R. J. (2005). Alice in Genderland. iUniverse.com.

Ogas, O. (1994, March 9). Spare parts: New information reignites a controversy surrounding the Hopkins gender identity clinic. *City Paper* (Baltimore), 18(10), cover, 10–15.

Oppenheim, G. (1979). Meyer's survey draws fire from leading authorities. *Transition,* 11.

Ostow, M. (1953). Transvestism. Letter to the editor. *Journal of the American Medical Association, 152*(16), 1553.

Prince, C. V. (1973). Sex vs. gender. In D. Laub and P. Gandy (Eds.), *Proceedings of the Second International Symposium on Gender Dysphoria Syndrome,* pp. 20–24. Palo Alto, CA: Stanford University Medical Center.

Prince, C. V. (1997). Seventy years in the trenches of the gender wars. In B. Bullough, V. Bullough, & J. Elias (Eds.), *Gender blending,* pp. 469–477. Amherst, NY: Prometheus Press.

Prince, V. (1978). The "transcendents" or "trans" people. *Transvestia, 16*(96), 81–92. Reprinted in 2005 in *International Journal of Transgenderism, 8*(4), 39–46.

Prior, J. C., & Elliott, S. (1998). Hormonal therapy of gender dysphoria: The female-to-male patient. In D. Denny (Ed.), *Current concepts in transgender identity,* pp. 297–313. New York: Garland.

Raymond, J. G. (1980). Paper prepared for the National Center for Health Care Technology on the social and ethical aspects of transsexual surgery. Rockville, MD: National Center for Health Care Technology.

Richards, R., & Ames, J. (1983). *Second serve: The Renée Richards story.* New York: Stein & Day.

Rodriguez-Madera, S., & Toro Alfonso, J. (2005). Gender as an Obstacle in HIV/AIDS Prevention: Considerations for the development of HIV/AIDS prevention efforts for male-to-female transgenders. *International Journal of Transgenderism, 8*(2–3), 113–122.

Roscoe, W. (Ed.). (1988). *Living the spirit: A gay American Indian anthology.* New York: St. Martin's Press.

Roscoe, W. (1990). *The Zuni man-woman.* University of New Mexico Press.

Roscoe, W. (1998). *Changing ones: Third and fourth genders in Native North America.* New York: St. Martin's Press.

Rosenfeld, C., & Emerson, S. (1998). A process model of supportive therapy for families of transgender individuals. In D. Denny (Ed.), *Current concepts in transgender identity,* pp. 391–400. New York: Garland Publishing.

Rothblatt, M. (1994). *The apartheid of sex: A manifesto on the freedom of gender.* New York: Crown Publishers.

Rudacille, D. (2005). *The riddle of gender: Science, activism, and transgender rights.* New York: Pantheon Books.

Rudd, P. (1989). *My husband wears my clothes: Crossdressing from the perspective of a wife.* Katy, TX: PM Publishers.

Scholinski, D. (1997). *The last time I wore a dress.* New York: Riverhead Books.

Schrang, E. (1998). Male-to-female feminizing genital surgery. In D. Denny (Ed.), *Current concepts in transgender identity,* pp. 315–333. New York: Garland Publishing.

Silicone use: Illicit, disfiguring, dangerous. (2003, July 2). Medical Advisory. San Francisco, CA: Gender Education & Advocacy, Inc. http://www.gender.org/advisories/silicone.html.

Sondegaard, G. (1994, Winter). Neutral ground: Transgender Tuesday at the Tom Waddell Clinic. *Transsexual News Telegraph, 1*(2), 10–11.

Sperber, J., Landers, S., Lawrence, S. (2005). Access to Health Care for Transgendered Persons: Results of a Needs Assessment in Boston. *International Journal of Transgenderism, 8* (2/3), 75–91.

Stone, A. R. (as Sandy Stone) (1991). The empire strikes back: A posttranssexual manifesto. In J. Epstein & K. Straub (Eds.), *Body guards: The cultural politics of gender ambiguity,* pp. 280–304. New York: Routledge.

Stone, C. B. (1977). Psychiatric screening for transsexual surgery. *Psychosomatics, 18*(1), 25–27.

Stryker, S. (2001). Introduction. In C. Jorgensen, *Christine Jorgensen: A personal autobiography.* San Francisco: Cleis Press.

Tayleur, C. (1994). Transsexuals and addiction: The unacknowledged crisis. *Chrysalis: The Journal of Transgressive Gender Identities, 1*(7), 11–14.

Taylor, T. (1996). *The prehistory of sex: Four million years of human sexual culture.* New York: Bantam Books.

Taylor, V., & Rupp, L. J. (2004). Chicks with dicks, men in dresses: What it means to be a drag queen. In Schacht, S.P., & Underwood, L. (Eds.), *The drag queen anthology: The absolutely fabulous but flawlessly customary world of female impersonators,* pp. 113–133. Binghamton, NY: Haworth Park Press.

Troka, D., Lebesco, K., & Noble, J. (Eds.). (2003). *The drag king anthology.* New York: Harrington Park Press.

Tucker, Duncan (Director). *TransAmerica* [Motion Picture]. (2005). United States: IFC Films.

Ulrichs, K. H. (1994). *The riddle of "man-manly" love: The pioneering work on male homosexuality.* Vols. 1 and 2. (Michael A. Lombardi-Nash, translator). Buffalo, NY: Prometheus Press.

Van, J., Maupin, A., & Stryker, S. (1996). *Gay by the bay: A history of queer culture in the San Francisco Bay area.* San Francisco: Chronicle Books.

Varnell, P. (1996, December). "Woman trapped as man"—or unable to accept being gay? *Pittsburgh's Out,* 18.

Vasey, P. (2000, December). Is Gender Identity of Childhood a mental disorder? Sex Roles. www.findarticles.com/p/articles/mi_m2294/is_2000_Dec/ai_75959827.

Walworth, J. (1998a). *Transsexual workers: An employer's guide.* Los Angeles: The Center for Gender Sanity.

Walworth, J. (1998b). *Working with a transsexual: A guide for coworkers.* Los Angeles: The Center for Gender Sanity.

Whitam, F. (1997). Culturally universal aspects of male homosexual transvestites and transsexuals. In B. Bullough, V. Bullough, & J. Elias (Eds.), *Gender Blending,* pp. 189–203. Amherst, NY: Prometheus Press.

Wiedeman, G. H. (1953). Letter to the editor. *Journal of the American Medical Association,* 152(12), 1167.

Wilchins, R. A., Lombardi, L., Priesing, D., & Malouf, D. (1997, April 13). GenderPac First National Survey of Transgender Violence. New York: Gender Public Advocacy Coalition.

Williams, M. (1999, September 29). Transsexuals tell of botched surgeries from former doctor. Associated Press.

Williams, W. L. (1986). *The spirit and the flesh: Sexual diversity in American Indian culture.* Boston: Beacon Press.

Wilson, B. (2004, 1 December). Northwestern U. concludes investigation of sex researcher, but keeps results secret. The Chronicle of Higher Education.

Wilson, K. (1998, June). The disparate classification of gender and sexual orientation in American psychiatry. 1998 Annual Meeting of the American Psychiatric Association, Workshop IW57, Transgender Issues, Toronto, Ontario Canada, June 1998. Available at http://www.transgender.org/gidr/papers.html.

Wilson, K. (2000). Gender as illness: Issues of psychiatric classification. In E. Paul (Ed.), *Taking sides: Clashing views on controversial issues in sex and gender,* pp. 31–38. Guilford, CT: Dushkin McGraw-Hill. Available at http://www.transgender.org/gidr/papers.html.

Wilson, K., & Hammond, B. (1996, March). *Myth, stereotype, and cross-gender identity in the DSM-IV.* Association of Women in Psychology Feminist Psychology Conference, Portland, OR, March 1996. Available at http://www.transgender.org/gidr/papers.html.

Xavier, J., Sharp, C., & Boenke, M. (2004). *Our trans children* (4th ed.). Washington, DC: Parents and Friends of Lesbians and Gays.

Chapter Nine

PHYSICAL THERAPY AND SEXUAL HEALTH

Talli Yehuda Rosenbaum

Physical therapists are trained to provide treatment to restore function, improve mobility, relieve pain, and prevent or limit permanent physical disabilities of patients suffering from injuries or disease (Bureau of Labor Statistics, U.S. Dept. of Labor, 2004). As community health professionals, physical therapists are involved in health and fitness education and promoting wellness. Sexual health is an integral component to overall wellness, and sexual activity a valued human activity. Physical therapists in various settings have an important role in promoting sexual health and treating dysfunction, through a specialized area called *pelvic floor rehabilitation.*

The pelvic floor muscles are the slinglike muscles that span across our bottom area and circle the pelvis. These muscles support the internal organs and promote bowel and bladder continence. Normal function of the pelvic floor musculature is essential in maintaining appropriate function of the pelvic organs, as well as optimal sexual functioning. This muscle group has a lifting action to aid in support and control, and relaxes and releases for voiding and sexual penetration. When the function of the pelvic floor is disrupted, due to weakness, known as *hypotonus* and/or excessive tightness, known as *hypertonus,* pain and sexual disorder may result. Physical therapy treatment offers a variety of direct and indirect interventions, utilizing manual techniques, exercises and equipment in the treatment of pelvic floor dysfunction, thereby enhancing sexual functioning. Physical therapists in a variety of rehabilitation settings may be involved in improving sexual health, as the pelvic floor is not the only area in the body that affects sexuality.

REHABILITATION AND ORTHOPEDICS

Ideally, engaging in comfortable and enjoyable sexual activity requires the ability to feel, touch, and move. Physical disability, orthopedic injury, neurological impairments or the presence of pain are all conditions that potentially affect sexual function. Physical therapists in a variety of treatment centers, both inpatient and outpatient, encounter patients with these conditions.

Treatment is geared towards the restoration of the ability to function and perform activities of daily living (ADLs) independently and painlessly. Treatment should include assessment of sexual function. Assessment first requires asking the relevant questions. Many health professionals, including doctors and nurses as well as physical therapists, have not been properly trained to address issues of a sexual nature. In some cases, health professionals may harbor their own feelings of embarrassment or hesitation to discuss sexuality and project these feelings on to their patients. Health professionals may also mistakenly assume that sexuality is not a concern due to advanced age, disability, or marital status. Consider the following example:

> Mrs. N was a 71-year-old, married female who underwent a total hip replacement operation due to chronic degenerative hip arthritis. After surgery, she was transferred to the hospital rehabilitation unit where she began twice daily physical therapy treatments. At the bedside after her surgery, a nurse provided her with instruction regarding the specific, postoperative protocol directed by her orthopedic surgeon. This protocol provided distinct instruction regarding what movements were prohibited for several weeks after the surgery. This included raising her hip past 90 degrees of bending, or bringing it too far out to the side or rolling inward. During the course of physical and occupational therapy she was instructed in functional activities including how to get up off the toilet or a chair, how to climb and descend stairs and how to properly bathe and shower. She personally met with the orthopedic surgeon briefly after surgery and had contact with the medical social worker to plan her discharge needs in addition to her regular contact with the nurses and therapy staff.
>
> On the last day of physical therapy before being discharged home, Mrs. N. confided to her physical therapist that there was one concern that remained unaddressed. She did not know whether or not she was permitted to have sexual intercourse. She stated that when she questioned the orthopedist about it, he made some sort of joke without actually answering her question. Mrs. N.'s physical therapist was glad that the subject was brought up by the patient but also realized she and the

rehabilitation staff had been remiss in not providing that information along with the teaching of the functional ADLs. She spent the rest of the session instructing Mrs. N. in positions to comfortably and safely continue sexual relations.

The above example unfortunately describes a medical norm, rather than an exception. A recent survey of orthopedic physicians demonstrated that 80 percent of surgeons reported they rarely or never discuss sexual activity with their patients who have had hip replacement surgery. Of surgeons who stated they did discuss this topic, 96 percent spent five minutes or less on the subject (Dahm, Jacofsky, & Lewallen, 2004).

Physical therapists are frequently involved in community wellness. Promotion of health and fitness takes the form of back pain prevention programs in the workplace, and lectures and fitness assessments in various settings. Pelvic floor awareness programs have recently begun to appear in the programs of hospitals and women's health clinics in the United States and abroad. These programs include teaching knowledge and awareness of bladder and bowel continence, as well as awareness of the existence of the pelvic floor and techniques for maintaining optimal strength and fitness of the pelvis.

FEMALE SEXUAL HEALTH AND THE PELVIC FLOOR

The pelvic floor refers to a group of muscles and connective tissues, including ligaments and fascia, which connects from the pubic bone in the front to the coccyx bone at the back. These muscles attach around the entire perimeter of the pelvis, like a shallow bowl. Muscle contraction results in a lifting action. The function of the pelvic floor is to provide a system of support for the organs of the pelvis and a system of voluntary control of the bowel and bladder. The pelvic floor muscles (PFMs) comprise a striated, skeletal muscle group, that is under voluntary control and is important in maintaining urinary and fecal continence as well as in providing support to the bladder, rectum and, in women, the uterus (see Figure 9.1).

The muscles of the pelvic floor consist of superficial muscles, including the bulbocavernous and ischiocavernous muscles, which are active during sexual activity and act directly on the clitoris, and the deeper muscles known collectively as the "levator ani" (LA) muscles, which consist of the pubococcygeous and iliococcygeus. The levator ani act to lift up the pelvic organs and are active in straining during defecation (Markwell, 2001). The LA muscles

Figure 9.1
Pelvic Floor Muscles

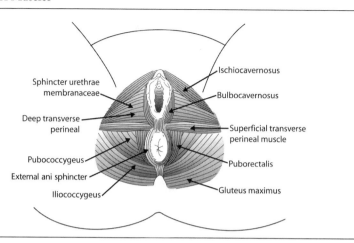

Sphincter urethrae membranaceae

Deep transverse perineal

Pubococcygeus

External ani sphincter

Iliococcygeus

Ischiocavernosus

Bulbocavernosus

Superficial transverse perineal muscle

Puborectalis

Gluteus maximus

Drawing does not represent exact anatomic proportions.

contract during sexual intercourse leading to genital responses that improve sexual function (Shafik, 2000). The puborectalis (PR) muscles act with the external anal and urethral sphincters, to close the urinary and anal openings, to contract the sphincters and prevent urinary or fecal leakage. All these muscles together comprise the PFM, which is under voluntary control and is important in sexual function, in maintaining urinary and fecal continence, allowing ease of bowel emptying, and in providing support to the pelvic organs.

It is apparent from the anatomical and physiological makeup of the pelvic floor, that optimal pelvic floor function is crucial in maintaining a healthy sexual life. Muscles that are overactive and high in tonal activity, for example, may cause narrowing of the vaginal entry, preventing vaginal penetration or rendering it painful. Pelvic floor muscles which are weak or de-conditioned, may provide insufficient activity necessary for vaginal friction or blood flow, and may even inhibit orgasmic potential (Graber & Kline-Graber, 1979).

Physiological demands on the woman's body throughout the female life cycle, particularly on the pelvic floor, may influence sexual function in many areas. Pregnancies and deliveries place a particular strain on the body in general and the pelvic floor specifically. During pregnancy, the abdominal muscles stretch, which increases pressure on the pelvic floor muscles. Returning to strenuous activities such as lifting, straining, heavy exercise and running before the abdominal and pelvic floor muscles have regained their strength, further compromises their integrity. During and after menopause, decreases in estrogen levels also affect the integrity of the pelvic floor, and it is during this period where many women begin to feel the effects of pelvic floor weakness. These effects may include urinary stress incontinence, a condition that is characterized by a loss of urine when there is an increase in intra-abdominal pressure, as in coughing, laughing or sneezing. Other common effects of pelvic floor weakness are prolapse. A prolapse occurs when a downward force on the pelvic organs causes them to slip down from the pelvis toward the vaginal cavity. Prolapse of the bladder, uterus or rectum may occur over time as a combined result of straining due to child-bearing, chronic constipation and/or excessive heavy lifting, combined with progressive weakening of the pelvic floor muscles (Swift, Pound & Dias, 2001).

Lower urinary tract symptoms (LUTS) are characterized by symptoms of urinary frequency (excessive need to urinate), dysuria (pain or difficulty with urination), urinary incontinence, and feelings of urgency. These symptoms have been found to have a close association with weakness of the pelvic floor muscles. Recent studies have indicated that impaired sexual arousal is significantly associated with LUTS and that 40–46 percent of women with LUTS suffer from impairment in their sex lives (Salonia et al., 2004).

Unfortunately, awareness of the existence of the pelvic floor muscles is low, even among the physically fit. Physical education curricula in schools do not generally include pelvic floor muscle education and even today, most fitness studios and gyms do not specifically provide training programs for the pelvic floor muscles as they do the arms, legs, buttocks and abdominals. Pelvic floor muscle contraction is an essential component of core stabilization programs and their inclusion should be determined before undertaking such a program.

Most women are only first made aware of these muscles when they are in advanced pregnancy and are being instructed by childbirth educators to do "Kegels." These are pelvic floor contractions named for Dr. Arnold Kegel an obstetrician who developed a system for strengthening these muscles in the 1950s. In order to help the woman identify how to activate her pelvic floor muscles when doing Kegels, she is asked to notice what muscles she would use to stop the flow of urine. While this may be an effective cue to teach women to identify the pelvic floor muscles, women today are cautioned that they should not use "stop-flow" contractions as an exercise to strengthen their muscles, as this may lead to a urinary tract infection. Kegel's research created the guidelines for focusing on endurance through a sustained 10 second muscle contraction and a full 10 second release. He also created the perineometer, which was a vaginal device connected to a pressure gauge. His research noted improved success for pelvic floor rehabilitation with his monitored system on a regular basis. Noteworthy is his acknowledgement that sexual dysfunction may be a result of pelvic floor muscle imbalance. His research documented improved sexual function, (especially with respect to sexual pain and orgasm problems) following pelvic floor muscle rehabilitation (Kegel, 1952).

Along with the abdominal muscles, the pelvic floor muscles are the muscles most affected by pregnancy and childbirth and therefore, affect most women. Even women who have not given birth have a pelvic floor that can be weakened by repetitive lifting, smoking (due to coughing; see Bump & McClish, 1994), or straining due to chronic constipation; or athletics that include high impact activities, such as running and jumping, for example.

Specifically, sexual function may be affected in women with pelvic floor dysfunction. Women with hypertonus have muscles that are shortened, and they may experience painful intercourse and decreased genital arousal. Women with excessive weakness may also complain of decreased genital arousal and orgasm. Women with LUTS, often report associated decreases in sexual interest and discomfort during sex. Many women fear loss of urine during sexual activity or upon orgasm. Consider the following example:

> Mrs. L is a 45-year-old interior designer and mother of three. She is an energetic and busy woman, who presented to her physician complaining of incontinence when she coughed, laughed, or sneezed. Her physician referred her to physical therapy to strengthen her pelvic floor muscles. The physical therapist evaluated Mrs. L and inquired about her urinary habits, exercise regime, and questioned her about her sexual function. Mrs. L appeared quite relieved and stated that she had in fact been refraining from sexual intercourse with her husband the past few months. She admitted that it was because she had begun to leak urine when she would orgasm. She was questioned as to whether it was possible that what she was describing was female ejaculate; however, she stated it was most definitely urine. After three months of physical therapy she stated that she no longer leaked urine and no longer needed a pad. She was however, most pleased that she had resumed sexual intercourse with her husband and no longer leaked urine.

Pelvic floor muscle training has been demonstrated to improve quality of life and sexual function in women with urinary stress incontinence (Bo, Talseth, & Vinsnes, 2000). Pelvic floor rehabilitation to strengthen weakened pelvic floor muscles is designed to increase awareness of the muscles of the pelvic floor, including learning to differentiate between those muscles that act to lift the internal organs (pubococcygeous, the key muscle of the levator ani) and those that provide sphincter closure (puborectalis and external anal sphincter). This may be accomplished through learning proper breathing, awareness of the location of the muscles and how to contract them and exercises to strengthen them.

Biofeedback (surface EMG) is an additional intervention for pelvic floor rehabilitation. It is an updated version of Kegel's perineometer and will be described in more detail in the treatment section of this chapter. Biofeedback is accomplished by inserting a sensor probe into the vagina. The patient is asked to contract the muscles around the probe and the muscle activity produced is displayed on a computer monitor. The patient can view a line graph that shows resting levels, strength and endurance. Training screens can utilize graphs or other animations, such as concentric rings that close and open with muscle contraction and release. This activity allows the patient to receive feedback regarding the quality of her contraction. By attempting to raise the height of the line graph, she increases her work capacity, thereby strengthening her muscles. She can also learn to recognize how to best release her muscles using the same feedback monitor.

Another physical therapy tool is electrical stimulation of the pelvic floor. This is accomplished by inserting a probe into the vagina and providing an electrical pulse which contracts the pelvic floor muscles. Providing an electrical stimulus directly to the muscles provides awareness to patients who are too weak or lack the ability to isolate these muscles on their own. Once they gain the awareness of the muscles through the electrical stimulation, they can then begin to strengthen them on their own. Providing a low frequency electrical pulse to the puborectalis muscles also helps to decrease symptoms of urinary urgency and frequency, through a reflex, which causes the smooth muscles of the bladder to relax (Murray, 1984; Sand, 1996).

MALE SEXUAL HEALTH AND THE PELVIC FLOOR

Awareness of the pelvic floor and its relationship to healthy sexual function may be even less prevalent in men than in women. The male pelvic structures are well supported by the prostate gland, and therefore LUTS, due to pelvic floor weakness is less common. Men who do experience LUTS generally do so because of aging and/or growth of the prostate, which may obstruct the urethra, where the urine exits. LUTS is also related to decreases in sexual function in aging men (Rosen et al., 2004).

Because the male pelvic floor does not undergo the transitions and stresses that the childbearing female's does, it is less implicated in sexual dysfunction. However, the pelvic floor has an important role in male sexual function and the pelvic floor muscles are active in normal erectile and ejaculatory function. Pelvic floor dysfunction has been implicated in male erectile dysfunction (Dorey, 2004) and early ejaculation (Piediferro, Colpi, Castiglioni, & Scroppo, 2004) and the efficacy of physical therapy to strengthen the pelvic floor muscles to improve these conditions has been studied (Dorey et al., 2004). One study demonstrated that a pelvic floor muscle rehabilitation program may be a noninvasive alternative for the treatment of patients with erectile dysfunction caused by obstructed blood flow from the veins, known as *venous occlusion* (Van Kampen et al., 2003).

Men can also develop painful pelvic floor muscle conditions, which may be related to hypertonus. Situations creating pelvic pain, such as trauma, prostatitis, or surgery may leave men with difficulties to diagnose conditions related to the muscle dysfunctions. This may impact their sexual function. The same physical therapy pelvic floor rehabilitation techniques that are used for women may also be applied to men. When using biofeedback or electrical stimulation, the probe is inserted into the patient's anus, or surface electrodes placed directly on the skin around the anus may be used.

THE ROLE OF PHYSICAL THERAPY IN FEMALE SEXUAL DYSFUNCTION

More often than not, sexual dysfunction results from a combination of anatomic, physiologic and psychosocial components. In the past, women experiencing difficulties with sex would consult a physician, who upon finding no physical evidence of disease or injury would treat the problem as psychological. Today, there is a greater understanding that optimal sexual function results from the balance of physical and psychological health, with emotional and relational satisfaction. One important but often overlooked element is that of musculoskeletal function. The condition of the bones and muscles of our body greatly affects how we function sexually. Pelvic floor muscle dysfunction has been associated with decreased libido, arousal, and vaginal lubrication (Berman et al., 1999). Low libido, vaginal dryness, painful intercourse, and decreased sexual satisfaction are reported in women with urinary incontinence (Handa, Harvey, Cundiff, Siddique, & Kjerulff, 2004). It has been proposed (Wurn, 2004) that difficulty in reaching orgasm in women with dyspareunia (painful intercourse) was related to decreases in visceral, bony and soft tissue mobility and demonstrated that manual treatment improved orgasmic ability. The most common dysfunction related to the musculoskeletal system is dyspareunia.

Sexual Pain Disorders

Traditionally, sexual pain disorders are classified as *dyspareunia* and *vaginismus* (see volume 2, chapter 12). *Dyspareunia* means "painful intercourse." It may describe a situation where there is pain with initial penetration, during thrusting, or after coitus is completed. It may manifest as pain at the entry to the vagina, known as superficial dyspareunia, or the pain may be deeper in to the pelvis, a condition known as deep dyspareunia. Dyspareunia has long baffled both the medical and psychological communities in terms of its origins and causes. Another confusing issue is the nomenclature and the tendency to overlap this condition with chronic pelvic pain, vulvar pain, and vulvar vestibulitis syndrome (Pukall, Payne, Kao, Khalifé, & Binik, 2005). While vaginismus and dyspareunia frequently coexist, the current classification of sexual pain disorders recognizes them as two separate entities. Vulvar pain and vulvar vestibulitis are categorized under the heading *dyspareunia*.

Vaginismus has been traditionally described as a condition of vaginal muscle spasm preventing sexual intercourse. While the physiological phenomenon of vaginal muscle spasm in response to attempted penetration has never been well documented (Reissing, Binik, Khalifé, Cohen, & Amsel, 2004), vaginismus is traditionally described as a contraction of the outer third of the vaginal muscles in response to penetration (American Psychiatric Association, 2000) and has been purported to result from a variety of possible psychological and emotional causes (i.e., sexual inhibitions due to repression, religion, or resentment toward men) (LoPiccolo, 1984; Masters & Johnson, 1970). A recently proposed definition of *vaginismus* is "the persistent or recurrent difficulties of the woman to allow vaginal entry of a penis, a finger, and or any object despite the woman's expressed desire to do so. There is often phobic avoidance, involuntary pelvic floor muscle contraction, and anticipation/fear/experience of pain. Structural abnormalities must be ruled out/addressed" (Basson et al., 2004).

This recent definition of vaginismus describes a phenomenon of penetration avoidance, which often correlates with fear of pain due to the actual physical perception of pain. It has not been empirically evidenced that patients with vaginismus present with pelvic floor "spasm," but muscle hypertonus has been documented (Reissing et al., 2004). It has also been suggested that vaginal muscle contraction at the time of attempted penetration represents an overall sympathetic response triggered by anxiety (Van der Velde & Everaerd, 2001). Whatever the mechanism, when the muscles of the vagina are tight, the ability to allow comfortable penetration is affected. Vaginal friction is increased, which narrows the vaginal opening, or *interoitus,* and perpetuates dyspareunia (Abramov, Wolman, & David, 1994). This is a frequent cause of unconsummated union and is discussed in a separate section of this chapter.

Recently it has been suggested that sexual pain disorders should be viewed primarily as pain disorders that affect sex, rather than disorders which are intrinsically sexual in nature (Binik, Meana, Berkley, & Khalifé, 1999). In a clinical setting, it is quite difficult to differentially diagnose sexual pain disorders. Patients with vaginismus are not only unable to have sex, but most often are unable to allow penetration of a tampon, or allow a gynecological exam to occur. Not only are their sex lives affected but also their ability to have standard medical exams which may affect their overall health. Therefore, it is often difficult to ascertain if underneath all that anxious behavior lies a painful disorder. For this reason, vaginismus often overlaps with dyspareunia, and the value of attempting to separate these entities has been questioned (De Kruiff, Ter Kuile, Weijenborg, & Van Lankveld, 2000).

The most common cause of dyspareunia affecting approximately 15 percent of pre-menopausal women is *vestibulodynia,* more commonly referred to as vulvar vestibulitis syndrome (VVS), a condition identified and named in the mid-1980s by the International Society for the Study of Vulvar Disease (ISSVD). The defining criteria used to diagnose vestibulitis are (Friedrich, 1988)

1. Pain with attempted penetration
2. Pain at points along the vestibule (vaginal entry) with cotton swab touch
3. Erythema (redness) of varying degrees

VVS is a subset of vulvodynia. Vulvodynia describes a condition of chronic and diffuse burning, stinging, and discomfort of the vulva that occurs spontaneously and without provocation. Vulvodynia is a chronic pain condition that interferes with sexual activity.

The causes of VVS are multifactorial, and they involve the nervous system, musculoskeletal system, immune system, and vascular system. On a cellular level, findings at the vulvar vestibule of VVS patients include increased mast cells, indicating chronic inflammation (Bornstein, Sabo, Goldshmid, & Abramovici, 2002), increased nociceptors, pain receptors, and increased vascularity (Bohm-Starke, Hiliges, & Brodda-Jansen, 2001). Genetic findings include variation of interleukin-1 receptor antagonist and melanocortin-1 receptor genes (Witkin, Gerber, & Ledger, 2002). This variation affects the ability to fight inflammation and may explain why certain women are more vulnerable to recurrent bacterial and yeast infections. Though not a defining criterion, often a woman with VVS will present with the inability to allow penetration due to the anticipation or genuine experience of pain.

Unconsummated Unions

The terms *unconsummated unions* or *unconsummated marriage* refer to a sociological phenomenon rather than a specific sexual dysfunction. Unconsummated unions/marriages may result from a variety of factors ranging from lack of sexual knowledge, education, or preparation to sexual dysfunction in one or both partners to simply a lack of desire to have sexual intercourse.

Unconsummated marriages may exist in unions where sexual expression, or at least sexual intercourse, within the marriage is not a component of the relationship. Marriages that take place for convenience or companionship, or marriages where one or both partners is homosexual, may be examples of unconsummated marriages by choice.

When a married couple is unable to have sexual intercourse, despite the desire to do so and despite various and repeated efforts, this is a source of a great deal of distress. However, the term "unconsummated marriage" is a limited one in that it only describes married couples and is therefore useful in a sociological and legal context, but not as a descriptive term of sexual dysfunction. The term *unconsummated union* would more accurately describe the inability of a couple, married or otherwise, to complete the act of sexual intercourse, despite the desire and attempts to do so, and where this is a source of distress to both partners.

While statistics regarding the prevalence of unconsummated marriage are not documented, it has been estimated that 1 percent of all couples presenting to infertility clinics had not consummated their marriage. It is also unclear whether the majority of these situations can be attributed to lack of knowledge, male sexual dysfunction, or female dysfunction. Literature describing this phenomenon has pointed to cultural factors and stresses the importance of an educational and interdisciplinary approach to treatment (Ribner & Rosenbaum, 2005; see also volume 3, chapter 11).

Women presenting with sexual pain disorders, in particular vaginismus and primary vulvar vestibulitis may have never been successful in achieving sexual intercourse due to a combination of pain and anxiety. Often they become "stuck" in a relationship status quo such that when the pain and muscle hypertonus are no longer present and they are physically able to allow intercourse, they continue to be held back by the notion that completing the act may change them or the relationship. There are many implications involved in suddenly possessing the tools to be able to consummate a long-term relationship that has been devoid of sexual intercourse. In addition to seeking a physical cure to the sexual dysfunction responsible for the lack of consummation, couples therapy providing tools to making this transition is a critical component of treatment.

PHYSICAL THERAPY TREATMENT OF SEXUAL PAIN DISORDERS

Anna is a tall attractive 26-year-old lawyer. She relates that she began to feel something was wrong with her when at age 14, she could not succeed in inserting a tampon. She recalls her two best girlfriends standing outside the bathroom door giving her instructions, but it was simply too painful, and it just seemed "terribly unnatural for something as large as a tampon to enter such a tiny hole." She decided to let it go when, at age 17, she felt ready to begin to have sexual intercourse with her boyfriend. They had been together for two years, and had done "everything but." She trusted him, felt comfortable with him, and had gone on birth control pills and felt she was mature enough and ready to take this step. While she was prepared that the first time may be uncomfortable, she was completely unprepared for how she responded. She simply did not let her boyfriend enter her. Each time he tried, she would close her legs in fear and anxiety. This too, she let go, until her third year of college. She and her high school boyfriend became "just friends" and she avoided dating.

When she finally did meet someone she wanted to have sex with, again she was unable to allow him to penetrate her. She continued to be unable to use tampons, and when she tried to see a gynecologist, she could not undergo the exam. She was diagnosed with vaginismus. She

(Continued)

(Continued)

began counseling, which consisted of discussions. At first the discussions were helpful. She learned about her anatomy, and was given instruction to go home and insert a finger in her vagina. However, she still couldn't have intercourse due to the pain. She continued in therapy to talk about her feelings toward sex, her family, and her religious beliefs, but she didn't think this was advancing her. In fact, she felt that the problem wasn't really psychological at all.

Finally, Anna heard about a physical therapy clinic that specialized in treating painful intercourse. She began physical therapy. The therapist showed her a mirror, and instructed her in inserting a small dilator. At first, she was extremely fearful, but after a few times, she saw that it wasn't so bad. She also allowed the physical therapist to insert the dilator as well. The therapist worked with her on slightly larger dilators until reaching the one that was about the size of an erect penis. This was difficult and painful, but with gentle stretching of the vaginal opening that the therapist did and showed her to do at home, she was finally able to insert it. After eight sessions of physical therapy, Anna was able to have intercourse. She owes her success to the physical therapy, which provided her with practical, hands-on treatment to get over her anxiety.

The physical therapy approach to treatment of women with complaints of inability to have intercourse, or painful intercourse, includes taking a detailed history, performing a physical exam, and providing a treatment plan consistent with the goals of the patient. Treatment tools utilized by the physical therapist range from the educational, providing anatomical and physiological information; cognitive behavioral, particularly with vaginal dilators; rehabilitative, as in pelvic floor muscle strengthening and relaxation with tools such as biofeedback; and palliative treatment methods to decrease pain and improve tissue mobility. Manual techniques including massage, stretching, soft tissue and bony mobilizations are important components of treatment. The physical therapy intervention generally consists of evaluation and treatment with education and cognitive behavioral therapy, exercises, manual therapy techniques and modalities including pelvic floor biofeedback, electrical stimulation, and sometimes ultrasound (Rosenbaum, 2005).

History

The physical therapy intervention begins with taking a detailed medical, gynecological, and sexual history. The history can reveal if there was a relationship between the timing of symptoms and a preceding sequence of events. Obviously a history of sexual abuse can be a strong trigger. However, a history of dysmenorrhea (painful menstruation), urinary tract infections, vaginal infections, and musculoskeletal injury can all contribute to muscle hypertonus. Other situations include complications or difficulty healing from abdominal surgery (including hysterectomy and Cesarean delivery), and following pelvic cancer surgery and treatment. The history includes gathering information regarding the patient's chief complaint with which she presents. In most cases, patients with vaginismus seek treatment when it becomes apparent that this condition interferes with sexual intercourse and the ability to have sexual intercourse is the goal of treatment. The inability to allow penetration extends to other nonsexually related functional activities as well, such as inserting a tampon or undergoing a gynecological exam. Moreover, patients with a burning vulva may primarily be seeking relief of their symptoms and may or may not even be sexually active. Whether sexual activity is a goal of treatment is determined together with the patient.

When the presenting complaint is pain with penetration or attempted penetration, a thorough pain assessment is necessary. It is important to determine where and when the pain occurs. The pain description helps determine direction for physical examination and treatment. It is important to determine if the pain is superficial or deep, if it occurs with arousal or orgasm, and if the pain can be alleviated and how.

It is also important to ask about urinary symptoms such as frequency and urgency and about bowel dysfunction or pelvic pain. Often, other chronic pain conditions occur together with vulvar pain syndromes. These may include chronic pelvic pain; irritable bowel syndrome; interstitial cystitis, a syndrome characterized by bladder pain; urinary urgency and frequency; and dyspareunia (Doggweiler-Wiygul & Wiygul, 2002; Jamieson & Steege, 1996). The common factor in all these conditions appears to be the existence within the muscles of the pelvic floor of tender areas known as "trigger points." Pressure applied to these points reproduces the patient's symptoms and triggers radiating pain (Travell & Simons, 1992). These conditions are related to muscle hypertonus and should be addressed concurrently.

Observation and Musculoskeletal Examination

The patient is observed breathing normally and asked to demonstrate diaphragmatic breathing. Conditions of anxiety, for example, are often manifested by shallow breathing. This places abnormal pressures on the body and can perpetuate conditions of tightness in the pelvic floor. Often it will be noted that these patients are holding in their abdominal muscles as well. Careful assessment is made of the strength, length, and mobility of the pelvic and lumbar joints as well as the surrounding musculature of the pelvis and hips. A typical musculoskeletal presentation of patients with vaginismus is tight hip flexors and adductors, muscles related to posture of "pulling in" and interestingly, they are commonly found to present with weak, undeveloped pelvic floor muscles when asked to perform an active contraction. This may occur even if there is hypertonus of the muscles that close the sphincters. Generally, only a physical therapist trained in urogynecological rehabilitation has the skill to determine the activity and functional ability of the various muscles of the pelvic floor.

Vulvar and Pelvic Floor Examination

The physical therapist's assessment of the vulva differs from a gynecological examination. Both the external and internal exam focuses on the mobility and integrity of the muscular, fascial, and connective tissue components. The vulvar and pelvic floor exam consists of the following:

1. Observation of the vulva, perineum, and anus to note areas of redness, raised areas, scar tissue, or edema
2. Palpation to note areas of tenderness to touch
3. Internal exam to assess pelvic floor muscle tension and tightness, tone, range of motion, and hymen presence and thickness
4. Assessment of internal muscle trigger points
5. Determination of the integrity of the pelvic organs and possible presence of prolapse of the bladder, uterus, or rectum and
6. Anorectal internal exam (when indicated by the history)

Pelvic floor muscle tone is assessed by both manual examination and sEMG (surface electromyography) assessment with a vaginal probe. Studies of the pelvic floors of patients with VVS have found they present with pelvic floor hypertonus and decreased resting and working level muscle stability (Glazer, 1998). Pelvic floor hypertonus had been associated with other dyspareunia related conditions such as interstitial cystitis (IC), levator ani syndrome and proctalgia fugax, a condition of puborectalis tightness, which is related to painful defecation (Kotarinos, 2003). Pelvic floor muscle assessment determines muscle tone when asking for a contraction, and when asking the muscle to rest, how strong the muscle can work, how long it takes for the muscle to contract and to get back to a resting state, and how well the muscle can stay contracted without letting go.

Physical Therapy Treatment

Physical therapy treatment is focused on restoring mobility, decreasing pain, and improving overall function. Physical therapists treating patients suffering from illness or disease address the sensory, inflammatory, neurological, and musculoskeletal aspects of the disease, and their effect on function. The specific techniques chosen for treatment are guided by the findings of the history and examination, and are standards of practice utilized for other regions of the body. Physical therapy treatment may include, but is not limited to the following components:

1. Setting of treatment goals with patient
2. Providing a home program of exercise and behavioral therapy
3. Manual therapy
4. Exercise
5. Biofeedback
6. Electrical Stimulation
7. Ultrasound and other modalities.

Setting of Treatment Goals

Prior to embarking on a treatment program, it is crucial to discuss goal setting with the client. Some women may be very focused on the ability to have pain-free sex, but this may not be the case for other women, who may consider pain relief their primary goal. The goal assessment also provides the patient with an explanation of the treatment and with options regarding what works best for her considering her schedule and the amount of time and energy she wishes or is able to invest. For example, some patients with urinary urgency and frequency may want to address this concurrently while some women may not be bothered by these particular symptoms. When pain-free sexual intercourse is the goal, discussion may ensue regarding other aspects of improvement in sexual function. Was sexual intercourse ever pleasurable and is the ability to enjoy and derive pleasure from intercourse a goal of the patient? Are there other areas of difficulty in sexual function, such as decreased interest, and genital and subjective arousal and to what extent are they related to the pain? Are there difficulties in the relationship that either predate the pain or have resulted from it? Goal setting includes determining what the possible benefits will be of the physical therapy treatment along with referral to appropriate professional colleagues to help address the psychosocial components.

Home Program and Behavioral Therapy

The patient is instructed in self-care including avoidance of irritants such as synthetic garments and detergents, as well as feminine products. Depending on the presentation, she may be instructed in baths with oils such as lavender, tea tree, and sea buckthorn, natural oils known for their anti-inflammatory qualities.

In conditions of pain due to local inflammation, reduced sensory pain threshold, neuropathic conditions, or a combination thereof, sensory rehabilitation provides relief of symptoms by raising pain threshold and "accustomizing" the affected area to touch. Patients with VVS have been found to demonstrate reduced pain threshold and more acute pain perception with touch (Granot, Friedman, Yarnitsky, & Zimmer, 2002; Pukall, Binik, Khalifé, Amsel, & Abbott, 2002).

Patients with VVS often demonstrate behaviors of avoidance regarding allowing direct touch or contact to the area, which hypersensitizes the area even more. Introduction of daily light touch by the patient herself with appli-

cations of vitamin E oil provides the therapeutic benefits of increasing pro-
prioception and body awareness, and decreasing local tissue hypersensitivity.

In conditions whereby there is associated voiding dysfunction, such as urinary frequency and urgency, the patient is asked to keep a bladder diary and
is taught timed voiding, in order to allow greater bladder capacity with less
frequent need to void. In these cases, she is also instructed in avoidance of
bladder irritants, such as caffeine and bladder irritating foods.

In conditions of superficial dyspareunia, introital tightness, or vaginismus,
the patient may be instructed in home use of vaginal dilators and in therapeutic exercise including deep breathing, relaxation, and pelvic floor conditioning
as well as independent manual stretching.

Manual Therapy

Various hands-on techniques are applied to treat musculoskeletal abnormalities, postural and skeletal asymmetries and soft tissue immobility. Trigger
points are discrete, focal, hyperirritable spots located in a taut band of skeletal muscle (Alvarez & Rockwell, 2002; Simons & Travell, 1983; Travell &
Simons, 1992). They produce pain locally and in a referred pattern and often
accompany chronic musculoskeletal disorders. The application of trigger point
massage in the pelvic area and transvaginally has been described in the treatment of pelvic pain and interstitial cystitis (Weiss, 2001) and for the treatment of vulvar pain syndromes (Fitzgerald & Kotarinos, 2003). Additional
techniques include massage, connective tissue and scar tissue release. Osteo-
pathic techniques such as visceral and urogenital manipulation, taught to
physical therapists in advanced training courses, are effective techniques as
well (Baral, 1993). Other techniques available to the physical therapist treating musculoskeletal dysfunction associated with pelvic and vulvar pain include
muscle energy techniques, strain-counterstrain, contract/relax, and passive and
resisted stretching. These mobilization and soft tissue techniques are designed
to normalize postural imbalances, improve blood circulation in the pelvic and
vulvar area, and improve pelvic and vulvar mobility.

Dilators are used not only to help overcome penetration anxiety but to
stretch the vaginal openings. Patients are given very specific guidance in using
the dilators, including proper positions that facilitate greater opening of the
vaginal entrance. Perineal dilators designed for pre-delivery perineal stretching in women hoping to avoid *episiotomy*, or stitches, is useful for stretching
the vaginal opening as well. They are also useful as a means to get used to
the touch sensation and learn active release of the muscle. Dilators come in a
series of gradually increasing sizes.

Exercise

Therapeutic exercises are designed to strengthen weak muscles, stretch tight
muscles, improve mobility and flexibility, increase endurance and decrease

pain. Sexual activity, which requires some amount of physical stamina as well as muscle strength, may be hampered by physical limitations and, often, general as well as specific pelvic exercises are indicated. Relevant to dyspareunia, specific exercises are taught to improve circulation, increase healing of the vulva and pelvis, and increase mobility of the vagina. In the case of vaginismus, often certain muscle contraction patterns are noted, such as hips together and rotated inward. Often the inner thighs are very tight and need stretching, simply to be able to maintain comfort in a lying down, legs-apart position. Finally, the patient is instructed in proper performance of pelvic floor muscle exercise. Research has shown that verbal instruction alone does not produce effective results and that only 30–50 percent of women respond to verbal instruction with proper isolation and contraction of the pelvic floor muscles (Bump, Hurt, Fantl, & Wyman, 1991). Furthermore, for pelvic floor muscle exercises to be effective, it is important not just to contract muscles, but also to coordinate the contraction with proper breathing, timing, and simultaneous recruitment of other core postural muscles.

Pelvic Floor Biofeedback

Pelvic floor biofeedback is based on the use of the perineometer developed by Dr. Arnold Kegel. The technology is similar to that utilized during EKGs for examining heart muscle function. Pelvic floor surface EMG (sEMG) biofeedback involves insertion of a probe into the vagina, which measures the activity of the pelvic floor muscles and displays it in graph form on the computer monitor (for illustrations of biofeedback machines see www.thoughttechnology. com). The patient is then able to visualize the activity of her muscles and learn to relax them as well as strengthen, stabilize and coordinate them. The value of biofeedback in treatment of voiding dysfunction and urinary incontinence is well documented (Jundt, Peschers, & Dimpfl, 2002; Weatherall, 1999). The application of biofeedback in the treatment of vulvar pain syndromes was first explored by Glazer, who noted that the baseline sEMG of women with vulvar pain and VVS differed from women with pelvic floor dysfunction related to conditions such as prolapse and urinary incontinence. He found the treatment with biofeedback helped improve pain and restore sexual function in women with VVS (Glazer, Rodke, Swencionis, Hertz, & Young, 1995). The goals of sEMG biofeedback are to normalize pelvic floor muscle tone, decrease hypertonus and improve contractile and resting stability.

When appropriate, the client is instructed in the use of a home EMG biofeedback unit. This can help to increase sensory awareness for improving exercise efficiency. Hypertonus and tightness conditions can also be accompanied by weakness. Therefore, building strength and endurance for repetitive exercise may add to the resilience toward activity, including intercourse.

Electrical Stimulation and Other Modalities

Other modalities available to the physical therapist include pelvic floor electrical stimulation. This can be delivered directly transvaginally, or used externally such as with interfential current. Use of pelvic floor electrical stimulation has been studied in the treatment of levator ani hypertonus and pelvic pain (Fitzwater, Kuehl, & Schrier, 2003) and reported to successfully improve pelvic floor muscle strength and reduce pain in the treatment of VVS (Nappi et al., 2003). The use of perineal ultrasound, the application of deep heat produced by frequency waves, for the treatment of dyspareunia has also been reported on in the literature (Hay-Smith, 2000).

THE MIND-BODY APPROACH TO TREATMENT OF SEXUAL PAIN DISORDERS

Successful treatment of sexual pain disorders requires a comprehensive approach. VVS, for example, has been shown to be a multifactorial but primarily physiological disorder (Bornstein, Zarfati, Goldik, & Abramovici, 1999). Various studies failed to link VVS with childhood sex abuse or history of trauma (Dalton, Haefner, Reed, Senapati, & Cook, 2002; Edwards, Mason, Phillips, Norton, & Boyle, 1997) or demonstrate a primary psychological cause for vulvar pain (Meana, Binik, Khalifé, & Cohen, 1997). However, several studies have linked VVS with psychological distress (Brotto, Basson, & Gehring, 2003; Sackett, Gates, Heckman-Stone, Kobus, & Galask, 2001) including increased states of depression and anxiety as well as sexual distress (White & Jantos, 1998) and conclude it is important to address psychological and sexual distress in women with vestibulitis (Danielsson, Sjoberg, & Wilkman, 2000; Gates & Galask, 2001; Nunns & Mandal, 1997). Although physical therapists are not psychologists or social workers, the therapeutic benefit of physical therapy treatment far surpasses only the physical.

Throughout treatment, the patient is encouraged and given practical tools to overcome her fear and anxiety and is given hands-on direction with activities that sex therapists and counselors are traditionally able only to discuss, such as insertion of dilators. Practical suggestions for dealing with decreased libido and arousal are part of treatment; however, when the need for psychological treatment is identified the patient should be referred for therapy. An interdisciplinary approach, in which communication between therapists enhances the results of both treatments, is superior to simply multidisciplinary treatment, where practitioners may be working with the client independently.

CONCLUSION

Although physical therapy is a relatively new profession in the world of sexual health, the contribution of physical therapists is extremely valuable. Physical therapists in various settings can be involved in educating, rehabilitating, and treating individuals who wish to enhance their sexual function.

REFERENCES

Abramov, L., Wolman, I., & David, M.P. (1994). Vaginismus: an important factor in the evaluation and management of vulvar vestibulitis syndrome. *Gynecological and Obstetrical Investigations, 38,* 194–197.

Alvarez, D. J., & Rockwell, P. G. (2002). Trigger points: diagnosis and management. *American Family Physician, 65*(4), 653–660.

American Psychiatric Association. (2000). *Diagnostic and statistical manual of mental disorders* (4th ed.-TR). Washington, D.C.: American Psychiatric Association.

Baral, J. (1993). *Urogenital Manipulation.* Seattle: Eastland Press.

Basson, R., Leiblum, S., Brotto, L., Derogatis, L., Fourcroy, J., Fugl-Meyer, K., Graziottin, A., Heiman, J. R., Laan, E., Meston, C., Schover, L., van Lankveld, J., & Weijmar Schultz, W. (2004). Revised Definitions of Women's Sexual Dysfunction. *Journal of Sexual Medicine,* Issue 1, Volume 1, 40–48.

Berman, J. R., Berman, L. A., Werbin, T. J. Flaherty, E. E., Leahy, N. M., & Goldstein, I. (1999). Clinical evaluation of female sexual function: Effects of age and estrogen status on subjective and physiologic sexual responses. *International Journal of Impotence Research, 11*(Suppl. 1), S31–8.

Binik, I., Meana, M., Berkley, K., & Khalifé, S. (1999). The sexual pain disorders: Is the pain sexual or the sex painful? *Annual Review of Sex Research, 10,* 210–235.

Bo, K., Talseth, T., & Vinsnes, A. (2000). Randomized controlled trial on the effect of pelvic floor muscle training on quality of life and sexual problems in genuine stress incontinent women. *Acta Obstetrica et Gynecologia Scandinavica, 79*(7), 598–603.

Bohm-Starke, N., Hilliges, M., & Brodda-Jansen, G. (2001). Psychophysical evidence of nociceptor sensitization in vulvar vestibulitis syndrome. *Pain, 94*(2), 177–183.

Bornstein, J., Zarfati, D., Goldik, Z., & Abramovici, H. (1999). Vulvar vestibulitis: Physical or psychosexual problem? *Obstetrics and Gynecology, 93,* 876–880.

Bornstein, J., Sabo, E., Goldshmid, N., & Abramovici, H. (2002). A mathematical model for the histopathologic diagnosis of vulvar vestibulitis based on a histomorphometric study of innervation and mast cell activation. *Journal of Reproductive Medicine, 9,* 742.

Brotto, L. A., Basson, R., & Gehring, D. (2003). Psychological profiles among women with vulvar vestibulitis syndrome: a chart review. *Journal of Psychosomatic Obstetrics and Gynaecology, 24*(3), 195–203.

Bump, R. C., Hurt, W. G., Fantl, J. A., & Wyman, J. F. (1991). Assessment of kegel pelvic muscle exercise performance after brief verbal instructions. *American Journal of Obstetrics and Gynecology, 165,* 322–329.

Bump, R., & McClish, D. (1994). Cigarette smoking and pure genuine stress incontinence of urine. A comparison of risk factors and determinants between smokers and non-smokers. *American Journal of Obstetrics and Gynecology,170*(2), 579–582.

Bureau of Labor Statistics, U.S. Department of Labor, Occupational Outlook Handbook, 2004–05 Edition, Bulletin 2540. Superintendent of Documents, U.S. Government Printing Office, Washington, DC.

Dahm, D. L., Jacofsky, D., & Lewallen, D. G. (2004). Surgeons rarely discuss sexual activity with patients after THA: A survey of members of the American Association of Hip and Knee Surgeons. *Clinical Orthopedics and Related Research, 428,* 237–240.

Dalton, V. K., Haefner, H. K., Reed, B. D., Senapati, S., & Cook, A. (2002). Victimization in patients with vulvar dysesthesia/vestibulodynia. Is there an increased prevalence? *Journal of Reproductive Medicine, 47*(10), 829–834.

Danielsson, I., Sjoberg, I., & Wikman, M. (2000). Vulvar vestibulitis: Medical, psycho-sexual and psychosocial aspects, a case-control study. *Acta Obstetricia et Gynecologia Scandinavica, 79,* 872–878.

De Kruiff, M. E., Ter Kuile, M. M., Weijenborg, P., & Van Lankveld J. J. (2000). Vaginismus and dyspareunia: Is there a difference in clinical presentation? *Journal of Psychosomatic Obstetrics and Gynaecology, 21*(3), 149–155.

Doggweiler-Wiygul, R., & Wiygul, J. P. (2002). Interstitial cystitis, pelvic pain, and the relationship to myofascial pain and dysfunction: A report on four patients. *World Journal of Urology, 20*(5), 310–314.

Dorey, G. (2004). Pelvic floor exercises as a treatment for men with erectile dysfunction *Nursing Times, 100*(12), 65–67.

Dorey, G., Speakman, M., Feneley, R., Swinkels, A., Dunn, C., & Ewings, P. (2004). Randomised controlled trial of pelvic floor muscle exercises and manometric biofeedback for erectile dysfunction. *British Journal of General Practice, 54*(508), 819–825.

Edwards, L., Mason, M., Phillips, M., Norton, J., & Boyle, M. (1997). Childhood sexual and physical abuse. Incidence in patients with vulvodynia. *Journal of Reproductive Medicine, 42*(3), 135–139.

Fitzgerald, M. P., & Kotarinos, R. (2003). Rehabilitation of the short pelvic floor. II: Treatment of the patient with the short pelvic floor. *International Urogynecology Journal, 14,* 269–275.

Fitzwater, J. B., Kuehl, T. J., & Schrier, J. J. (2003). Electrical stimulation in the treatment of pelvic pain. *Journal of Reproductive Medicine, 48*(8), 573–577.

Friedrich, E. G. (1988). Therapeutic studies on vulvar vestibulitis. *Journal of Reproductive Medicine, 33,* 514–517.

Gates, E. A., & Galask, R. P. (2001). Psychological and sexual functioning in women with vulvar vestibulitis. *Journal of Psychosomatic Obstetrics and Gynaecology, 22,* 221–228.

Glazer, H. (1998). Electromyographic comparisons of pelvic floor in women with dysesthetic vulvodynia and asymptomatic women. *Journal of Reproductive Medicine, 43,* 959–962.

Glazer, H., Rodke, G., Swencionis, C., Hertz, R., & Young, A. W. (1995). Treatment of vulvar vestibulitis syndrome with electromyographic biofeedback of pelvic floor musculature. *Journal of Reproductive Medicine, 40,* 283–290.

Graber, G., & Kline-Graber, G. (1979). Female orgasm: role of the pubococcygeus muscle. *Journal of Clinical Psychiatry, 40,* 348–351.

Granot, M., Friedman, M., Yarnitsky, D., & Zimmer, E. Z. (2002). Enhancement of the perception of systemic pain in women with vulvar vestibulitis. *British Journal of Obstetrics and Gynecology, 109,* 863–866.

Handa, V. L., Harvey, L., Cundiff, G. W., Siddique, S. A., & Kjerulff, K. H. (2004). Sexual function among women with urinary incontinence and pelvic organ prolapse. *American Journal of Obstetrics and Gynecology, 191*(3), 751–756.

Hay-Smith, E. J. (2000). Therapeutic ultrasound for postpartum perineal pain and dyspareunia. *Cochrane Database of Systemic Reviews (2),* CD000945.

Jamieson, D., & Steege, J. (1996). The prevalence of dysmenorrhea, dyspareunia, pelvic pain and irritable bowel syndrome in primary care practices. *Obstetrics and Gynecology, 1,* 55–58.

Jundt, K., Peschers, U. M., & Dimpfl, T. (2002). Long-term efficacy of pelvic floor re-education with EMG-controlled biofeedback. *European Journal of Obstetrics, Gynecology and Reproductive Biology, 105*(2), 181–185.

Kegel, A. (1952). Sexual functions of the pubococcygeus muscle. *Western Journal of Surgery, Obstetrics and Gynecology* (October issue), 521–524.

Kotarinos, R. K. (2003). Pelvic floor physical therapy in urogynecologic disorders. *Current Women's Health Report, 3*(4), 334–339.

LoPiccolo, J. (1984). Treating vaginismus [a video]. Chapel Hill, NC: The Sinclair Institute.

Markwell, S. J. (2001). Physical therapy management of pelvi/perineal and perianal pain syndromes. *World Journal of Urology, 19,* 194–199.

Masters, W. H., & Johnson, V. E. (1970). *Human sexual inadequacy.* Boston: Little, Brown & Co.

Meana, M., Binik, Y.M., Khalifé, S., & Cohen, D. (1997). Biopsychosocial profile of women with dyspareunia. *Obstetrics and Gynecology, 90,* 583–589.

Murray, K. H. (1984). Treatment of motor and sensory detrusor instability by electrical stimulation; and Re: The neurophysiological basis of bladder inhibition in response to intravaginal electrical stimulation. *Journal of Urology. 131*(2), 356.

Nappi, R. E., Ferdeghini, F., Abbiati, I., Vercesi, C., Farina, C., & Polatti, F. (2003). Electrical stimulation (ES) in the management of sexual pain disorders. *Journal of Sex and Marital Therapy, 29*(Suppl, 1), 103–10.

Nunns, D., & Mandal, D. (1997). Psychological and psychosexual aspects of vulvar vestibulitis. *Genitourinary Medicine, 73,* 541–544.

Piediferro, G., Colpi, E. M., Castiglioni, F., & Scroppo, F. I. (2004). Premature ejaculation. 3. Therapy. *Archives of Italian Urology and Andrology, 76*(4), 192–198.

Pukall, C. F., Binik, Y. M., Khalifé, S., Amsel, R., & Abbott, F. V. (2002). Vestibular tactile and pain thresholds in women with vulvar vestibulitis syndrome. *Pain, 96,* 196–175.

Pukall, C. F., Payne, K. A., Kao, A., Khalifé, S., & Binik, Y. M. (2005). Dyspareunia. In: Balon, R., & Segraves, R. T. (Eds.). *Handbook of Sexual Dysfunction,* 249–272. New York: Taylor & Francis.

Reissing, E. D., Binik, Y. M., Khalifé, S., Cohen, D., & Amsel, R. (2004). Vaginal spasm, pain, and behavior: An empirical investigation of the diagnosis of vaginismus. *Archives of Sexual Behavior, 33,* 5–17.

Ribner, D., & Rosenbaum, T. Y. (2005). Evaluation and treatment of unconsummated marriage in Orthodox Jewish couples. *Journal of Sex and Marital Therapy, 31*(4), 341–353.

Rosen, R., Altwein, J., Boyle, P., Kirby, R.S., Lukacs, B., Meuleman, E., O'Leary, M. P., Puppo, P., Chris, R., & Giuliano, F. (2004). Lower urinary tract symptoms and male sexual dysfunction: the multinational survey of the aging male (MSAM-7). *Progressive Urology, 14*(3), 332–344.

Rosenbaum, T. Y. (2005). Physiotherapy treatment of sexual pain disorders. *Journal of Sex and Marital Therapy, 31*(4), 329–340.

Sackett, S., Gates, E., Heckman-Stone, C., Kobus, A. M., & Galask, R. (2001). Psychosexual aspects of vulvar vestibulitis. *Journal of Reproductive Medicine, 46*(6), 593–598.

Salonia, A., Zanni, G., Nappi, R. E., Briganti, A., Deho, F., Fabbri, F., Colombo, R., Guazzoni, G., Di Girolamo, V., Rigatti, P., & Montorsi, F. (2004). Sexual dysfunction is common in women with lower urinary tract symptoms and urinary incontinence: Results of a cross-sectional study. *European Urology, 45*(5), 642–648.

Sand, P. K. (1996). Pelvic floor stimulation in the treatment of mixed incontinence complicated by a low-pressure urethra. *Obstetrics and Gynecology, 88,* 757–760.

Shafik, A. (2000). The role of the levator ani muscle in evacuation, sexual performance, and pelvic floor disorders. *International Urogynecological Journal, 11,* 361–376.

Simons, D. G., & Travell, J. G. (1983). Myofascial origins of low back pain. 3. Pelvic and lower extremity muscles. *Postgraduate Medicine, 73,* 99–105, 108.

Swift, S. E., Pound, T. & Dias, J. K. (2001) Case-control study of etiologic factors in the development of severe pelvic organ prolapse. *International Urogynecology Journal,* 187–192.

Travell, J. & Simons, D. (1992). *Myofascial pain and dysfunction: The trigger point manual.* (Vol. 2). Baltimore: Williams and Wilkins.

Van der Velde, J., & Everaerd, W. (2001). The relationship between involuntary pelvic floor muscle activity, muscle awareness and experienced threat in women with or without vaginismus. *Behavior Research and Therapy, 39,* 395–408.

Van Kampen, M., De Weerdt, W., Claes, H., Feys, H., De Maeyer, M., & Van Poppel, H. (2003). Treatment of erectile dysfunction by perineal exercise, electromyographic biofeedback, and electrical stimulation. *Physical Therapy, 83*(6), 536–543.

Weatherall, M. (1999) Biofeedback or pelvic floor muscle exercises for female genuine stress incontinence: a meta-analysis of trials identified in a systematic review. *BJU International, 83*(9), 1015–1016.

Weiss, J. M. (2001). Pelvic floor myofascial trigger points: manual therapy for interstitial cystitis and the urgency-frequency syndrome. *Journal of Urology, 166,* 2226–2231.

White, G., & Jantos, M. (1998). Sexual behavior changes with vulvar vestibulitis syndrome. *Journal of Reproductive Medicine, 43*(9), 783–789.

Witkin, S. S., Gerber, S., & Ledger, W. J. (2002). Influence of interleukin-1 receptor antagonist gene polymorphism on disease. *Clinical Infectious Diseases, 34*(2), 204–209.

Wurn, B. F. (2004). Increasing orgasm and decreasing dyspareunia by a manual physical therapy technique. *Medscape General Medicine, 6*(4), 47.

Recommended Resources

American Physical Therapy Association Section on Women's Health, http://www.womenshealthapta.org.

Dr. Glazer's Web site, http://www.vulvodynia.com.

The International Pelvic Pain Society, http://www.pelvicpain.org.

National Vulvodynia Association, http://www.nva.org.

Talli Y. Rosenbaum's Web site, http://www.physioforwomen.com.

The V-Book: The Doctor's Complete Book to Vulvovaginal Health by Elizabeth Stewart and Paula Spencer (2002).

The Vulvodynia Survival Guide by Howard Glazer & Gae Rodke (2002).

Chapter Ten

UNDERSTANDING FAMILY PLANNING, BIRTH CONTROL, AND CONTRACEPTION

Carey Roth Bayer

A variety of definitions exist for the terms family planning, birth control, and contraception. Regardless of which definition one uses, each of the terms refers to methods of planning for whether or not to have children. Some of the methods protect against sexually transmitted infections (STIs). For clarity, the term, family planning, will be used throughout this chapter. Also, to view illustrations of many of the methods discussed in this chapter, visit the following Web site: http://www.managingcontraception.com/managingcontraception.pdf.

Family planning methods have been in existence throughout history. A few of the early methods used included coitus interrupts or penile withdrawal before ejaculation; wiping out the vagina after intercourse; inserting honey, pepper, and/or animal dung in the vagina as barriers to semen; women holding their breath at the time of ejaculation; women jumping backwards seven times after intercourse; men donning condoms made of animal intestines; and, women inserting oiled paper or beeswax into the vagina as cervical caps (Wikipedia 2005; Potts & Campbell, 2002). As myths were debunked and scientists discovered more about the biology of the human body, family planning methods were refined. Scientists began to understand the menstrual cycle at the beginning of the twentieth century, which revolutionized family planning altogether. By the early 1900s, rubber condoms, cervical caps, diaphragms, spermicides, and intrauterine devices (IUDs) were being used to prevent pregnancy, and Ludwig Haberlandt was collaborating with a pharmaceutical company in Budapest on the possibility of an oral contraceptive (Potts & Campbell, 2002). The first oral contraceptive pills came on the market in the United States in 1960 (Crooks & Baur, 1999). The late 1900s and early 2000s gave rise to a variety of other family planning methods including injectable hormones, hormonal implants, intrauterine systems, vaginal rings, transdermal patches or patches placed on the skin, and different types of oral contraceptive pills. Family planning methods continue to be revised and refined as scientists make new discoveries in the human body. New methods such as hormonal contraceptives for men, as well as microbicides or agents used to kill bacteria, protozoa, viruses, and fungi, particularly those causing STIs such as the human immunodeficiency virus (HIV), are currently under development (Sitruk-Ware, 2005).

Family planning methods are complex. With all the methods available today, it is easy to see how one can get confused. The effectiveness rates reported in this chapter are the percentages of women in the United States experiencing an unintended pregnancy while using a particular method both typically and perfectly. The goal throughout this chapter is to provide you with an easily understandable breakdown of the family planning methods currently available in the United States. Methods differ around the world due to science, politics, religion, research, finances, availability, and values. In this chapter, only those approved in the United States will be addressed due to space limitations.

The next sections are broken down in order from least invasive methods to most invasive methods, starting with fertility awareness methods and ending with sterilization. The chapter concludes with a discussion of potential future methods, as well as discussions on partner communication, method choice, and prevention of STIs. With all the methods currently available, communication among partners, discussion of STI prevention, and consistent method use are all vital components of family planning method selection.

FERTILITY AWARENESS

Fertility awareness methods, sometimes referred to as natural family planning (NFP), are methods that involve identification of the fertile days of a woman's menstrual cycle. Identification of fertile days can be done through counting cycle days, measuring body temperature, testing mucus, and monitoring urine. Once the fertile days are identified, sexual intercourse is avoided during the fertile timeframe, also known as periodic abstinence. In order to become fertile, ovulation or the release of an egg from a woman's ovary must occur. Fertility awareness methods do not require drugs, physical devices, or medical personnel for implementation. The effectiveness of abstinence or delaying sexual intercourse alone and unintended pregnancy is 0 percent for perfect use and the percentage is unknown for typical use (Hatcher et al., 2004). The fertility awareness methods discussed in this section include the calendar or rhythm method, basal body temperature, cervical mucus, lutenizing hormone (LH) surge, symptomthermal method, lactational amenorrhea, and coitus interruptus or penile withdrawal.

Calendar or Rhythm Method

The calendar or rhythm method is used to determine the number of fertile days of a woman's menstrual cycle based on past cycle lengths (Grimes, Gallo, Grigorieva, Nanda, & Schultz, 2005). Since it is difficult to identify the exact day of ovulation due to changes in menstrual cycles, it is easier to identify the fertile phase. The fertile phase may begin three to five days before ovulation and ends 24 hours after ovulation. When using the fertility awareness methods, one must take into account that sperm can survive inside the body from two to seven days after intercourse (Hatcher et al., 2004).

Ovulation is calculated by tracking the menstrual cycle for 6 to 12 months, particularly noting the first day of vaginal bleeding. The number of days in a cycle is calculated as the first day of bleeding one month to the first day of bleeding in the next month. Once the cycle length is calculated, one can approximate ovulation and the fertile phase. The fertile phase is determined by subtracting 18 from the shortest cycle length and subtracting 11 from the longest cycle length (Hatcher et al., 2004). For example, if a woman's cycle ranged from 24 days to 36 days, her fertile phase would run from day 6 to day 25. Those women with cycles ranging from 28 days to 30 days would have fertile phases from day 10 to day 19. Once the fertile phase is identified, in order to prevent pregnancy intercourse is either avoided during that timeframe or another method is used. Though intercourse is avoided during the fertile phase, other forms of intimacy can still continue. The effectiveness of the calendar or rhythm method and unintended pregnancy is 9 percent for perfect use and 25 percent for typical use (Hatcher et al., 2004).

Basal Body Temperature

The basal body temperature method, like the calendar method, is another means of determining the fertile phase in a woman's cycle. A woman's resting body temperature drops slightly just before ovulation and increases 0.4°F–1.0°F following ovulation (Crooks & Bauer, 1999; Hatcher et al., 2004; Jones, 1997; Strong, DeVault, Sayad, & Yarber, 2005). The resting body temperature must be measured every morning before getting out of bed since activity can affect the body temperature. Use of either a digital or basal body temperature thermometer is important to detect the small temperature changes. Strong et al. (2005) recommend tracking the basal body temperature for 6 to 12 months to learn the woman's temperature pattern. Intercourse should be avoided from the onset of menstruation until three days after the temperature rise, but other forms of intimacy may continue. The effectiveness of the basal body temperature method and unintended pregnancy is 3 percent for perfect use and 25 percent for typical use (Hatcher et al., 2004).

Cervical Mucus

Another method for determining fertility is the cervical mucus method. Cervical mucus changes in color and consistency at different time points in the menstrual cycle. Cervical mucus is scant or undetectable after menstruation, as well as in the unfertile post-ovulation time period. However, just before ovulation, the mucus is cloudy, sticky, and yellow or white. The mucus at ovulation changes to wet, clear, slippery, and stretchy, like a raw egg white. This facilitates conception by allowing the sperm to migrate easier into the uterus and fallopian tubes to meet the egg. After ovulation, the mucus becomes thick, sticky, and cloudy. Abstinence or another method should be used as soon as the woman notices any cervical secretions. Intercourse may resume four days after the ovulation mucus (wet, clear, slippery, stretchy) occurs. A woman can check cervical mucus by inserting a finger in the vagina to feel the secretions, observing toilet paper after wiping the vulva, or checking the inside of the underwear. Hatcher et al. (2004) recommend monitoring cervical secretions for several months to determine the cervical mucus pattern. The effectiveness of this method and unintended pregnancy is 3 percent for perfect use and 25 percent for typical use (Hatcher et al., 2004).

Lutenizing Hormone Surge

Monitoring for the LH surge is another way of predicting ovulation. This method is used predominantly by those couples actually trying to get pregnant. Testing for the LH surge is accomplished through the use of ovulation predictor kits used to test a woman's urine midcycle during the most probable time for ovulation. The kits are similar to home pregnancy tests where a woman urinates either into a cup for dipping the test strip or directly onto the test strip. The test strip indicates whether or not the woman is experiencing a LH surge. Ovulation occurs approximately 36 hours after the LH surge (Gaines, 2005). While it is possible that this method could be used to determine days to avoid intercourse, the method can get expensive as a new ovulation prediction kit needs to be purchased each month. The kits are available over-the-counter at a variety of stores.

Symptothermal Method

The symptothermal method is a combination of at least two fertility awareness methods, usually the basal body temperature method and the cervical mucus method, used to detect fertility. Additional indices of ovulation used with this method include: breast tenderness; vaginal spotting, slight discharge of blood from the vagina; mittelschmerz, one-sided lower abdominal pain at ovulation; feelings of heaviness or abdominal swelling; changes in libido; and changes in cervical texture, position, and dilation (Hatcher et al., 2004; Jones, 1997; Strong et al., 2005). Before and during ovulation, the cervix is moist, soft, and opens; however, after ovulation occurs, the cervix closes, drops, and becomes firm. It is possible for a woman to use all of the fertility awareness methods discussed above to determine not only when she ovulates, but also when she is least likely to get pregnant after intercourse. Using multiple methods to determine when to abstain from intercourse is more effective for preventing pregnancy than using any one method alone. Regardless of the method(s) chosen, intimacy can continue, even when abstaining from intercourse. The effectiveness of the symptothermal method and unintended pregnancy is 2 percent for perfect use and 25 percent for typical use (Hatcher et al., 2004).

Lactational Amenorrhea

The lactational amenorrhea method (LAM) is a method that can be used by mothers who are exclusively or nearly exclusively breastfeeding their babies. In order for the woman to be protected from pregnancy using the LAM, her baby must be less than six months old, her menstrual periods cannot have returned, and her baby must get at least 85 percent of feedings—both day and night—from her breast milk (Hatcher, Rinehart, Blackburn, Geller, & Shelton, 2001). When the baby sucks on the mother's nipples, the mother experiences a surge in prolactin, which stops estrogen production and ovulation (Hatcher et al., 2004). If at any point the mother does not meet the three criteria mentioned, she should consider the use of another method. Most postpartum health practitioners recommend using additional types of birth control when a woman chooses to have intercourse again after childbirth, even though she is breastfeeding. Jones (1997) recommends avoiding the use of oral combination pills when lactating because they cause breast milk suppression and the steroids in them can enter the breast milk. However, the impact of hormonal contraception on quality and quantity of breast milk remains controversial (Truitt, Fraser, Grimes, Gallo, & Schulz, 2003). Many health practitioners prescribe oral contraceptives once lactation is firmly established. The effectiveness of LAM and unintended pregnancy in the first six months of breastfeeding is 0.5 percent for perfect use and 2 percent for typical use (Hatcher et al., 2004).

Coitus Interruptus or Penile Withdrawal

Coitus interruptus or penile withdrawal is not a fertility awareness method, but another method that requires no drugs or devices. When using withdrawal, the penis is completely withdrawn from the vagina before ejaculation occurs. Preejaculatory fluid containing sperm is secreted from the penis prior to ejaculation. It is important to remember that whether preejaculate or ejaculate, both contain sperm that when deposited in or near the vagina, can swim to fertilize an egg. This method takes control on the man's part to ensure that he completely withdrawals when the urge to continue with intercourse is often strong. The effectiveness of coitus interruptus or penile withdrawal and unintended pregnancy is 4 percent for perfect use and 27 percent for typical use (Hatcher et al., 2004).

BARRIER METHODS

The next section of this chapter focuses on barrier methods. Barriers are defined as methods that block the sperm from reaching the egg. Two different types of barriers are discussed in this chapter, mechanical barriers and chemical barriers. The mechanical barriers covered include male condoms, female condoms, cervical caps, diaphragms, Lea's shield, and sponges. The chemical barriers discussed include spermicidal creams, films, foams, jellies, suppositories, and tablets. Though the dental dam is not used for intercourse, it is still a mechanical barrier—used for STI prevention during oral-vaginal or oral-anal contact. All of these methods are non-hormonal methods.

Male Condom

Male condoms are mechanical barriers made of latex, polyurethane, or lamb intestine. They are used not only as a barrier preventing the sperm from uniting with the egg, but also as a barrier for preventing STIs. The condom is rolled on a fully erect penis prior to intercourse or ejaculation. If the condom has a reservoir at the top, hold this between two fingers (to prevent air entrapment) as the condom is applied to the glans of the penis. Be sure to determine ahead of time which side of the condom touches the glans before you roll it down the shaft of the penis. Once intercourse is complete, hold the rim of the condom and carefully withdraw the penis from the vagina before loss of erection. Dispose of the condom and wash any areas of the body that came in contact with bodily fluids.

Condoms may also be used during oral or anal penetration for STI prevention as pregnancy cannot occur during oral or anal activities. If either partner has a latex allergy, latex condoms should not be used. Care should be taken when using lamb intestine condoms as they may not provide the same STI protection as latex or polyurethane condoms (Hatcher et al., 2004). Condoms may be used alone or with any other family planning methods. If condoms are the primary method being used, the couple should have knowledge of emergency contraception (EC) in case the condom should break or slip during intercourse. The effectiveness of condoms and unintended pregnancy is 2 percent for perfect use and 15 percent for typical use (Hatcher et al., 2004).

Female Condom

Like the male condom, the female condom is also a mechanical barrier. The female condom is a polyurethane sheath with a flexible ring attached to both the open and closed ends. The ring on the closed end is used to insert the condom into the vagina. The ring on the open end is used to help hold the condom in place outside the vagina during intercourse. Though the condom is lubricated on both the interior and exterior, Strong et al. (2005) do not recommend using both a male and female condom together as the male condom adheres to the female condom when the penis is inserted for intercourse.

Female condoms provide protection from STIs and can be placed in the vagina up to eight hours before intercourse. They are intended for one-time use only. In order for a woman to use a female condom, she must be comfortable touching her genitals and inserting the condom deep into her vagina, eventually fitting it against the cervix. The effectiveness of female condoms and unintended pregnancy is 5 percent for perfect use and 21 percent for typical use (Hatcher et al., 2004). Both male and female condom application can be built into lovemaking activities.

Cervical Cap

The cervical cap also known as the FemCap is a silicone rubber, latex-free device that fits around the cervix and looks like a thimble with a brim. The cap functions as a mechanical barrier preventing the sperm from swimming through the cervical os. Spermicide is placed on both sides of the thimble-like device which fits against the cervix and acts as a chemical barrier. The cap comes in three sizes and must be prescribed by a medical practitioner after determining the number of pregnancies the woman has had.

Once the cap is inserted around the cervix, the woman or her partner should check for correct positioning by sliding a finger around the cap to check for an adequate cervical seal. The cap should be inserted 15 minutes prior to sexual arousal and stay in position for at least 6 hours after intercourse (FemCap, 2005). However, it can be inserted up to 6 hours before intercourse and stay in for up to 48 hours after intercourse (Hatcher, et al., 2004). Upon removal, the cap should be thoroughly cleaned. It can be reused for up to two years. The woman may need to be refitted for a different size cap after pregnancy due to changes in the size of the cervix. The effectiveness of this method and unintended pregnancy for nulliparous women (women who have not given birth to a child) versus parous women (women who have given birth to a child) is 9 percent for perfect use and 16 percent for typical use (nulliparous), and 26 percent for perfect use and 32 percent (parous) (Hatcher, et al., 2004).

Diaphragm

The diaphragm is a mechanical barrier similar to the cervical cap. However, the diaphragm differs in a variety of ways. The flexible latex or silicone barrier looks more like a bowl than a thimble. It, too, must be fitted to each woman. Resizing may be required after pregnancy or with a 20 percent weight fluctuation (Hatcher et al., 2004). Before the diaphragm can be inserted into the vagina and secured around the cervix, spermicide must be placed on the rim and inside the dome of the diaphragm. When inserted into the vagina, the side of the dome containing spermicide should face up toward the cervix. The pubic bone and vaginal wall hold the device in place, covering the cervix. The device should be inserted not more than six hours before intercourse and must remain in place for at least six hours after intercourse. The diaphragm must be removed within 24 hours of placement, unlike the cervical cap, which can remain in place for up to 48 hours. The effectiveness of this method and unintended pregnancy is 6 percent for perfect use and 16 percent for typical use (Hatcher et al., 2004).

Like the cervical cap, the diaphragm is reusable for up to two years. The device should be washed with soap and water, dried, and stored in a dry, cool location. Care should be taken to inspect the diaphragm for any holes or tears before and after each use. The diaphragm may be used for multiple rounds of intercourse without removing it, but a condom should be used as well for the second and each subsequent round since spermicide should not be used more than once in 24 hours (Hatcher et al., 2004).

Lea's Shield

Lea's shield is another mechanical barrier similar to both the cervical cap and the diaphragm. The main difference amongst the three methods is that the shield does not require fitting. It is held in place by the vaginal walls, not the cervix or pubic bone (Lea's Shield, 2004). A one-way valve on the device maintains a tight seal between the vaginal walls and the device. Like the cap and diaphragm, spermicide is used with the shield as well, to create a chemical barrier in addition to a mechanical one for any sperm that enter the vagina. The shield can be inserted any time before intercourse, but must remain in place for at least eight hours after intercourse. A woman can reuse the shield after cleaning with mild soap. The shield should be replaced with the first signs of deterioration. The effectiveness of this method and unintended pregnancy is 9 percent for perfect use and 16 percent for typical use in nulliparous women, and 26 percent for perfect use and 32 percent for typical use in parous women (Hatcher et al., 2004).

Sponges

The sponge is the only family planning device that is both a mechanical and chemical barrier. The device not only blocks the cervix, but it also has a spermicide built in that releases spermicide for over 24 hours after insertion. The sponge is inserted like the cap, diaphragm, and shield; however, no additional spermicide is needed with the sponge. Just before insertion, wet the device with tap water to activate the spermicide. When inserted, the dimple in the sponge fits securely around the cervix. The sponge may be inserted up to 24 hours before intercourse and can stay in place for a maximum of 30 hours. No additional methods are needed with multiple acts of intercourse since the sponge provides continuous protection during that timeframe. Like the cap, diaphragm, and shield, the sponge must remain in place for at least six hours after intercourse (Allendale Pharmaceuticals Inc., 2005; Kuyoh, Toroitich-Ruto, Grimes, Schulz, & Gallo, 2003). The sponge was recently re-released on the market for public consumption without prescription (in September 2005). The effectiveness of the sponge and unintended pregnancy is 9.7–12.7 percent for perfect use and 15.3–18.7 percent for typical use (Allendale Pharmaceuticals Inc., 2005).

Spermicidal Creams, Films, Foams, Jellies, Suppositories, and Tablets

Spermicides are chemical barriers that work by attacking the sperm body and flagella or tail, and reducing its ability to swim; therefore, preventing the sperm from reaching the cervical os. Spermicides are made in a variety of forms including vaginal creams, films, foams, jellies, suppositories, and tablets. As mentioned earlier in the chapter, the sponge also has a spermicide built into the device. Some condoms are available with spermicide already in place. When using spermicide alone, either the woman or her partner should insert the spermicide in the vagina as close to the cervix as possible.

Spermicides should be inserted anywhere from 15 minutes to one hour before intercourse. Hatcher et al. (2004) note that spermicides inserted greater than an hour before intercourse may drip out of the vagina. Also, intercourse should be completed within 60 minutes of spermicidal application. Care should be taken to observe for any vaginal, oral, or anal irritation. Should irritation occur, spermicidal use should be stopped and another family planning method used instead.

Nonoxynol-9 (N-9) is the spermicide available in the United States. Of note "vaginal spermicides are not effective in preventing cervical gonorrhea, Chlamydia, or HIV infection" (Hatcher et al., 2004, p. 149). Controversy exists over whether spermicides actually enhance the transmission of HIV (Grimes, 2003; Van Damme et al., 2002). In light of these concerns, the World Health Organization (2003) recommends that high-risk women having frequent intercourse with multiple partners should not use products containing N-9. Also, N-9 may cause genital irritation in some women. The effectiveness of spermicides alone and unintended pregnancy is 15 percent for perfect use and 29 percent for typical use (Hatcher et al., 2004).

Dental Dams

The dental dam is a latex shield placed over the vulva and perineum as a safer sex barrier in oral-vaginal sex (Bailey, Farquhar, Owen, & Whittaker, 2003). The dam may also be used in oral-anal activities. Though this method is not used for vaginal intercourse to prevent pregnancy, it does provide a barrier preventing STI transmission from the mouth to the genitals and vice versa. The dams come in various flavors, shapes, colors, and sizes. For those with latex allergies, the latex dams should be avoided. Care should also be taken to ensure that only one side of the dam is used and that the dam is not flipped over and reused for additional sexual activities. Dental dams should be discarded after one use to prevent transmitting bacteria from one body part to another.

ORAL HORMONAL METHODS

Oral hormonal methods are often referred to as either oral contraceptives (OCs) or "the pill." They are a common method used amongst women in the United States. "Although sterilization is the most prevalent method of contraception overall, oral contraceptives are the most widely used reversible method and also the most commonly used method among young women" (Davis & Castaño, 2004, p. 297). Since the inception of the OC approximately 40 years ago, many varieties of OCs have been developed. Throughout this section the following OCs will be discussed: combination oral contraceptives (COCs), progestin-only contraceptives or progestin-only pills (POPs), and emergency contraceptives (ECs).

Combination Oral Contraceptives

Combination oral contraceptives are pills containing various amounts of estrogen and progestin. The combination of hormones suppresses ovulation through negative feedback of the pituitary gland; thickens cervical mucus, making it difficult for sperm to swim through the cervical os; and alters the endometrium, reducing the likelihood of implantation (Duramed Pharmaceuticals, Inc., 2003;

Hatcher et al., 2004; Organon, 2003; Organon (a), 2004). COCs contain a variety of both estrogen and progestin dosages to accommodate the individualized hormonal needs of each woman. Women on COCs should take those with the least amount of hormones compatible with their needs (Wyeth, 2004).

Not only do the dosages vary, but so do the regimens for taking the pills. The regimens range from 20 to 21 day cycles to 28 day cycles to even 13 week cycles. Women using the 20–28 day pill cycles will generally have menstrual bleeding while taking the placebo or "inactive" pills. Women using the 13 week pill cycles will only have menstrual bleeding four times a year during week 13 while taking the "inactive" pills. It is possible that the timing and duration of menstrual cycles will change based on the dose and cycle length of the COC being used. Women are also cautioned that break through bleeding (intermenstrual bleeding, during the time of the cycle which is usually without bleeding), may occur while taking COCs.

Women considering using COCs need to be committed to taking the pill every day at the same time for the method to be most effective. Those women who have any of the following should not take COCs: a current pregnancy, a smoking habit, age greater than 35 years, high blood pressure, diabetes, high cholesterol, obesity, or frequent headaches. Women with kidney, liver, or adrenal disease should not take the COC, Yasmin (drospirenone and ethinyl estradiol), since it contains the progestin, drospirenone. Drospirenone may increase potassium in the woman causing serious heart and health problems (Berlex, 2004). COCs do not provide protection from STIs. The effectiveness of COCs and unintended pregnancy is 0.3 percent for perfect use and 8 percent for typical use (Hatcher et al., 2004).

Progestin-Only Oral Contraceptives

Progestin-only pills (POPs) are oral contraceptives that contain only progestin. POPs are also called minipills. The dose of progestin in POPs is lower than the dosage of progestin in COCs and the hormonal pills are taken continuously during the 28 day cycle. Like the COCs, POPs prevent pregnancy by thickening cervical mucus, diminishing sperm motility, suppressing ovulation, and thinning the endometrium, inhibiting implantation (Hatcher et al., 2004). Women on POPs may experience decreased menstrual bleeding. Those taking POPs at the same time every day may experience amenorrhea or no menstrual bleeding.

POPs have fewer side effects and health risks than COCs, but are also less effective (Strong et al., 2005). The main advantage with POPs is that most women can use them. Those women prohibited from using COCs due to the estrogen are still candidates for POPs. POP users must take pills at the same time each day otherwise the POPs may not be as effective for preventing pregnancy. Women using POPs, like those using COCs need to remember that neither oral contraceptive provides protection from STIs. If an STI is suspected, a condom should be used in addition to the pill. The effectiveness of POPs and unintended pregnancy is 0.3 percent for perfect use and 8 percent for typical use (Hatcher et al., 2004).

Emergency Contraception

Emergency contraceptive (EC) methods are those methods used to prevent pregnancy in an emergency situation after intercouse, specifically if condoms break, devices fail, products expire, or after rape. The EC methods available in the United States are high dose POPs, COCs, and insertion of a copper intrauterine device (IUD). High dose POPs and COCs are the most common methods used as EC. Though the copper IUD is an option, it is not used as frequently due to cost and the expectation that the woman will continue using the IUD (Hatcher et al., 2004).

High dose POPs and COCs must be taken within five days of unprotected intercourse, but should be taken as soon as possible. The copper IUD can be inserted up to eight days after unprotected intercourse, though; it too should be inserted as soon as possible. Antinausea medication should be administered before the use of high dose COCs as the dose of estrogen may induce vomiting. Additional side effects of EC use may include breast tenderness and irregular bleeding. The high dose OCs work by disrupting normal follicular development and maturation, blocking the LH surge, and inhibiting ovulation if taken before ovulation. If taken after ovulation, the high dose OCs have little effect on ovarian hormonal production and endometrial maturation (Hatcher et al., 2004). The use of an IUD for EC works by interfering with implantation of the fertilized egg in the uterus. All three of these methods work to prevent pregnancy; however, they are ineffective if implantation of the fertilized egg has already occurred.

HORMONAL APPLICATION METHODS

Hormonal application methods are some of the newest contraceptive methods on the market today. These methods are applied to the skin like a band-aid and absorption of the hormones occurs by passing through the skin, also known as a transdermal method. The specific hormonal method discussed in the next section is the transdermal contraceptive patch.

Transdermal Contraceptive Patch

The transdermal contraceptive patch, also known as "the patch," was approved in the United States in the early twenty-first century. The patch works much like COCs by primarily inhibiting ovulation since it contains both estrogen and progestin (Ortho-McNeil, 2005). The patch also alters the cervical mucus and endometrium, similar to both COCs and POPs. The main difference between the COCs and the patch is that the patch is an adhesive affixed to the skin on a weekly basis. The patch is changed once a week for three weeks. The fourth week is a "patch-free" week in order for menstruation to occur. The patch should be applied to the abdomen, buttocks, upper outer arm, or the upper torso—excluding the breasts. The site should be rotated with each patch change.

Since the patch releases estrogen and progestin, the possible side effects are similar to those of the COCs. One main difference is that any woman weighing over 198 pounds should consider an alternative contraceptive method as the patch may not be as effective for these women (Ortho-McNeil, 2005). The effectiveness of this method and unintended pregnancy is 0.3 percent for perfect use and 8 percent for typical use (Hatcher et al., 2004).

HORMONAL INJECTABLE METHODS

Hormonal injectable methods are hormones administered as an injection into the buttock or upper arm to prevent pregnancy. Currently, the only injectable method available in the United States is Depo-Provera (depot medroxyprogesterone acetate, DMPA). Lunelle (estradiol and medroxyprogesterone), another injectable method given monthly, is no longer available and may not return to the market (Hatcher et al., 2004). The hormonal injectable discussed in the next section is Depo-Provera.

Depo-Provera

Depo-Provera, a hormonal injection, is administered every three months to prevent pregnancy. The injection works by suppressing ovulation, thickening cervical mucus, slowing tubal and endometrial mobility, and thinning the endometrium (Pharmacia & Upjohn, 2004). DMPA is a long-acting family planning method. Women must return to their health care practitioners promptly every three months to continue contraceptive coverage. For those wishing to get pregnant after stopping DMPA, it may take 10–12 months before pregnancy can occur.

Women are advised not to use DMPA long-term because it may cause calcium loss in bones leading to osteoporosis or porous bones at risk of breaking (Pharmacia & Upjohn, 2004). Menstrual bleeding may be irregular and some users may stop menstruating altogether. One of the most common side effects of DMPA is weight gain. Women have gained anywhere from 2.75 to 5 pounds per year while on the injections. Like the other hormonal methods,

DMPA does not protect against STIs. The effectiveness of DMPA and unintended pregnancy is 0.3 percent for perfect use and 3 percent for typical use (Hatcher et al., 2004).

INSERTABLE HORMONAL METHODS

As demonstrated thus far, hormonal methods are administered in a variety of ways. The vaginal ring (VR) and intrauterine system (IUS) are two of the newer insertable hormonal methods available today. Throughout the next section both the VR and IUS are discussed as insertable hormonal methods.

Vaginal Ring

The hormonal vaginal ring contains an estrogen and progestin like COCs. Vaginal rings prevent pregnancy primarily by inhibiting ovulation, though they also cause changes in the cervical mucus and endometrium making fertilization and implantation difficult (Organon (b), 2004).

The VR cycle is similar to the patch cycle. The VR is inserted once a week for three weeks and no ring is inserted the fourth week to allow for menstruation. At the same time each week, the old ring should be removed and a new one placed. If the VR is outside the vagina for greater than three hours, pregnancy prevention may not be as effective and an alternate family planning method should be used (Organon (b), 2004). While the VR is in place, it releases a continuous dose of hormones.

The VR is inserted into the vagina and pushed as far back in the vagina as possible. On rare occasions the VR has been expelled or fallen out. Should this occur, rinse the VR with cool to lukewarm water and reinsert it into the vagina within three hours. In order for the VR to be effective, it must be in place continuously for three weeks.

Since the VR contains both estrogen and progestin, women who smoke are not advised to use the VR. The more common side effects of VRs are vaginal infection or irritation, vaginal discharge, headache, weight gain, and/or nausea (Organon (b), 2004). The VR does not provide protection against STIs. Before selecting this method, the woman should be comfortable with inserting a VR in the vagina. The effectiveness of this method and unintended pregnancy is 0.3 percent for perfect use and 8 percent for typical use (Hatcher et al., 2004).

Intrauterine System (IUS)

The hormonal intrauterine system is small, plastic, and T-shaped, containing a stem filled with the hormone levonorgestrel, a progestin (Strong et al., 2005). When the IUS is inserted in the uterus, it continually releases the hormone. The IUS helps prevent pregnancy by thickening the cervical mucus and thinning the endometrium. Once inserted, the IUS prevents pregnancy for up to five years (Berlex, 2004a). After five years, the IUS must be removed, but a new one can be reinserted.

The IUS is both inserted and removed by a trained healthcare professional. Before inserting the IUS, the healthcare professional should confirm that the woman is not currently pregnant or has a history of any ectopic pregnancies, pregnancies outside the uterus. Then, nonsteroidal anti-inflammatory drugs (NSAIDs) should be administered. NSAIDs are helpful in decreasing the discomfort the woman may experience with insertion of the IUS through the cervical os into the uterus. Once the IUS is inserted, the woman should be able to feel with her fingers two small strings hanging in the vagina, just below the cervix. It is important for the woman to occasionally check herself to ensure the strings are present, thus confirming that the IUS is in the correct place. This should be done particularly after menstruation. If the woman feels more of the IUS than just the strings, it is not in the right place and will need to be removed by a healthcare professional.

Some of the most common side effects of the IUS are cramping, dizziness, and fainting with insertion. After insertion, the woman may experience bleeding irregularities ranging from no menstruation to spotting and heavy bleeding (Berlex, 2004a). The IUS, like the rest of the hormonal family planning methods, does not provide protection from STIs. The effectiveness of the IUS and unintended pregnancy is 0.1 percent for both perfect use and typical use (Hatcher et al., 2004).

NONHORMONAL INTRAUTERINE METHODS

Nonhormonal intrauterine methods are those devices inserted into the uterus to prevent pregnancy. The IUS was discussed in the previous section. The main difference between the IUS and the intrauterine device (IUD) is the presence of hormones. The IUD does not contain hormones. Currently, only the Copper T IUD and the hormone releasing IUS are available in the United States (Hatcher et al., 2004; Kaunitz, 2005). The next section discusses the IUD.

Intrauterine Device

The intrauterine device (IUD) is a small, flexible, T-shaped plastic device with copper on both the arms and stem (FEI Women's Health, 2005). The IUD works by preventing the sperm from reaching or fertilizing the egg, as well as by preventing implantation of the fertilized egg in the uterus. Unlike many of the other methods discussed, the IUD does not prevent ovulation. A healthcare professional must insert the IUD. The insertion process parallels the IUS insertion process. The main difference between the IUD and IUS beside the presence of hormones is the duration of protection. The IUD provides 10 years of protection compared to the 5 years provided by the IUS. Like the IUS, the IUD must be removed 10 years after it is placed. If the woman would like to continue use of the IUD, a new one can be inserted when the old one is removed.

The most common side effects of the IUD are pain and fainting with insertion and/or removal, heavy bleeding between menstrual periods, and occasionally skipping a menstrual period. On rare occasions, partial or total uterine perforation may occur on insertion. It is also possible that the IUD may be expelled during the menstrual cycle (FEI Women's Health, 2005). The woman will need to feel for the two strings that hang just below the cervix in the vagina to ensure the IUD is in the correct place. The IUD does not provide protection from STIs. The effectiveness of the IUD and unintended pregnancy is 0.6 percent for perfect use and 0.8 percent for typical use (Hatcher et al., 2004).

STERILIZATION

Sterilization is a permanent family planning method available for both women and men that involves a surgical intervention making the reproductive organs incapable of producing or delivering viable sperm and eggs (Strong et al., 2005). For all practical purposes, sterilization should be considered as an irreversible family planning method. In the next section female sterilization methods and male sterilization methods are discussed.

Female Sterilization

Female sterilization can occur in a variety of ways. The most common female sterilization method is a tubal ligation or "tube tying." During a tubal ligation, the fallopian tubes are surgically cut, clipped, banded, or burned. By blocking the fallopian tubes, the egg released from the ovary cannot reach the uterus, and sperm entering the cervix and uterus cannot reach the egg. Tubal ligations are performed using a variety of surgical techniques. The techniques differ based on the approach to reach the fallopian tubes. Some physicians make surgical incisions through the abdomen, while others reach the tubes through the vagina and cervix. The procedures utilizing abdominal incisions are called laparoscopies or minilaparotomies. Procedures performed through the vagina and cervix are called culpotomies or culdoscopies. Each procedure has advantages and disadvantages which should be discussed with a physician.

When tubal ligation is used for female sterilization, menstruation continues since the uterus and ovaries are unaffected. In some cases the uterus or ovaries need to be removed for medical reasons. These procedures are called hysterectomies and oophrectomies. If the uterus and/or ovaries are removed, menstruation will cease, which is called surgical menopause.

A new female sterilization technique available is called Essure. The Essure procedure entails placing small, flexible micro-inserts into the fallopian tubes. Once the microinserts are in place, body tissue grows into them causing the blockage of the tubes (Conceptus, 2004). The woman must use an alternative family planning method for the first three months after the micro-insert placement since it may take up to three months for the tissue to block the tubes.

Regardless of which female sterilization method is being considered, the woman must remember two important points. First, female sterilization is permanent. While some procedures can be reversed, reversal is costly and failure rates are high (Hatcher et al., 2004). Second, sterilization does not protect against STIs. Counseling to ensure family completion or the desire for no (more) children must be undertaken prior to sterilization. The effectiveness of female sterilization and unintended pregnancy is 0.5 percent for both perfect use and typical use (Hatcher et al., 2004).

Male Sterilization

Male sterilization is a permanent family planning method for men that is achieved by preventing the sperm from entering the seminal fluid. The sperm are blocked through a procedure called a vasectomy. During a vasectomy, the vas deferens are cut or burned. This procedure is done through incision(s) in the scrotum (Strong et al., 2005) or by piercing the scrotal skin with metal forceps (Hatcher et al., 2004) to reach the vas deferens. Like the female sterilization methods, there are advantages and disadvantages to the various techniques. The techniques, as well as the side effects, should be discussed with a physician prior to sterilization.

Vasectomies do not affect a man's ability to become erect or ejaculate. Because sperm can live in the man's reproductive system for days to weeks after the vasectomy, an alternative family planning method should be used until his semen has been confirmed as sperm-free. Males should undergo the same counseling as women considering sterilization to confirm that families are complete and no (more) children are desired. Men should also remember that sterilization is considered permanent and does not protect against STIs. Though reversals can be performed, there is no guarantee that fertility will return. The effectiveness of male sterilization and unintended pregnancy is 0.10 percent for perfect use and 0.15 percent for typical use (Hatcher et al., 2004).

FUTURE FAMILY PLANNING METHODS

Jones (1997) noted that the ideal contraceptive would be:

1. Highly effective
2. Virtually free of side effects

3. Not require conscientious adherence to the method
4. Long-acting
5. Reversible
6. Help prevent transmission of sexually transmitted disease
7. Inexpensive
8. Used by either sex if possible
9. Not interfere with sexual satisfaction. (p. 284)

A method fulfilling all these criteria does not exist. However, family planning method development continues today. The following family planning methods in development are discussed in the next section: oral contraceptives, transdermal methods, vaginal rings, implants, intrauterine devices, quinacrine sterilization, male contraceptive delivery systems, vaccines, and microbicides.

Oral Contraceptives

Two specific types of new oral contraceptives are in development. Lower dose combined oral contraceptives with 15 micrograms of ethinyl estrodial are being used in Europe (Hatcher et al., 2004). Another OC in development is one containing folic acid since many pregnancies occur due to the incorrect usage of the OCs. Adequate levels of folic acid are needed to prevent neural tube defects in developing fetuses. Since mothers often have an inadequate intake of folic acid and unintended pregnancies do occur even when taking OCs, an OC with folic acid has the potential to prevent the birth of children with disabilities secondary to neural tube defects (Kaunitz, 2005).

Transdermal Methods

In addition to the contraceptive patch, two other transdermal methods, the transdermal gel and transdermal spray, are in development. Nomegestrol acetate (NES) is a nonandrogenic progestin that is inactive when taken orally, but potent when administered through non-oral methods. The NES methods are being developed because they do not have the side effects of acne, oily skin, and changes in lipid profiles that the methods with androgenic progestins do (Sitruk-Ware, 2005). The gel and sprays in development contain NES, which aids in inhibiting ovulation.

Vaginal Rings

Four new vaginal rings are in development: the Progering, NES/EE ring, NES ring, and CDB-2914 or VA-2914 rings. The duration of action for the Progering is six months continuously. The NES/EE ring provides one year of contraceptive coverage while the NES ring provides six months of coverage. The duration of action for the CDB-2914 or VA-2914 rings is three months continuously. These rings in development provide a longer duration of protection than the current vaginal ring available on the market.

Implants

Norplant was an implantable contraceptive system that was first approved in 1983, but is no longer available in the United States. The system of six rods containing levonorgestrel (LNG) were implanted beneath the skin of the upper arm and provided protection for five to seven years depending on the age and weight of the woman (Hatcher et al., 2004; Wyeth Laboratories, 2003). Wyeth Laboratories stopped distributing Norplant due to the difficulties reported when healthcare providers were trying to remove the implants from patients (Sitruk-Ware, 2005).

Though Norplant is no longer available, two new implants have been developed, Jadelle and Implanon. Jadelle is a two-rod implant containing LNG, which provides coverage for five years (Sitruk-Ware, 2005). Implanon is a single-rod implant containing the progestin etonogestrel (ENG), which is effective for three years (Organon (c), 2003). All of the implants must be removed when their duration of effectiveness is over, though new implants can be inserted at the time of removal. At this time, none of the implants are available on the United States' market.

Intrauterine Devices

GyneFix Copper IUD is the new IUD in development. GyneFix differs from the existing IUDs in that it is frameless. The string containing six copper sleeves is embedded in the top of the uterus and protrudes through the cervix for monthly monitoring (Hatcher et al., 2004). The concept behind the GyneFix development was that uterine size differs in each woman. The current IUDs with frames often do not fit women and migrate or are expelled from the uterus (GyneFix, n.d.). GyneFix is effective for five years and has a lower expulsion rate due to its frameless structure. It is currently unavailable in the United States.

Quinacrine Sterilization

Quinacrine sterilization (QS) is a nonsurgical method of permanent sterilization. Seven pellets of the drug quinacrine are inserted into the uterus with an applicator similar to the ones used to insert IUDs. Once the pellets are inserted, they dissolve, seep into the fallopian tubes, and cause scarring in the tubes. The scarring prevents the sperm from reaching the egg. The process is repeated an additional one to two times at monthly intervals (Informed Consent Working Group, 2003). Quinacrine is not currently approved by the

United States Food and Drug Administration (FDA) for use as a sterilization method.

Male Contraceptive Delivery Systems

The male contraceptive delivery systems in development include subdermal implants, orals and injections, orals and implants, and implants and injections (Sitruk-Ware, 2005). Many of these methods work by combining norethisterone enanthate (NETE) and testosterone undecanoate (TU) to suppress the production of sperm. In some cases, the men experienced azoospermia or no sperm present in their ejaculate (Meriggiola et al., 2005). A nonhormonal method of male sterilization in development includes an injection of a temporary polymer into the vas deferens to block sperm (Strong et al., 2005).

Vaccines

Contraceptive vaccines are in development for both women and men. Three specific types of vaccines are being studied: those that target the gamete (sperm and egg) production; those that target the gamete function; and those that target the gamete outcome (Naz, 2005). For gamete production, the specific targets are gonadotropin releasing hormone, follicle-stimulating hormone, and lutenizing hormone. For gamete function, the specific targets are the zona pellucida proteins and sperm antigens, and for gamete outcome the specific target is human chorionic gonadotropin (hCG). The vaccine furthest along in the development process is the hCG vaccine, a gamete outcome vaccine. Men and women may be sensitized to their own sperm and egg cells through the contraceptive vaccines (Strong et al., 2005).

Microbicides

While the main focus of this chapter has been on pregnancy prevention methods, one major concern when choosing a method is the protection against not only pregnancy, but also STIs. New methods are in development to fight STIs more effectively, specifically microbicides. Microbicides are agents used to kill microbes (bacteria, fungi, viruses, etc.). A variety of microbicides are in development to fight STIs including: BufferGel, PRO 2000 0.5 percent and 2 percent, Carraguard, Savvy, and Ushercell (Balzarini & Van Damme, 2005; Sitruk-Ware, 2005). These microbicides are in the form of vaginal gels. The categories of microbicides in development range from non-specific to more specific to highly specific for HIV. Microbicides that function as spermicides as well, may not be available for another 5–10 years (Hatcher et al., 2004). A breakthrough in microbicidal development could have a huge impact on decreasing HIV transmission, particularly in underdeveloped countries where HIV rates are high and medical care is not readily available.

SUMMARY

The purpose of this chapter was to give a broad overview of the family planning methods available in the United States today. As demonstrated throughout the chapter, a plethora of methods are in existence with many more in development. The chapter progressed through minimally invasive methods to maximally invasive methods, and finished with a look at the future of family planning. With all the family planning methods available, one might think that unintended pregnancy would be low; however, that is not the case. Choosing a family planning method or methods is not enough to prevent unintended pregnancy. Those methods must be communicated between partners and used correctly every time. Correct and consistent method use is the key to effective family planning.

The majority of the methods discussed do not protect against STIs when used alone. It is not only important to communicate about method choice with partners, but also about STI protection. If in doubt whether a partner is at risk for transmitting a STI, make sure to use additional family planning methods that protect against STI transmission. The abundance of methods available can leave you feeling overwhelmed, however there are health practitioners available at doctors offices, university health systems, public health and family planning clinics. Once a method is chosen, family planning can be easy and effective with communication and consistent use.

REFERENCES

Allendale Pharmaceuticals Inc. (2005). *About the sponge.* Retrieved August 13, 2005, from http://www.todayssponge.com/howtouse.htm.

Bailey, J., Farquhar, C., Owen, C., & Whittaker, D. (2003). Sexual behavior of lesbians and bisexual women. *Sexually Transmitted Infections, 79,* 147–150.

Balzarini, J., & Van Damme, L. (2005). Intravaginal and intrarectal microbicides to prevent HIV infection. *Canadian Medical Association Journal, 172(4),* 461–464.

Berlex. (2004). Yasmin 28 tablets: Combination brief and detailed patient labeling. Montville, NJ: Berlex.

Berlex . (2000a). Mirena: Levonorgestrel-releasing intrauterine system: Patient information booklet. Montville, NJ: Berlex.

Conceptus. (2004). Essure: The non-incisional approach to permanent birth control: Patient information booklet. San Carlos, CA: Conceptus Incorporated.

Crooks, R., & Baur, K. (1999). *Our sexuality* (7th ed.). Pacific Grove, CA: Brooks/Cole Publishing Company.

Davis, A., & Castaño, P. (2004). Oral contraceptives and libido in women. *Annual Review of Sex Research, XV,* 297–320.

Duramed Pharmaceuticals, Inc. (2003). Seasonale: Package insert. Pomona, NY: Duramed Pharmaceuticals, Inc.

FEI Women's Health. (2005). Paragard T 380A intrauterine copper contraceptive: Patient package. Tonawanda, NY: FEI Products, LLC.

FemCap. (2005). Directions for use. Retrieved September 26, 2005, from http://www. femcap.com/directions.htm.

Gaines, D. (2005). Pros and cons of ovulation prediction kits (OPKs). Retrieved September 25, 2005, from http://health.discovery.com/centers/pregnancy/americanbaby/opks.html.

Grimes, D. (2003). Frequent daily use of nonoxynol-9 may increase the risk of HIV infection. *The Contraception Report, 13(4)*, 4–6.

Grimes, D., Gallo, M., Grigorieva, V., Nanda, K., & Schultz, K. (2005). Fertility awareness-based methods for contraception: Systematic review of randomized controlled trials. *Contraception, 75*, 85–90.

GyneFix. (n.d.). GyneFix: Prescribing information. Retrieved October 8, 2005. from http://www.contrel.be/GYNEFIX%20SPECIALISTS/prescribing_information.htm.

Hatcher, R., Rinehart, W., Blackburn, R., Geller, J., & Shelton, J. (2001). *The essentials of contraceptive technology.* Baltimore, MD: Johns Hopkins University School of Public Health, Population Information Program.

Hatcher, R., Zieman, M., Cwiak, C., Darney, P., Creinin, M., & Stosur, H. (2004). *A pocket guide to managing contraception 2004–2005 edition.* Tiger, GA: The Bridging the Gap Foundation. Informed Consent Working Group. (2003). Quinacrine sterilization (QS): Informed consent. *International Journal of Gynecology and Obstetrics, 83*(Suppl. 2), S147-S159.

Jones, R. (1997). *Human reproductive biology* (2nd ed.). San Diego, CA: Academic Press.

Kaunitz, A. (2005). Beyond the pill: New data and options in hormonal and intrauterine contraception. *American Journal of Obstetrics and Gynecology, 192*, 998–1004.

Kuyoh, M., Toroitich-Ruto, D., Grimes, K., Schulz, M., & Gallo, M. (2003). Sponge versus diaphragm for contraception: A Cochrane review. *Contraception, 67*, 15–18.

Lea's Shield. (2004). Common questions. Retrieved September 26, 2005. from http://www.leasshield.com/faq.htm.

Meriggiola, M., Costantino, A., Saad, F., D'Emidio, L., Morselli Labate, A., Bertaccini, A., et al. (2005). Norethisterone enanthate plus testosterone undecanoate for male contraception: Effects of various injection intervals on spermatogenesis, reproductive hormones, testis, and prostate. *The Journal of Clinical Endocrinology & Metabolism, 90(4)*, 2005–2014.

Naz, R. (2005). Contraceptive vaccines. *Drugs, 65*(5), 593–603.

Organon. (2003). Cyclessa: Physician insert. West Orange, NJ: Organon USA Inc.

Organon (a). (2004). Desogen: Package insert. West Orange, NJ: Organon USA Inc.

Organon (b). (2004). Nuvaring: Physician's insert. West Orange, NJ: Organon USA Inc.

Organon (c). (2003). Implanon: Implant for subdermal use: Standard. West Orange, NJ: Organon USA Inc.

Ortho-McNeil. (2005). Ortho Evra: Prescribing information. Raritan, NJ: Ortho-McNeil Pharmaceutical, Inc.

Pharmacia & Upjohn. (2004). Depo-Provera contraceptive injection: Patient labeling. Kalamazoo, MI: Pharmacia & Upjohn Company.

Potts, M., & Campbell, M. (2002). History of contraception. *Gynecology and Obstetrics, 6* (8), *1–27*. Retrieved September 9, 2006, from http://big.berkeley.edu/ifplp. history.pdf.

Sitruk-Ware, R. (2005). Delivery options for contraceptives. *Drug Discovery Today, 10*(14), 977–985.

Strong, B., DeVault, C., Syad, B., & Yarber, W. (2005). *Human sexuality: Diversity in contemporary America* (5th ed.). NY: McGraw-Hill.

Truitt, S. T., Fraser, A. B., Grimes, D. A., Gallo, M. F., & Schulz, K. F. (2003). Combined hormonal versus nonhormonal progestin-only contraception in lactation. *Cochran Database Syst Rev. 2003*, (2), CD003988.

Van Damme, L., Ramjee, G., Alary, M., Vuylsteke, B., Chandeying, V., Rees, H., et al. (2002). Effectiveness of COL-1492, a nonoxynol-9 vaginal gel, on HIV-1 transmission in female sex workers: A randomized controlled trial. *Lancet, 360*, 971–977.

Wikipedia (September 22, 2005). Birth control. Retrieved September 24, 2005, from http://en.wikipedia.org/wiki/Family_planning.

World Health Organization. (2003). *WHO/CONRAD technical consultation on nonoxynol-9.* Geneva, Switzerland: World Health Organization.

Wyeth. (2004). Aless-28 tablets: Information for the patient. Philadelphia, PA: Wyeth Pharmaceuticals Inc.

Wyeth Laboratories. (2003). Norplant system: Levonorgestrel implants: Prescribing information. Philadelphia, PA: Wyeth Laboratories.

Chapter Eleven

SEXUALLY TRANSMITTED INFECTIONS

Raven James

In this chapter, a variety of sexually transmitted infections (STIs, formerly known as sexually transmitted diseases [STDs]) are discussed. The shift in terminology to *STI* resulted from the mind-set that many of these infections are not diseases, and that the term *infection* more accurately and inclusively describes their etiology. *STI* will be the terminology used in this chapter.

The United States has the highest rate of STIs of any industrialized nation. Sexually active youth in the United States account for about half of all the new cases of annual infections. More than half of all Americans will get a STI at some point in their lifetime (American Social Health Association [ASHA], 2005).

STIs have been in existence for centuries. Some of these infections are curable (bacterial); others are not (viral). With the growing rates of STIs and emergence of new types of viral infections over the last few decades, the implications for treatment and prevention of STIs have become more complex and frustrating for educators and providers alike.

Most individuals will present with sexual risk and infection over the course of their lives. The information presented here is intended to assist readers in making informed decisions about sexual choices they are likely to encounter and in talking to sexual partners about STIs, testing and prevention. This important process of knowledge and intervention is crucial for initiating, developing and maintaining healthy relationships and lifestyles.

The CDC estimates that 19 million new infections occur each year, almost half of them among young people ages 15–24 (Weinstock, Berman & Cates, 2004). The number of documented AIDS cases in the United States is over 900,000 with approximately 40,000 new HIV infections each year (Centers for Disease Control [CDC], 2004). Although AIDS diagnosis and deaths are lower than in previous times, the decrease has more to do with treatment intervention than rates of infection. STIs and HIV disproportionately impact the health of African Americans and Latino's as compared with Whites. Here is a brief summary of some STI statistics in the United States:

- Chlamydia is the most prevalent bacterial STI with approximately three million new cases annually. The highest infection rates are in 15–19 year olds (CDC, 2006).
- In 2004, 929,462 chlamydia cases were reported (CDC, 2004a).
- Gonorrhea is the second most commonly reported infectious disease in the United States, with 330, 132 cases reported in 2004 (CDC, 2004a).
- Trichomoniasis is the most common curable STI in young, sexually active women. An estimated 7.4 million new cases occur each year in women and men (CDC, 2006b).
- Over the past four years the syphilis rate in the United States has been increasing, mainly in metropolitan areas with large populations of men who have sex with men (CDC, 2004a).
- Nationwide, at least 45 million people ages 12 and older, or one out of five adolescents and adults, have had HSV infection (CDC, 2006d).
- Every year, about 5.5 million Americans acquire genital HPV infection (CDC, 2006e).
- As of 2001, an estimated 3.9 million Americans have chronic Hepatitis C (Hepnet.com, 2006).

Despite of the high incidence of STIs, knowledge levels are low in adolescents, adults, and their health care providers. Continuing to ignore the existence and risk of STIs will not make the problem disappear. By educating students and other health care professionals and ourselves, we can help find ways to intervene, prevent, and treat STIs.

Many factors contribute to the epidemic of STIs in the United States. Having multiple partners and sexual contact with no barriers is a major reason for the high incidence of STIs in adolescence and early adulthood (Feroli & Burstein, 2003). Lack of adequate public health measures and limited access to treatment also contribute to this major health problem (volume 3, chapter 1). It is common for physicians and nurse practitioners to be reluctant to ask questions about their patient's sexual behaviors, and thereby to lose opportunities for STI-related counseling, diagnosis and treatment. A nationally representative survey of 3,390 U.S. adults, ages 18–64, found that only 28 percent reported being asked about STIs during routine medical checkups (Tao, Irvin, & Kassler, 2000). Another national survey that examined sex, alcohol and STIs found that problematic drinking among men and women can increase the risk for STI (Erikson & Trocki, 1994).

The majority of persons with STIs are asymptomatic (have no symptoms) and unaware of their infections. This contributes to the spread of STIs. Commonly, women and men will not experience any symptoms, despite having an infection. In this instance, a person may unknowingly infect another person with a STI. Often, infected individuals are embarrassed to seek treatment or talk to their partner about being infected, exacerbating the situation. In the prevention section, we will learn tips for talking to a partner about STIs, as well as tips for safer sex practices.

STIs can be broken down into two categories, bacterial and viral. The bacterial STIs are curable; the viral STIs are incurable although antiviral drugs are being developed at this time despite efforts to develop drugs to treat viral infections. The following sections will discuss bacterial STIs, viral STIs, common vaginal infections, and prevention strategies. Causes, symptoms and complications, diagnosis, and treatments will be covered for each infection. Most of the factual information regarding the infections discussed in this chapter is based on The Centers for Disease Control and Prevention (CDC) treatment guidelines. If you need more information, it is recommended that you contact your local health department, or call CDC Information. This information can be located in the Resource section at the end of this chapter. These services can answer questions, provide free literature or refer you to a local clinic for testing and treatment.

BACTERIAL INFECTIONS

CHLAMYDIA—Chlamydia is a sexually transmitted infection caused by the bacterium, *Chlamydia trachomatis*.

Incidence and Transmission

Chlamydia is the most common STI in the United States (CDC, 2006). Any sexually active person can be infected with chlamydia. Most often, chlamydia is found in younger people who have multiple sex partners. Because the cervix (opening to the uterus) of teenage girls and young women is not fully matured, they are at particular risk for infection if sexually active. Chlamydia is spread through oral, vaginal, or anal sexual contact. It can also be transmitted from mother to infant during childbirth.

Young women who use oral contraceptives are at particular risk for developing chlamydia infection if exposed (Ivey, 1997). Part of the reason for this is that young women are thinking about birth control, and neglect to use protection against chlamydia infection, such as condoms or dental dams (see chapter 10 of this volume). Research has also identified douching as a risk factor for chlamydia infection (Peters et al., 1992; Sievert & Black, 2000). Douching one or more time per month can adversely affect the normal bacterial levels of the vagina (lactobacilli) that help maintain a healthy vaginal environment, thus increasing susceptibility to bacterial agents (Ness et al., 2003).

Symptoms and Complications

Symptoms of Chlamydia, if present, generally appear in men and women in about two weeks after infection. However, most individuals (both men and women), show no symptoms, thus the infection is also known as a "silent" disease. Symptoms of chlamydia for both males and females include a discharge, and discomfort urinating (urethritis). Females may experience lower abdominal pain, fever, nausea, pain during intercourse, bleeding between menstrual periods and general malaise. A newborn that has been infected by the mother may contract neonatal pneumonia or neonatal conjunctivitis (pink eye).

People who do not experience symptoms are at risk for developing complications of chlamydia. Most complications from chlamydia affect women and stem from Pelvic Inflammatory Disease (PID). PID will develop in about 40 percent of women untreated for chlamydia, and can cause chronic pelvic pain, ectopic pregnancies, infertility, permanent damage to the fallopian tubes and surrounding tissue and the need for hysterectomies. Women infected with chlamydia are up to five times more likely to become infected with HIV, if exposed (CDC, 2006).

Complications of chlamydia in men are rare. Sometimes, infection can spread to the epididymis (the tube that carries sperm from the testes) and cause pain, fever and rarely, sterility.

Diagnosis and Treatment

Chlamydia is diagnosed with two types of laboratory tests. One test involves collecting a specimen from an infected site (penis or cervix) to directly test for the bacterium; the other is a urine test that can accurately detect the bacteria. Chlamydia is treated with antibiotics such as doxycycline, azithromycin, amoxicillin, ofloxacin, and erythromycin (all generic names). A single dose of azithromycin or doxycycline (twice daily) are the most commonly used treatments and are taken by mouth.

Past infection does not give immunity to chlamydia. In fact, previous infections can allow complications to occur more rapidly. All sex partners should be tested and treated, if necessary. Infected persons should abstain from sexual contact until they and their sexual partners have completed treatment, otherwise re-infection is likely.

GONORRHEA—Gonorrhea is an infection caused by the bacterium *Neisseria gonorrhoeae.*

Incidence and Transmission

The bacterium that causes gonorrhea can multiply easily in warm, moist areas of the body, including the reproductive tract, the cervix, uterus, urinary tract as well as the eyes, throat, mouth and anus. Gonorrhea is a very common infectious disease. Approximately 700,000 Americans will become infected each year with gonorrhea (CDC, 2006a).

Any sexually active person can become infected with gonorrhea. Most often, gonorrhea is found in younger people (ages 15–30) who have multiple sex partners. Gonorrhea is reported more frequently from urban areas rather than from rural areas. Gonorrhea is spread through sexual contact between penis, vagina, mouth, or anus. It can also be transmitted from mother to child during childbirth. Touching infected genitals, and then the eyes can also pass gonorrhea. Re-infection can occur if the treated person comes into contact with the bacterium again.

Symptoms and Complications

In males, symptoms usually appear two to seven days after infection but may take as long as 30 days to begin. Symptoms include a burning sensation while urinating, or a white, yellow or green discharge from the penis. Sometimes men with gonorrhea experience painful or swollen testicles. About ten to fifteen percent of men will not show any symptoms, but they are still at risk for developing complications as well as unknowingly passing the infection to others.

In females, the symptoms of gonorrhea are often mild, and about 80 percent of infected women will not show any symptoms. Often, when a woman is infected with gonorrhea, the symptoms are so general they may be mistaken for a bladder or vaginal infection and may go undetected. Symptoms in women include a discharge, a painful or burning sensation while urinating, or bleeding between menstrual periods. As with men, asymptomatic women are at risk for complications and infecting others.

Symptoms of rectal infection in both men and women include discharge, anal itching, soreness, bleeding, or painful bowel movements. Rectal infection may also be asymptomatic. Infections in the throat may cause soreness, but mostly are asymptomatic as well.

Complications of untreated gonorrhea infection in women include PID, which can lead to chronic abdominal pain, fever, infertility, and increased risk of ectopic pregnancy or damage to the fallopian tubes and surrounding tissue. In men, gonorrhea can cause epididymitis, a painful condition of the testicles that can lead to infertility if left untreated. Without treatment, gonorrhea can also affect the prostate and can lead to scarring inside the urethra, making urination difficult.

Gonorrhea can spread to the joints or blood. This condition can be life threatening. People infected with gonorrhea are more likely to contract HIV, if exposed. HIV-infected persons with gonorrhea are more likely to transmit HIV to another person (CDC, 2006a).

A pregnant woman with gonorrhea may infect her baby as it passes through the birth canal during delivery. The infection in newborns can cause blindness, joint infection, or a life-threatening blood infection. Treatment of pregnant women is recommended as soon as it is detected to reduce the risk of infection and these complications to the newborn. Pregnant women should not be treated with quinolones or tetracyclines; they should be treated with a recommended or alternate cephalosporin. Women who cannot tolerate a cephalosporin should be administered a single, 2-gram dose of spectinomycin intramuscularly (CDC Treatment Guidelines, 2002).

Diagnosis and Treatment

Several laboratory tests are available to diagnose gonorrhea. A medical worker can do a swab test and obtain a sample for testing from the infected parts of the body (cervix, urethra, rectum, or throat) and send the sample to a laboratory for analysis. A urine test can be used is the bacterium is present in the cervix or urethra. A Gram stain is a quick laboratory test that can be done in a medical office, allowing bacterium to be seen under a microscope. The Gram stain is more accurate for men than for women.

Gonorrhea is treated with penicillin or other antibiotics in pill form or by injection into the buttocks. All strains of gonorrhea are curable, but this infection is becoming more and more resistant to many standard medications. Commonly, gonorrhea and chlamydia infection can occur together, in which case antibiotics for both infections are usually given together.

SYPHILIS—Syphilis is primarily a sexually transmitted infection caused by the bacterium *Treponema pallidum.*

Incidence and Transmission

Syphilis has been called "the great imitator" because so many of the signs and symptoms are similar to other diseases. Although rates of syphilis infection have decreased in women, rates amongst men are 3.5 times those of women. In 2002, the incidence of infectious syphilis in the United States was highest in women 20 to 24 years of age and men 35 to 39 years of age (CDC, 2006c).

Syphilis is spread by sexual contact with an infected individual through direct contact with syphilis sores. Sores occur mainly on the external genitals, vagina, anus, or in the rectum. Sores can also occur on the mouth and lips. Transmission by sexual contact requires exposure to moist lesions of the skin or mucus membranes. Transmission of the organism occurs through vaginal, anal or oral sex. Congenital syphilis is passed from mother to fetus.

Symptoms and Complications

The first sign of syphilis (primary stage) is usually a sore (called a chancre), that is painless and appears at the site of initial contact. There can be multiple sores possibly accompanied by swollen glands that develop within a week after the appearance of the initial sore. The time between infection with syphilis and the appearance of the first chancre can range from 10 to 90 days (average 21 days). The chancre is usually firm, round, small, and painless. The sore will last from three to five weeks, and will disappear by itself even if no treatment is received. Persons infected are still infectious to others, even though symptoms may come and go. If treatment is not received during this time, the infection progresses to the secondary stage.

Skin rash and mucous membrane lesions appear during the secondary stage of syphilis. These lesions and rashes can appear as the chancre is healing, approximately six weeks after the first sore appears. The rash may appear as red, rough reddish spots on the palms of the hands and feet (palmar rashes) and usually does not itch. The rashes may appear on other parts of the body (trunk, arms, and legs) and resemble other diseases; they may be so faint that they go unnoticed. Swollen glands, sore throat, spotty hair loss, weight loss, headaches, muscle ache and fatigue may also occur in this stage. The symptoms in this stage will disappear without treatment and the infection progresses to a latency stage.

The latent stage begins when the secondary symptoms disappear, and without treatment, there may be no noticeable symptoms for years. The person remains infected and infectious, and the disease continues to progress, causing damage to the internal organs, including the heart, brain, nerves, eyes, liver, bones and joints. Internal damage can take years to develop. Signs of late stage syphilis (tertiary stage) include paralysis, numbness, gradual blindness, dementia, and difficulty coordinating muscle movements. If left untreated, death may also occur.

The syphilis bacterium can infect the baby of a pregnant woman, causing stillborn babies, or one who dies shortly after birth. Depending on how long the pregnant woman has been infected, the baby may be born without signs or symptoms. If not treated immediately, the baby may develop serious problems, become developmentally delayed, have seizures, or die.

Diagnosis and Treatment

Diagnosis of syphilis is done one of two ways; some health care providers can examine material from a chancre using a special "dark-field" microscope, otherwise, a blood test will determine whether a person is infected with the bacterium. Antibodies will develop shortly after infection, and can be detected by the blood test. A low level of antibodies will remain in the blood for years after treatment, but health care providers can tell by the levels (titer) whether it is an active infection or one that has been treated.

Treatment for syphilis is simple in its early stages. A single injection of penicillin will cure a person who has had the infection for less than a year. Additional doses are necessary to treat a person who had had syphilis longer than a year. Other antibiotics are available to treat syphilis for those who are allergic to penicillin. Damage done by syphilis is not reversible, even though the bacterium can be cured, so early detection and treatment are important if someone has been infected with this particular bacterium.

NON-GONOCOCCAL URETHRITIS—Any inflammation of the urethra that is not caused by gonorrhea is called non-gonococcal urethritis or NGU.

Incidence and Transmission

It is believed that chlamydia and two other bacteria are primary causes of NGU (ASHA, 2006). NGU can also result from other infectious agents, allergic reactions to vaginal secretions or irritation from soaps, vaginal contraceptives or deodorant sprays.

NGU affects more men than women. Although NGU primarily produces symptoms in men, it is believed that women also carry the organisms that can cause NGU. The most common route of transmission is through vaginal intercourse. The bacteria can also be passed by mouth to penis sex, suggesting that oral factors and oral bacteria can also cause NGU (Lafferty, Hiltunen-Back, Reuwala, Neiman, & Paavonen, 1997).

Symptoms and Complications

Men who contract NGU often show symptoms similar to gonorrhea, including discharge from the penis and mild burning sensation during urination. The discharge is usually less pronounced than in gonorrhea. Women are often unaware of NGU infection unless informed by a male partner of his infection. There may be mild itching, or painful urination, but generally, symptoms are absent in women.

Symptoms usually disappear 2 to 3 months after infection without treatment, but the disease may still be present. If left untreated in women, it can cause cervical inflammation or PID; in men, it can spread to the prostate, epididymis, or both. In rare cases, untreated NGU can produce a form of arthritis.

Treatment

A single dose of azithromycin (generic) or a week of doxycycline (generic) usually clears NGU infection. All sexual partners should be examined and treated if necessary.

TRICHOMONIASIS—This bacterial STI is caused by the single-cell protozoan parasite, *Trichomoniasis vaginalis*.

Incidence and Transmission

There are an estimated 5 million American cases each year of Trichomoniasis, also called "Trich." Transmission occurs through penis to vagina or vulva to vulva contact. The vagina is the most common site of infection in women and the urethra (urine canal) is the most common site of infection in men.

Symptoms and Complications

Symptoms in men are often absent. However, some men may have an irritation inside the penis, mild discharge, or slight burning after urination or ejaculation. Women may experience a frothy, yellow-green vaginal discharge with a strong odor. This may cause discomfort during intercourse, as well as itching of the female genital area. Rarely, abdominal pain may occur. Symptoms in women usually occur within 5–28 days after infection. Complications resulting from this infection can include increased susceptibility to HIV if exposed, an increase in the transmissibility of HIV, if infected, as well as early birth or low birth weight (under five pounds) in pregnant women (CDC, 2006b).

Diagnosis and Treatment

Trichomoniasis infection is diagnosed with a physical examination and a laboratory test. The parasite is more difficult to detect in men than in women. In women, the examination can reveal small red ulcerations on the vaginal wall or cervix.

Trichomoniasis is usually treated with the prescription drug, metronidazole (generic name), which is administered by mouth in a single dose. This treatment usually cures the infection. Both partners should be treated at the same time. Metronidazole can also be used by pregnant women.

VIRAL INFECTIONS

HERPES—Herpes is caused by the *Herpes simplex virus* (HSV).

Incidence and Transmission

There are eight different types of herpes viruses that can infect humans, the most common being the varcilla-zoster virus (VZV) that causes chicken pox, followed by Herpes simplex virus type 1 (HSV-1) and Herpes simplex virus type 2 (HSV-2). HSV-1 and HSV-2 are usually transmitted sexually, and show up as oral or genital herpes. HSV-1 typically appears as lesions or sores on or near the mouth, oral herpes (commonly called fever blisters or cold sores) and HSV-2 generally causes lesions or sores in the genital area (genital herpes). Although they are two different viruses, oral-genital transmission may occur. HSV-1 can be transmitted from the mouth to the genital area, and HSV-2 can be transmitted from the genitals to the mouth.

One hundred million Americans are estimated to be infected with oral herpes and 50 million with genital herpes (about one in every five persons) (Calvert, 2003; CDC, 2006d). Genital herpes affects more people worldwide than any other STI (Gershengorn & Blower, 2000). An estimated 1 million new cases each year occur in the United States.

Genital herpes can be transmitted through oral-genital, oral-anal, penile-vaginal, and penile-anal contact. Oral herpes can be transmitted through kissing or through oral-genital contact. A person who receives oral sex from partner who has oral herpes can develop genital herpes of either type 1 or type 2, depending on which the partner is infected with. Recent research indicates a shift in genital herpes being caused by HSV-1 herpes (Engelberg, Carrell, Krantz, Corey, & Wald, 2003).

Herpes is most contagious when the sores are present. Avoiding contact with the open lesions through touching, kissing, or intercourse is extremely important during this time. HSV can also be transmitted when there are no visible symptoms (Calvert, 2003; Wald et al., 2000). This is called "asymptomatic viral shedding," labeling the emission of infectious HSV onto body surfaces when there are no symptoms of herpes present. Many cases of herpes are transmitted when the infectious person is not aware of their symptoms (CDC, 2006d).

For prevention, it is recommended to use condoms or other barrier methods at all times, especially if you don't know your partner's status. For those who know they are infected, condoms, and other barrier methods are recommended, especially when visible lesions are present, but this is where talking to partners to decide together and educating yourself about the latest treatments are vital. As are support groups for those newly infected. In the prevention section, there is more information regarding condoms, barriers methods and their limitations. Information regarding support groups can be found in the resource section at the end of this chapter.

Symptoms and Complications

The incubation period of genital herpes is generally 2 to 14 days, and the symptoms last about 20 days. Some individuals do not experience any symptoms of herpes (Donovan, 2004), but are still infectious to their partners. The symptoms usually appear in the genital area as one or more small, red, painful bumps, called papules. The labia are the most common area affected in women. The papules develop into tiny painful blisters that contain a clear fluid. Once the blisters rupture, they form wet, painful open sores surrounded by a red ring. Infected individuals are highly contagious during this time. About 10 days after the papules appear; the open sore forms a crust and begins to heal, taking a good ten days or more.

Other symptoms of HSV include swollen lymph nodes in the groin area, fever, muscle aches and headaches. Women may experience vaginal discharge and sometimes painful urination, especially if the urine contacts the open sores. Sores can recur after healing. The herpes virus remains in a person's nerve endings and flare-ups may be triggered by stress, poor nutrition, depression, extended exposure to sunlight, menstruation in women or other genital infections.

Some individuals experience preliminary signs before outbreaks occur, called prodromal symptoms. When these signs appear, the infected person typically experiences viral shedding and should abstain from unprotected contact with a sexual partner. These indications include a tingling, burning, "pins and needles" or throbbing sensation in the areas where the sores appear. Engaging in unprotected sex with an infected person is a personal choice, which is why talking to partner(s) to decide jointly is important. Herpes *can* be transmitted with no symptoms at all

Complications from herpes are more serious for women than men and include an increased risk of developing cervical cancer and infection of a newborn if she is pregnant. HSV in and of itself does not cause cervical cancer, but acts as a cofactor in the progression of the disease (CDC, 2006d). A newborn can contract herpes in the birth canal, especially if open sores are present near delivery, and cesarean deliveries are recommended to avoid exposure. About 60 percent of untreated infected infants will die or be seriously affected (Corey & Handsfield, 2000).

Another serious complication of herpes can occur when the infected person transfers the virus to an eye after touching a virus-shedding sore. This can lead to a severe eye infection called ocular herpes. To avoid this risk, it is best to avoid touching the open sores, or to wash the hands thoroughly after contact with any sores.

Treatment

There is no cure for oral or genital herpes. Three different antiviral medications are available for treating herpes. Zovirax (generic name is Acyclovir) or Zorifax, is the cheapest and most commonly utilized medication and it is available in oral, topical or injectable forms. Oral acyclovir taken three times daily is the most common; injectable acyclovir is only used in severe cases, and the topical ointment is the least effective mode of this medication. Valtrex (generic name is Valacyclovir) and Famvir (generic name is Famciclovir) are two other oral medications recently available in the United States for treating herpes infection.

There are two main approaches to treating herpes, suppressive and episodic. Suppressive therapy is taken daily to prevent outbreaks and episodic therapy is used only when an outbreak occurs. Episodic therapy has been effective in reducing the total outbreak period and severity of pain during the outbreak. Suppressive therapy reduces but does not eliminate the frequencies of recurrences, and also reduces asymptomatic viral shedding, thus reducing the risk of transmitting the virus to a partner. Often, suppressive therapy is recommended for those persons who have six or more outbreaks per year.

Other measures may help reduce outbreaks or decrease pain and symptoms during an outbreak for the infected person. Taking aspirin can help reduce pain during outbreaks, or using topical anesthetics. Lifestyle choices are also important; reducing stress, improving nutrition, avoiding overexposure to sunlight, avoiding alcohol or other immune suppressing agents can help prevent outbreaks as these are all factors that can trigger outbreaks. Keeping herpes blisters clean and dry can help lesson secondary infection and facilitate healing. Wearing loose clothing can also help reduce irritation to the affected areas. For those who experience frequent outbreaks, being aware of the events preceding outbreaks (such as fatigue, stress, etc.) can assist in avoiding those that may trigger outbreaks.

HUMAN PAPILLOMAVIRUS (HPV) or GENITAL WARTS—Genital HPV infection is a sexually transmitted infection that is caused by *human papillomavirus*.

Incidence and Transmission

There are more than 100 different strains or types of human papillomavirus. More than 30 of these are sexually transmitted, and they can infect the genital area of men and women including the skin of the penis, vulva, anus or lining of the vagina, cervix, or rectum. Most people infected with HPV will not have any symptoms. Once a person is infected with HPV, they will always be infected, even if there are no visible symptoms.

Some of these viruses are called "high-risk" types and may cause abnormal Pap tests in women. They may also lead to cancer of the cervix, vagina, anus or penis. Others are called "low-risk" types and may cause mild Pap test abnormalities or genital warts. Genital warts are single or multiple growths or bumps that appear in the genital area, and are sometimes cauliflower shaped.

Genital HPV is primarily spread through genital contact with an infected person. As most HPV infections have no signs or symptoms, most infected persons are not aware that they are infected, yet they can transmit the virus to a sexual partner. It is rare for a pregnant woman to pass HPV to her baby during vaginal delivery, but if the woman and her physician are aware of the infection, cesarean section can be an option for reducing risk of transmission. A baby that is exposed to HPV very rarely develops warts in the throat.

Approximately 40 million people are currently infected with HPV in the United States (Sauder, Skinner, Fox, & Owens, 2003). At least 50 percent of sexually active men and women acquire genital HPV infection at some point in their lives. By age 50, at least 80 percent of sexually active women will have acquired genital HPV infection (CDC, 2006e). About 5.5 million Americans get a new genital HPV infection each year.

The virus lives in the mucous membranes and usually causes no symptoms. Most people who have a genital HPV infection do not know they are infected; some people develop visible genital warts, or have pre-cancerous changes in the cervix, vulva, anus, or penis. Very rarely, HPV infection results in anal or genital cancers. HPV types 6 and 11 are associated with cancers of the genitals and anus, and types 16 and 18 are linked more to cervical cancer, which is the second leading cause of death in women worldwide (O'Neill-Morante, 2000).

Symptoms and Diagnosis

Genital warts usually appear as soft, moist, pink, or flesh-colored swellings, usually in the genital area. They can be raised or flat, single or multiple, small or large, and are sometimes cauliflower shaped. The warts can appear on the vulva, in and around the vagina, in and around the anus, on the cervix, and on the penis, scrotum, groin, or thigh. After exposure to HPV though an infected person, genital warts can appear from a few weeks, to nine months, or never.

Genital warts are diagnosed by visible inspection. These warts may be removed by self-applied medication prescribed through a physician, or by medical treatments which include cryosurgery, where the warts are freeze-burned off in an outpatient procedure. People sometimes choose not to have treatment if the warts disappear on their own. No one treatment is better than another, but surgical removal of warts is usually done in cases where the warts are numerous and large. Removing the warts does not cure the virus, it only treats the symptoms. The warts can also come back, even years after removal.

HPV is usually diagnosed in women on the basis of an abnormal Pap smear. The Pap test screens for cervical cancer and pre-cancerous changes of the cervix in women. Many abnormal Pap tests are related to HPV infection. An HPV DNA test is available to confirm HPV infection in women and also to help health care providers decide if further tests or treatment are needed. The

HPV DNA test may be used in women over the age of 30, or with mild Pap abnormalities.

Treatment and Prevention

Treatments for HPV include the application of topical ointments such as Podifin (generic name is podofillin toxin), Aldara (generic name is imiquimod) cream, or trichloroacetic acid, and cryotherapy (freezing) with liquid nitrogen or cryoprobe. About 60–70 percent of people respond to these treatments, the other 20–30 percent of people experience recurrence after treatment (Abramowicz, 1994). As a result, many people need second or extended treatments with freezing or topical agents. Cauterization by electric needle, vaporization by carbon dioxide laser, or surgical removal of large or persistent warts may be necessary. There is increasing evidence that many people treated for visible genital warts also have subclinical or asymptomatic HPV infections, which are extremely difficult or impossible to eradicate (Gilbert, Alexander, Grosshans, & Jolley, 2003).

VIRAL HEPATITIS—Hepatitis literally means "inflammation of the liver." In the case of viral hepatitis, the liver becomes inflamed and affected by a virus. The three major types of viral hepatitis are hepatitis A, hepatitis B, and hepatitis C.

Incidence and Transmission

Hepatitis A virus (HAV) infects up to 200,000 Americans every year. It is transmitted through oral-fecal contact, which includes mouth to anus contact (rimming) or through food preparation from an infected person, contaminated water or shellfish. Homosexual men are at higher risk than other groups if they engage in anal intercourse or rimming (Hepnet.com, 2006).

Hepatitis B virus (HBV) infects over 140,000 people every year in the United States. Three to four thousand Americans die each year from cirrhosis and 1,000 from liver cancer due to HBV. About 30 percent of HBV cases are transmitted through heterosexual contact. HBV is 100 times more infectious than HIV (Human Immunodeficiency Virus). Body fluids that can transmit HBV are blood, semen, vaginal fluid and saliva.

Transmission of HBV usually occurs through the skin by needles contaminated with HBV (injection drug use or occupational exposure), but in rare cases has also been passed by hemodialysis, human bites, blood transfusion or transplant. HBV transmission through the mucosal membranes can occur through unprotected oral, vaginal or anal intercourse, from mother to infant via childbirth, blood on household items (toothbrushes or razors) and intranasal drug use (sharing straws for snorting).

Hepatitis C virus (HCV) infects over 150,000 Americans each year. An estimated 3.9 million Americans (about 2% of the entire population) have chronic HCV (Hepnet.com, 2006a). It has been estimated that 75–85 percent of substance users injecting for more than one year will become infected with HCV (Hepnet.com, 2006a). Each year, 8–10,000 Americans die of HCV-related cirrhosis or cancer of the liver.

Hepatitis C is a blood borne pathogen and is primarily transmitted through injection drug use, blood transfusions prior to 1992, clotting factor prior to 1987, occupational exposure for health-care workers, and mother to infant (5–10%). Infection occurs through unprotected sex where blood is present (such as menstruation, anal sex or rough sex), a history of STIs, tattooing or body piercing and intranasal cocaine use (snorting). Sixty percent of HCV cases are reported through injection drug use (IDU), 15 percent through sexual exposure, 10 percent through transfusion (before initial blood product screening in 1990), 5 percent through health care workers (HCW), hemodialysis and mother to child, and 10 percent report unknown risk (Hepnet.com, 2006a). Unknown risk refers to patients that cannot or will not identify any risk factors.

Symptoms and Complications

Symptoms of viral hepatitis vary from nonexistent to mild flu-like symptoms (poor appetite, nausea, diarrhea sore muscles, fatigue, headache) to an incapacitating illness characterized by high fever, vomiting and severe abdominal pain. One of the most notable signs of viral hepatitis is jaundice (yellowing of the whites of the eyes and/or skin). As the disease progresses, the liver enlarges and becomes tender, a person may experience chills, weight loss, develop a distaste for cigarettes and food, the urine darkens and the feces lightens.

With hepatitis A, initial symptoms (acute infection) occur about one week after infection. A person is infectious to others up to two weeks later. No chronic carrier or disease state develops from hepatitis A infection. Individuals will develop immunity after they clear the initial symptoms. Type A is rarely life-threatening. The incubation period is between 15 and 50 days, with 30 being the average. A blood antigen or antibody test is used to diagnose hepatitis A.

One-third of adults and 90 percent of children have no symptoms of HBV. Symptoms last 1–4 weeks to six months for those who develop them. Ten percent of adults do not clear symptoms, 30–50 percent of 1–5 year olds will not clear symptoms, and 80–90 percent of newborns will not clear symptoms. Of adults, 90–95 percent recover within 6 months and develop lifelong immunity. Fifty percent of those adults who do not clear the symptoms will develop acute liver disease.

Initial symptoms may be mild or absent for HCV. The virus is detectable two weeks to six months after infection. Standard blood tests for hepatitis C are the EIA (enzyme immunoassay), RIBA (recombinant immunoblot assay) and the PCR (polymerase chain reaction). The EIA is an inexpensive test that looks for HCV antibodies. If a person is immune compromised, they may test negative with this test but nonetheless be infected. Therefore, the RIBA is used to confirm a positive EIA test. The PCR, also used as a confirmatory test for the EIA, can detect low levels of HCV RNA in serum and is used to diagnose HCV in those who are immunosuppressed; PCR is the most specific test for infection but is expensive and not as available as the EIA and RIBA.

Out of every 100 people infected with HCV:

- 85 may develop long-term infection.
- 70 may develop chronic liver disease.
- 15 may develop cirrhosis over 20–30 years.
- 5 may die from cirrhosis or liver cancer. (Hepnet.com, 2006a)

Treatment and Prevention

At present, no specific therapy is known to be effective against HAV. Treatment usually consists of bed rest and increased fluids to prevent dehydration. The disease usually runs its course in a few weeks, although in cases of severe infection, complete recovery may take several months. HBV treatment is similar to HAV and generally runs its course in several weeks as well. In the case of chronic HBV infection, the antiviral drug interferon or lamivudine is used to treat the infection.

For those 70–80 percent of HCV who are chronic carriers of the virus, there are medications currently available for treatment. A combination therapy of antiviral drugs interferon and ribavarin has been shown to be relatively effective in controlling HCV (Colgan, Michocki, Greisman, & Moore, 2003). About 40 percent of people treated with this therapy actually remain free of the virus with no symptoms of liver disease, 5–12 years after treatment (Smith & Rockey, 2004). The yearly cost of this therapy is high (between $5,000 and $15,000), making its availability to the uninsured and poor a serious problem.

Primary prevention procedures of hepatitis A are as follows:

- hand-washing
- use of gloves when handling body fluids
- risk reduction for anal/oral sex (e.g., condoms, dental dams)
- vaccination of travelers to high incidence areas of hepatitis A with immune globulin

A safe and effective vaccine has been available for HBV since 1982 in the United States and in 1995; the U.S. Food and Drug Administration approved an effective and safe HAV vaccine as well. There is currently no available vaccine for HCV, although efforts are underway to develop one. Persons at high-risk for contracting HAV and HBV should consider getting immunized. These groups include health care workers, injection drug users and their partners, homosexual and bisexual men, heterosexually active persons with multiple partners, sexual partners or housemates of people infected with HAV or HBV, people with chronic liver disease and military personnel working in field conditions (CDC, 2002; Miller & Graves, 2000). In addition, the CDC recommends that all children be vaccinated against HBV.

Other prevention measures for HAV, HBV and HCV include safer sex practices. Prevention for HCV includes not sharing injection equipment, not sharing razors, toothbrushes or straws for snorting drugs. Health care workers, tattoo artists and body piercing shops should all follow standard health precaution practices to minimize the risk of exposure to any bloodborne pathogens.

HUMAN IMMUNODEFICIENCY VIRUS (HIV)—This virus can be sexually transmitted, passed through shared needles, or passed from mother to fetus or infant. HIV compromises the immune system and causes AIDS (Acquired Immune Deficiency Syndrome), a disease that destroys the immune system's ability to fight off diseases. HIV falls into a special category of viruses called retroviruses, so named because they reverse the usual order of reproduction within cells they infect, a process called reverse transcription.

Incidence and Transmission

Over 900,000 cumulative cases of AIDS have been reported in the United States through January 2004, and over 500,000 people have died since it was first discovered in 1981 (CDC, 2005). The number of persons living with HIV in the United States continues to increase. An estimated 1,039,00 to 1,185,000 people in the United States are currently living with HIV infection as of the end of 2003; most of them have not progressed to AIDS (CDC, 2005). The CDC (2005) estimates that 25 percent of all infected persons are not yet aware of their HIV-positive status.

Approximately 5 million new cases of HIV infections occur globally every year, and by January 2003 an estimated 42 million people were infected worldwide (UNAIDS, 2003). More than 3 million persons worldwide die annually from HIV disease and AIDS (CDC, 2005). A projected 45 million additional people worldwide will become infected by 2010 unless health professionals succeed in mounting drastically expanded global prevention efforts (UNAIDS, 2003).

HIV is most commonly passed from one person to another through blood semen, vaginal fluids and breast milk. Other internal body fluids, such as cerebral fluid or spinal fluid can be infectious, but in general, only a surgeon or possibly an Emergency Medical Technician (EMT) would be at risk to exposure from those fluids. Any body fluid that has visible blood can pose a risk for HIV exposure from the blood.

The virus is very fragile outside the human body; it needs a warm, moist environment to survive in. Generally, once a body fluid that can transmit HIV is dried, it is no longer infectious for HIV. Other viruses, such as Hepatitis C, can survive in dried blood for many days, so it is good practice to minimize any exposure to another person's blood.

Sexual transmissions of HIV from one person to another include oral, vaginal, and anal sex. In the United States, AIDS cases attributable to heterosexual transmission are accelerating (CDC, 2005; Watkins, 2002). Heterosexual contact has always been the primary mode of transmission worldwide, especially in Africa and Asia (Ahmed et al., 2003; Betts, 2001). Of the more than 42 million people infected with HIV worldwide, approximately 70 percent were infected through heterosexual contact, 10 percent are men who have sex with men (MSM), and the rest were infected through mother-to-child transmission, injection drug use, and contaminated blood supplies (Murphy, 2003). In Africa, where most of HIV infections occur, the vast majority of infections are acquired through heterosexual transmission.

HIV is also easily transmitted through blood contaminated needles shared by injection drug users (IDU). Injection drug use was also referred to as intravenous drug use (IVDU), but drugs can be injected under the skin (also called skin-popping), so the term IDU is utilized to be more inclusive of other needle-using behaviors (including steroids). Anyone who shares blood contaminated needles is at risk for HIV exposure and/or infection.

The virus can also be transmitted from mother to fetus through pregnancy, childbirth, or breast feeding. Mother to child transmission (MTCT) occurs most often through the birthing process, where blood and vaginal secretions can pass through mucous membrane of the infant's eyes, nose or mouth. In recent years, mandatory testing of pregnant women and treatments during pregnancy has decreased the incidence of MTCT transmission where they are used. HIV medications can be administered to an infected mother during the second and third trimester of pregnancy, during delivery, and to the baby for several months after birth, which reduces the risk of MTCT transmission from 25–30 percent to below 10 percent (CDC, 2004b).

Rarely, HIV transmission can occur from receiving a blood transfusion. The American Red Cross began testing the blood supply for HIV in 1985 and as of 1996, the risk for contracting HIV infection in the United States from a blood transfusion is estimated to be 1 in 676,000 or less than 2 in a million (Williams et al., 1997). HIV can usually be detected in an infected person after about 21 days of infection. Behavioral screening of donors before blood donation also helped to decrease the incidence of HIV in the blood supply. A person may also choose to auto-donate blood for elective surgery for high-risk surgeries in the event they may require blood to further reduce any risk.

Donating blood is not a risk factor for HIV transmission in the United States as blood banks, the Red Cross, and other blood collection centers use sterile equipment and a new disposable needle with each donor. Unfortunately, U.S. procedures for safeguarding the blood supply are not practiced globally. According to the World Health Organization (WHO), more than two-thirds of the world's countries fail to ensure safe blood supplies for their population (Crossette, 2000).

The actual route of entry for HIV into a person's body is through a break in the skin, or through a person's mucous membrane. Mucous membranes line the wet areas of our bodies, including the eyes, inside of the nose, inside of the mouth, vagina, anus and the tip of the penis. If any of these areas are exposed to one of the fluids that can infect a person, the virus has a way to enter the body. Viruses and bacteria can pass through the mucous membrane and into the blood stream via our capillaries. It is believed that mucosal transmission is less effective than transmission through cuts or micro cuts in the skin and mucous membranes (AIDSINFONET.org, 2005).

Just because a person is exposed to HIV does not mean he or she will become infected with the virus. Often, it takes more than one exposure to a virus before someone becomes infected (Koopman, 1996; Royce, Sena, Cates & Cohen, 1997; Vernazza, Eron, Fiscus & Cohen, 1999). It depends on how much virus is present in the body fluid (virulence), how frequent the exposure, the route of entry, and what type of resistance the person at risk has to infection. HIV infection is most likely during the seroconversion process (see diagnosis section), where viral loads are very high (Koopman, 1996; Royce, Sena, Cates, & Cohen, 1997; Vernazza, Eron, Fiscus, & Cohen, 1999). This formula can be illustrated as follows:

VIRULENCE X EXPOSURE

Resistance

With respect to prevention of HIV infection (especially if someone has a new partner) the problem with this equation is that there is no way of knowing by looking at someone whether or not they have HIV, let alone how much virus is in their body fluids if they become exposed through sexual behaviors.

Blood contains the highest amount of HIV, followed by semen, vaginal fluid and breast milk. Individuals are safer to go on the assumption that potential partners are infected with HIV or STIs, until they find out otherwise. This way, safer sex measures can be practiced until both partners are tested, and discuss the boundaries of the relationship; otherwise, there will be risk for HIV or other infections.

Tests are available that can determine the actual amount of virus a person has in the blood after they have become infected—called a viral load test. The test measures how many viruses are present in a milliliter of blood. A viral load of less than 50 virus per milliliter of blood is undetectable by the test. This does not mean a person has cleared HIV, only that the test is not sensitive enough to measure lower amounts of the virus. These tests are utilized in treatment to measure the efficacy of anti-HIV medications. In general, the higher the viral load, the greater the chance of transmitting the virus (Koopman, 1996; Royce, et al., 1997; Vernazza, et al., 1999). When a person is in later stages of HIV disease, or AIDS, it is more likely for viral loads to be higher. Surprisingly, when a person is newly infected, before HIV antibodies appear in the blood, viral activity is also quite high. Some experts believe that infections of HIV during this primary infection stage accounts for a large portion of HIV cases worldwide.

Diagnosis

HIV antibodies can usually be detected about 3–4 weeks after initial infection, but this may take 3–6 months, depending on the type of testing used. The process of developing antibodies is called seroconversion. During the time it takes to seroconvert, a person will test HIV negative because enough HIV antibodies have not yet been produced by the immune system to show up on the antibody test. Once the infected person seroconverts, they will then test positive for the virus. Standard blood tests used to detect HIV include the ELISA (Enzyme-Linked Immunosorbent Assay) and Western Blot. Rapid tests are becoming more widely utilized; for example a finger stick sample of blood can provide test results that are 99.6 percent accurate in as little as twenty minutes (Food and Drug Administration, 2002). Another test, called OraSure, uses an abrasive swab that scrapes off a small sample of the membrane inside the cheek in the mouth. The oral specimen must be sent to a laboratory, and results are usually available in a week. Another rapid test by OraSure, called OraQuick, uses a drop of blood from finger stick whole blood specimens. Test results are available in twenty minutes and are 99.6 percent accurate (Food and Drug Administration, 2002).

Many states offer free, anonymous HIV testing. This type of testing is used to encourage people to be tested that might normally be uncomfortable to be tested otherwise. Some anonymous test sites allow a person to convert their anonymous test result to a confidential one if they receive a positive test in order to facilitate referral for medical follow-up. Confidential testing is always done in a physician's office, and a medical record is then kept on file of the test results. Some life insurance applications require confidential HIV tests be done prior to obtaining coverage.

For a test site near you, visit the National HIV Testing Resource at www. hivtest.org. For service in English or en español you can call either: 1–800-CDC-INFO or 1–800–342–2437. The lines are open 24 hours a day, seven days a week. For the Deaf and Hard-of-Hearing TTY Service, call 1–888–232–6348, or go online to the Web site of American Social Health Association at www.ashastd.org.

Symptoms and Complications

As with many viruses, HIV often causes flu-like symptoms within a few days to weeks of initial infection. Not all people will experience symptoms, and the symptoms will vary with intensity and severity from person to person. Symptoms include, fever, swollen lymph nodes, diarrhea, nausea, muscle aches, skin rashes, and loss of appetite. These initial symptoms are signs that a virus is present and the symptoms will diminish with time. Months or years may pass before secondary symptoms occur.

Secondary symptoms are similar to initial symptoms, but will be more severe, persist over time and be unrelated to other illnesses. These symptoms include marked weight loss (usually 10% or more of a persons total body weight), skin rashes, fatigue, persistent diarrhea, chronic cough, oral candidiasis, severe vaginal yeast infections, repeated fevers, swollen glands in multiple sites that may be very large in size, and drenching night sweats. Oral candidiasis or oral thrush is a yeast infection of the mouth. It is common for infants to develop this condition as their immune systems are not fully developed, but an otherwise healthy adult does not commonly experience this condition. Often, infected persons are diagnosed at this stage because the repeated, persistent symptoms tip off physicians that there may be an immune disorder.

As HIV continues to replicate in the body and destroy healthy cells, the immune system loses its capacity to protect against a variety of infections. After the initial infection, a person is classified as asymptomatic, where they are infected with HIV and are not experiencing any obvious symptoms of the disease. HIV is present, although they may not even be aware that they are infected; during this time they may unknowingly infect others. The incubation period for AIDS (from the point of infection until medical diagnosis of the disease) can range from 8 to11 years in adults, with the median being about 10 years. A small percentage of infected persons have remained symptom free for much longer periods of time. Another group of AIDS diagnosed individuals have had known HIV infection for over 20 years, thanks to early diagnosis and treatment (Table 11.1).

Table 11.1
Progression of HIV Disease

Initial Infection	Asymptomatic	Symptomatic	AIDS
1–3 months	Up to 10 years years or longer	May last 3–5 years or longer once symptoms appear	CD4 < 200 1 of 26 opportunistic infections
Antibodies can usually be detected during this time		Fever Diarrhea Swollen glands Weight loss Thrush Night sweats Fatigue Nausea	Lymphomas Pulmonary TB PCP CMV Herpes zoster Toxoplasmosis Kaposi's sarcoma Invasive cervical cancer Recurrent pneumonia Other

As HIV continues to multiply and invade healthy cells in an infected person's body, the immune system loses its ability to defend itself against opportunistic infections. Opportunistic infections are infections caused by organisms that usually do not cause disease in a healthy person. However, they affect individuals with poorly functioning or suppressed immune systems. People who progress to AIDS can develop a range of serious, life-threatening complications. The most common, most deadly and most preventable one is a pneumonia caused by a bacterium that normally inhabits a person's lungs, *Pneumocystis carinii.* Some other opportunistic infections associated with HIV are severe fungal infections that can cause a type of meningitis, tuberculosis, salmonella illness (bacterial disease), toxoplasmosis (caused by a protozoan) and encephalitis (viral infection of the brain). The body is also vulnerable to cancers, such as lymphoma, cervical cancer and Kaposi's sarcoma (a common cancer of men with AIDS), which causes skin lesions and affects the internal organs as well.

Treatment

There is currently no cure for HIV infection. The goals of medical treatment for HIV disease are to slow down the progression of the virus, reduce the amount of virus in the bloodstream, prevent opportunistic infections, prolong life and reduce the incidence of symptoms.

The first class of drugs that were developed to fight HIV is called nucleoside reverse transcriptase inhibitors. There are currently twelve of these medications available on the American market for treating HIV. Another class of drugs that block the same step of the cycle, but in a different way, is called non-nucleoside reverse transcriptase inhibitors, or NNRTIs. Three of these drugs have been approved for treatment. The third class of available drugs used to treat HIV is called protease inhibitors (PIs). These drugs block the step where raw material

Table 11.2
Global AIDS Treatment Statistics

Region	Regional Estimates (Low- and Middle-Income Countries only) UNAIDS/WHO Estimates		
	People Receiving Treatment in June 2005	People Needing Treatment in June 2005	Treatment Coverage in June 2005 (%)
Sub-Saharan Africa	500,000	4,700,000	11
Latin America and the Caribbean	290,000	465,000	62
East, south, and southeast Asia	155,000	1,100,000	14
Europe and central Asia	20,000	160,000	13
North Africa and the Middle East	4,000	75,000	5
All developing and transitional countries	970,000	6,500,000	15

Source: www.avert.org/aidsdrugs.htm

for new HIV is cut into specific pieces. There are currently ten of these medications approved for treatment in the United States. The newest class of drugs includes fusion and attachment inhibitors. They prevent HIV from attaching to a cell by blocking the early step in the replication cycle. So far, one fusion inhibitor has been approved for treatment in the United States.

In June 2005, UNAIDS and the World Health Organization (WHO) estimated that 6,500,000 people in the developing and transitional countries were in need of antiretroviral (ARV) drug treatment for AIDS (AVERT, 2006). Of these, only 15 percent were receiving drugs. This chart presents data on access to antiretroviral treatment around the world. More data about AIDS drug access targets and results and the issues involved in providing treatment for millions can be found at AVERT.org (Table 11.2).

HIV uses an enzyme called reverse transcriptase that transcribes the viral RNA into DNA. HIV also encodes another enzyme, called protease (protein digesting), that is needed for its replication within the cells. Once HIV takes over the infected person's CD4 cells, it takes over the cells genetic material and reproductive capacity, producing more HIV to infect other cells. Anti-viral therapies attack and destroy HIV or inhibit the virus' ability to reproduce (see Figure 11.1).

Physicians must consider several issues before commencing drug therapy with a patient: the viral load (or amount of virus in a person's blood); the CD4

Figure 11.1
HIV Life Cycle

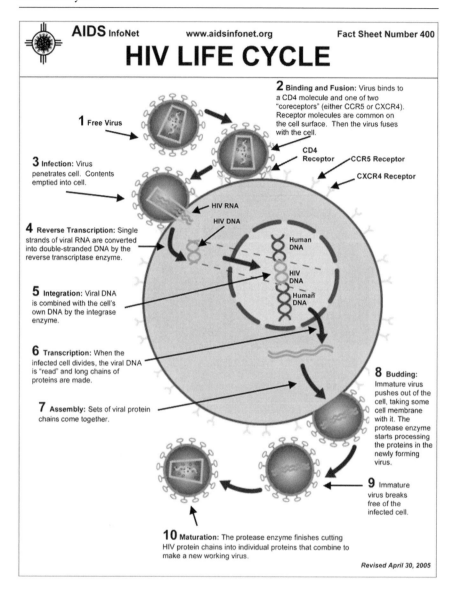

count; and any symptoms the patient is experiencing. CD4 cells are part of the immune system and are also known as T-helper cells or T-4 cells. In healthy people these cells help coordinate the immune system's response to disease and infection. Normal CD4 counts in healthy people not infected with HIV range from 600 to1200 cells per microliter of blood. Cumulative data supports initiation of therapy if the viral load is over 100,000 per milliliter of blood, if the CD4 count is below 350, or if the person is experiencing symptoms of HIV disease (Ahdeieh-Grant et al., 2003; CDC, 2002). Usually, several drugs are used in combination when treating for HIV, as it is more effective to interrupt the replication cycle of the virus when a combination of replication points are targeted by the specific medications. This combination of drugs usually consists of three or more medications also called triple drug therapy, highly active antiretroviral therapy (HAART) or the "AIDS cocktail."

Another issue a doctor and patient must consider when beginning drug therapy are the patient's ability to adhere to the drug regimen. When multiple medications are utilized, they must be taken on a regimented schedule that requires taking multiple pills at different time intervals, some on a full stomach, and others before eating. Complicated dosing schedules, drug toxicity, prophylactic medications taken to prevent opportunistic infections, combined with medications used to treat the side effects of other medications, along with supplements and/or vitamins makes for a complex, regimented schedule that can be very difficult for patients to adhere to. It is not uncommon for a person with HIV to be taking 30 or more pills daily.

If combination therapy is started and the patient does not adhere to the very specific regimen, it is likely that HIV will become resistant to the medications or mutate so that a whole class of drugs may not be effective for that individual for future treatment. Whenever HIV becomes resistant to medications over time, new medication combinations should be commenced. The initiation of combination therapy must be thoroughly discussed between patient and health provider and all the risks and benefits weighed. The success of combination treatment depends upon the ability of the infected individual to consistently and correctly adhere to complicated medication dosing schedules for long periods of time. Several studies have shown that rates of non-adherence to the regimen range from 37 to 70 percent (Murphy, Roberts, Martin, Marelich, & Hoffman, 2000).

STI as a Cofactor for HIV Transmission

Epidemiological evidence for STI as a cofactor for HIV transmission has emerged from several studies (Hayes & Schultz, 1992; Mortens, Hayes, & Smith, 1990; Pepin et al., 1989; Wasserheir, 1991). Separate and apart from behavioral risk factors, both the ulcerative STIs (syphilis, chancroid, and genital herpes) and the discharge STIs (gonorrhea, chlamydia and trichomoniasis) are associated with increased risk of HIV transmission. The ulcerative STIs increase risk 9-fold, and the discharge diseases from 3- to 5-fold (Wasserheir, 1991).

A number of explanations can be offered to account for the role of STIs as cofactors in vaginal transmission of HIV infection; the break down of protective epithelial layers of skin and mucosal surfaces leading to exposure of blood vessels, elimination of protective, normal vaginal flora, alteration of the acidic pH of the vagina, inflammation with the presence of CD4-positive target cells in the reproductive tract, to name a few (Hitchcock, 1996).

Given this brief analysis, it seems logical that prevention of STIs can assist in HIV prevention as well. Looking at the rates of STIs in the United States, it is increasingly apparent that there is a high infection rate that should not be ignored. Efforts to strengthen existing STI and HIV prevention programs and to develop new and creative ways to effectively control these treatable diseases could help in reducing new HIV infections.

Prevention

The only sure way to prevent HIV infection is to avoid all contact with any body fluids that can transmit the virus. For sexual transmission, this means abstinence from all sexual behaviors that involve the exchange of blood semen or vaginal fluids, involvement in a mutually monogamous relationship with an uninfected partner, or the correct, consistent use of barrier methods that will prevent the passage of the virus from one person to another. Barrier methods will be described in more detail at the end of this chapter.

For persons who inject substances, the following is recommended, listed in order from safest, to least safe:

Safest: Abstinence (quit using altogether), including drug treatment as part of process.

Next safest: Methadone maintenance (for heroin) or buprenorphine. Methodone produces a high; buprenorphine reduces cravings and withdrawal, with no high.

Next safest: Find an alternative method of using (i.e., snort or smoke the drug instead of injecting it).

Next safest: Don't share works (injection equipment). Each person has their own set of works.

Next safest: Use new needles every time for injection, either through a needle exchange program or in some states, a person can purchase syringes at a pharmacy without a prescription.

Next safest: Clean needles between sharing using CDC recommended guidelines for cleaning:

3X 3X 3X Method

1. Draw up clean water in syringe, shake for 30 seconds, squirt out water (repeat two more times).
2. Draw up bleach in syringe, shake for 30 seconds, squirt out bleach (repeat two more times).
3. Draw up clean water in syringe, shake for 30 seconds, squirt out water (repeat two more times).

Next safest: Lesser steps and times in cleaning methods. Some people use bleach first, than water, and only rinse and squirt for ten seconds once or twice. Anything is better than nothing.

Do not share cotton balls to stop bleeding, cookers to heat up drugs, ties to stop circulation, or anything that can pass blood from one person to another.

Accurate and up to date information about HIV and STIs is critical to halt its spread. But, as many people knew all along, information is not enough (Prochaska, DiClemente & Norcross, 1992). People need more than the facts—they need support in changing behaviors that put them at risk. Some effective strategies for HIV prevention are messages designed to teach people successful condom use strategies, such as how to negotiate condom use with partners who refuse to use condoms, attitudinal messages that clearly describe preventative outcomes of condom use, improving sexual communication, decreasing the number of sexual partners and increasing both overall knowledge of and skills in applying prevention tactics (Johnson, Carey, Marsh, Levin, & Scott-Sheldon, 2003).

PREVENTING SEXUALLY TRANSMITTED INFECTIONS

As was mentioned earlier, about half of all Americans will contract a STI at some point in their lifetime. With such a high incidence of infection, prevention of STIs is necessary to reduce risk behaviors and promote healthier lifestyles (see chapter 10 of this volume). Abstinence from sexual activity is the only 100 percent safe way to prevent acquiring a STI. Knowing your and your partner's personal sexual health status and negotiating a monogamous relationship is another way to reduce the risk of contracting a STI. For many people, however, it is stressful and embarrassing to discuss sexual matters, making disease prevention difficult to achieve. One study with 119 college couples found that most of the participants were unaware of their partner's past sexual experiences or risk behaviors (Seal, 1997).

The secrecy and shame associated with sexuality and STIs in particular, make communication regarding sexual risk and past behaviors most embarrassing. But the truth of the matter is that if sexual partners are not comfortable in discussing sexual risk with one another, they are at high risk for exposure and infection. Learning strategies to initiate discussion with a potential sex partner is essential in preventing STIs and making smart sexual decisions. The following are basic guidelines for preventing exposure to STIs.

Know Your Sexual Health Status

If you are currently uninvolved in a sexual relationship, getting tested for STIs is an important step to take. It is possible you may have a STI that you are unaware of, giving you the opportunity for treatment and secondary prevention, or peace of mind knowing that you are disease free.

Assess a Potential Partner's Risk

Once you know your own sexual health status, think about getting to know a person before you become sexual with them. Often, people neglect to ask questions regarding past relationships or have a conversation about sexual matters. Some people will not be truthful when answering questions, but observing a person over a period of time may give you an indication of whether or not you feel you can trust that person. By taking the time to get to know someone, you may even be able to get tested together before initiating sexual activity. If the person is someone you have not taken time to get to know, then using protection would be the next step.

Use Barrier Methods with a Partner

This includes male and/or female condoms for vaginal and anal intercourse, as well as condoms or barriers for oral intercourse as well. Condoms will prevent STIs when used correctly and consistently, but they are not 100 percent effective. For people who are new at using condoms, there can be a learning curve in using them correctly. If they are not used every time, they will be less effective. Some STIs, such as HPV or HSV can be on areas of the genitals where a condom does not cover, so if you or your partner has one of these viruses, it is important to be aware of whether and where your symptoms have occurred in order to reduce risk. In some instances, such as an outbreak of genital or oral herpes, abstaining from sexual activity or focusing on activities that do not involve the exchange of bodily fluids may be desirable.

Some persons have allergic reactions to latex, and if this is the case, condoms made of polyurethane should be substituted. The female condom is made of polyurethane as is the brand of male condoms, Avanti. Using a condom that causes an allergic reaction can actually increase the risk of infection if exposed, as the skin can become irritated or develop a rash as a result.

When using condoms, the following guidelines should be considered as well:

- Always use a water-soluble lubricant (K-Y jelly or Astroglide) with condoms, as dry condoms can cause friction and this can damage the mucous membranes, increasing risk.
- Never use oil-based lubricants with latex condoms. Latex is an oil-based product, and oil-based lubricants can cause the condom to break.
- Avoid using nonoxynol—9. Some condoms are lubricated with this spermicide, which may help prevent pregnancy, but it also can act as an irritant to the mucous membrane, which may actually increase risk of STIs.
- Check the packaging for expiration date and its condition. Outdated, worn-looking, brittle or torn packaged condoms should be discarded.
- Take care when opening the package that nothing tears the condom, such as teeth or jewelry.

- Store condoms in a cool, dry place, out of direct sunlight. Try not to keep condoms in glove compartments of cars, wallets or back pockets.

- Make sure you squeeze air out of the tip of the condom before it is rolled on, air pockets can cause friction, weakening the condom. Roll the condom out over the erect penis; do not unroll the condom first then try to put it on.

- Never use more than one condom (i.e., *no* double bagging). Two condoms can cause friction, weakening the condom.

- If a condom does break, stop and replace it immediately.

- After ejaculation, hold the condom at the base when withdrawing, to ensure the condom does not slip off. Then take the condom off.

- Never reuse a condom.

Reduce or Avoid Sexual Activity with Multiple Partners

As discussed earlier, multiple sexual partners increase the risk for many STIs. Reducing or avoiding sexual activity with multiple partners will reduce a person's exposure to STIs. Persons with multiple sexual partners should have routine STI examinations in order to assess for infections even when no symptoms are present.

Inform a Partner if You Have an STI

This may seem like a formidable task, but if you find out you have an STI while you are involved with another person, it is important that you inform them of your infection so they can get treated and you do not continue to put each other at risk. The stigma associated with having a STI can make this conversation difficult, but it is healthier to have the discussion than ignore it. Contracting a STI does not mean you are "bad" or "dirty." It simply means you have an infection that needs attention, like any other health condition would. Because so many STIs do not produce obvious symptoms, it is a common occurrence to discover months or even years after the fact, that you were infected with a STI.

Be honest in initiating the discussion. If you notice a discharge or bump, or sore, say so. Getting it checked out does not mean you or your partner was unfaithful; you may have had the infection and not known about it. The way you approach the subject can influence how your partner may react. Choose a time when you are both relaxed. Do not blame the other person; nothing will be gained from this approach. If you take an upfront, matter-of-fact tone, you may be able to resolve the matter in a caring way.

Try to be sensitive to your partner's feelings and reactions. It is understandable for someone to be angry or upset at this type of news. Being supportive and not reacting defensively to them may help you work through initial responses. Think about how you would feel if it was your partner telling you the same news.

In some instances, the local health department or health care providers can do partner notification. Some benefits of utilizing health department notification is that the person being notified will receive counseling to reduce further risk of exposure, treatment and testing options. Utilizing these services is beneficial when notifying past sexual partners is not practical for the infected person. Partner notification is crucial to treat infected persons and to curtail the spread of infections.

CONCLUSION

STIs are preventable if partners take precautionary measures and abstain from risky behaviors. Changing behavior is not always a matter of having correct information. A person's attitudes and beliefs toward sexuality will also influence how sexual decisions are made. Communication is an important tool in establishing and maintaining a healthy sexual lifestyle. When partners can discuss sexual histories, get tested prior to engaging in sexual activity and use recommended prevention measures when risk is identified, the chance of contracting STIs decreases proportionately.

REFERENCES

Abramowicz, M. (1994). Drugs for sexually transmitted diseases. *The Medical Letter, 36,* 1–6.

Ahdeieh-Grant, L., Yamashita, T., Phair, J., Detels, R., Wolinsky, S., Margolick, J., Rinaldo, C., & Jacobson, L. (2003). When to initiate highly active antiretroviral therapy: A cohort approach. *American Journal of Epidemiology, 157,* 738–746.

Ahmed, H., Mbwana, J., Gunnarsson, E., Ahlman, K., Guerino, C., Svenson, L., Mhalu, F., & Lagergard, T. (2003). Etiology of genital ulcer disease and association with human immunodeficiency virus in two Tanzanian cities. *Sexually Transmitted Diseases, 30,* 114–119.

AIDSINFONET. (2005). *How risky is it?* Retrieved December 19, 2005, from http://www.aidsinfonet.org/factsheet_detail.php?fsnumber=152.

American Social Health Association. (2005). *Overview fact sheet on sexually transmitted diseases.* Retrieved November 20, 2005, from http://www.ashastd.org.

American Social Health Association. (2006). *NGU (Nongonococcal Urethritis).* Retrieved May 3, 2006, from http://ashastd.org/learn/learn_ngu.cfm#1.

AVERT. (2006). *Who is getting AIDS drugs.* Retrieved February 22, 2006, from http://www.avert.org/aidsdrugs.htm.

Betts, A. (2001). Role of semen in female-t-male transmission of HIV. *Annals of Epidemiology, 11,* 154–155.

Calvert, H. (2003). Sexually transmitted diseases other than human immunodeficiency virus infection in older adults. *Clinical Infectious Diseases, 36,* 609–614.

Centers for Disease Control. (2002). Sexually transmitted diseases treatment guidelines, 2002. *Morbidity and Mortality Weekly Report, 51,* 36–82.

Centers for Disease Control. (2004). *HIV/AIDS surveillance report.* Retrieved December 28, 2004, from http://www.cdc.gov/hiv/stats/hasr1302/commentary.htm.

Centers for Disease Control. (2004a). *Trends in reportable sexually transmitted diseases in the United States, 2004.* Retrieved April 22, 2006, from http://www.cdc.gov/std/stats/04pdf/trends2004.pdf.

Centers for Disease Control. (2004b). Zidovudine for the prevention of HIV transmission from mother to infant. *Morbidity and Mortality Weekly Report 43*(16), *285–287.*

Centers for Disease Control. (2005). *HIV fact sheets.* Retrieved December 15, 2005, from http://www.cdc.gov/hiv/pubs/Facts/At-A-Glance.htm.

Centers for Disease Control. (2006). *Chlamydia—CDC fact sheet.* Retrieved April 22, 2006, from http://www.cdc.gov/std/Chlamydia/STDFact-Chlamydia.htm.

Centers for Disease Control. (2006a). *Gonorrhea—CDC fact sheet.* Retrieved April 22, 2006, from http://www.cdc.gov/std/Gonorrhea/STDFact-Gonorrhea.htm.

Centers for Disease Control. (2006b). *Trichomoniasis—CDC fact sheet.* Retrieved April 22, 2006, from http://www.cdc.gov/std/Trichomonas/STDFact-Trichomoniasis.htm.

Centers for Disease Control. (2006c). *Syphilis—CDC fact sheet.* Retrieved April 22, 2006, from http://www.cdc.gov/std/Syphilis/STDFact-Syphilis.htm.

Centers for Disease Control. (2006d). *Genital Herpes—CDC fact sheet.* Retrieved April 22, 2006, from http://www.cdc.gov/Herpes/STDFact-Herpes.htm.

Centers for Disease Control. (2006e). *Genital HPV infection—CDC fact sheet.* Retrieved April 22, 2006 from http://www.cdc.gov/HPV/STDFact-HPV.htm.

Colgan, R., Michocki, R., Greisman, L., & Moore, T. (2003). Antiviral drugs in the immunocompetent host. Part I. Treatment of hepatitis, cytomegalovirus, and herpes infections. *American Family Physician, 67,* 757–762.

Corey, L., & Handsfield, H. (2000). Genital herpes and public health: Addressing a global problem. *Journal of the American Medical Association, 283,* 791–794.

Donovan, B. (2004). Sexually transmissible infections other than HIV. *Lancet, 363,* 545–556.

Crossette, B. (2000). Two-thirds of nations fail to make sure blood supplies are safe. *The Oregonian,* April 7, A16.

Engelberg, R., Carrell, D., Krantz, E., Corey, L., & Wald, A. (2003). Natural history of genital herpes simplex virus type 1 infection. *Sexually Transmitted Diseases, 30,* 174–177.

Erikson, K. & Trocki, K. (1994). Sex, alcohol and sexually transmitted diseases: A national survey. *Family Planning Perspectives, 26,* 257–263.

Feroli, K. & Burstein, G. (2003). Adolescent sexually transmitted diseases. *American Journal of Maternal/Child Nursing, 28,* 113–118.

Food and Drug Administration. (2002). *FDA approves new rapid HIV test kit.* Retrieved December 19, 2002, from http://www.fda.gov/bbs/topics/NEWS/2002/NEW00852.html.

Gershengorn, H., & Blower, S. (2000). Impact of antivirals and emergence of drug resistance: HSV-2 epidemic control. *AIDS Patient Care and STD's, 14,* 133–142.

Gilbert, L., Alexander, L., Grosshans, J., & Jolley, L. (2003). Answering frequently asked questions about HPV. *Sexually Transmitted Diseases, 30,* 193–194.

Hayes, R. & Schultz, R. (1992). What proportion of HIV infections are attributable to genital ulcers in sub-Sahara Africa. (Abstract WD 4001). Presented at 8th International Conference on AIDS. Amsterdam, The Netherlands.

Hepnet.com. (2006). *Hepatitis A Infocenter.* Retrieved May 3, 2006, from http://hepnet.com/hepa.html.

Hepnet.com. (2006a). *Hepatitis C.* Retrieved May 3, 2006, from http://www.hepnet.com/hepc/hcvrisk.html.

Hitchcock, J. (1996). The witch within me. *Newsweek,* March 27, 16.

Ivey, J. (1997). The adolescent with pelvic inflammatory disease: Assessment and management. *Nurse Practitioner,* February, 78–91.

Johnson, B., Carey, M., Marsh, K., Levin, K., & Scott-Sheldon, L. (2003). Interventions to reduce sexual risk for human immunodeficiency virus in adolescents, 1985–2000. *Archives of Pediatric and Adolescent Medicine, 157,* 381–388.

Koopman, J. (1996). Emerging objectives and methods in epidemiology. *American Journal of Public Health, 86,* 630–632.

Lafferty, W., Hiltunen-Back, E., Reuwalda, T., Nieman, P., & Paavonen, J. (1997). Sexually transmitted diseases in men who have sex with men. *Sexually Transmitted Diseases, 24,* 272–278.

Miller, K., & Graves, , J. (2000). Update on the prevention and treatment of sexually transmitted diseases. *American Family Physician, 61,* 379–386.

Mortens, T., Hayes, R. & Smith, P. (1990). Epidemiological methods to study the interaction between HIV infection and other sexually transmitted diseases. *AIDS, 4,* 57–65.

Murphy, D., Roberts, K., Martin, D., Marelich, W., & Hoffman, D. (2000). Barriers to antiretroviral adherence among HIV-infected adults. *AIDS Patient Care and STD's, 14,* 47–58.

Murphy, E. (2003). Being born female is dangerous for your health. *American Psychologist, 58,* 205–209.

Ness, R., Hillier, S., Richter, R., Soper, D., Stamm, C., Bass, D., Sweet, R., Rice, P., Downs, J., & Aral, S. (2003). Why women douche and why they may or may not stop. *Sexually Transmitted Diseases, 30,* 71–74.

O'Neill-Morante, M. (2000). Human papillomavirus: A review of manifestations, diagnosis, and treatment. *Physician Assistant,* January, 19–25.

Pepin, J., Plummer, F., Brunham, B., Piot, P., Cameron, D., & Ronalds, A. (1989). The interaction of HIV infection and other sexually transmitted diseases: An opportunity for intervention. *AIDS 3,* 3–9.

Peters, S., Beck-Sague, C., Farshy, C., Gibson, I., Kubota, K., Solomon, F., Morse, S., Prochaska, P., DiClemente, C., & Norcross, J. (1992). In search of how people change: Applications to addictive behaviors. *American Psychologist, 47(9),* 1102–1114.

Royce, R., Sena, A., Cates, W., & Cohen, M. (1997). Sexual transmission of HIV. *New England Journal of Medicine, 336,* 1072–1078.

Sauder, D., Skinner, R., Fox, T., & Owens, M. (2003). Topical imiquimod 5% cream as an effective treatment for external genital and perianal warts in different patient populations. *Sexually Transmitted Diseases, 30,* 124–128.

Seal, D. (1997). Interpartner concordance of self-reported behavior among college dating couples. *Journal of Sex Research, 34,* 39–55.

Sievert, A., & Black, C. (2000). Behavior associated with *Neisseria gonorrhoeae* and *Chlamydia trachoimatis:* Cervical infection among young women attending adolescent clinics. *Clinical Pediatrics, 39,* 173–177.

Smith, A., & Rockey, D. (2004). Viral hepatitis C. *Lancet, 363,* 661.

Tao, G., Irvin, K. & Kassler, W. (2000). Missed opportunities to assess sexually transmitted diseases in U.S. adults during routine medical check-ups. *American Journal of Preventive Medicine, 18,* 109–114.

UNAIDS. (2003). *HIV/AIDS Statistics: Global trends in the epidemic.* Retrieved December 28, 2004, from http://www.sfaf.org/aboutaids/statistics/global.html.

Vernazza, P., Eron, J., Fiscus, S., & Cohen, M. (1999). Sexual transmission of HIV: Infectiousness and prevention. *AIDS, 13*(2), 155–166.

Wald, A., Zeh, J., Selke, S., Warren, T., Ryncarz, A., Ashley, R., Krieger, J., & Corey, L. (2000). Reactivation of genital herpes simplex virus type 2 infection in asymptomatic seropositive persons. *New England Journal of Medicine, 342,* 844–850.

Wasserheir, J. (1991). Epidemiological synergy: Interrelationships between HIV infection and other STD's. In L. Chen, L. *AIDS and women reproductive health,* 47–72. New York: Plenum Press..

Watkins, S. (2002). Demographic shifts change national face of HIV/AIDS. *SIECUS Report, 31,* 10–12.

Weinstock, H., Berman, S., & Cates, W. (2004). Sexually transmitted disease among American youth: Incidence and prevalence estimates, 2000. *Perspectives on Sexual and Reproductive Health, 36*(1), 6–10.

Williams, A., Thomson, R., Schreiber, G., Watanabe, K., Bethel, J., Lo, A., Kleinman, S., Hollingsworth, C., & Nemo, G. (1997). Estimates of infectious disease risk factors in U.S. blood donors. *Journal of the American Medical Association, 277,* 967–972.

Chapter Twelve

SEXUAL REHABILITATION AFTER CANCER

Ralph Alterowitz and Barbara Alterowitz

Many cancers and cancer treatments affect sexuality. Treating cancer patients and their partners presents a complex set of issues to the sex counselor or therapist.[1] Medical and psychological issues are added to any sexual issues a couple may have had before the cancer diagnosis and treatment. Some couples had perfectly happy and satisfying sex lives before cancers struck, and are suddenly faced with physical and psychological changes for which they were not prepared. In order to work effectively with couples affected by cancer, a therapist must be aware of the medical issues and the emotional effects of cancer and its treatments. Most references to couples apply regardless of the sexual orientation of the couple—heterosexual or same sex. In the case of a single individual without a steady partner, the therapist can explain many concepts to help the person be best prepared for effective functioning with a prospective partner.

Given the limitations, this chapter only deals with major diseases that have the potential to impair an individual and thereby the couple's relationship. Many treatments for pelvic cancers and some breast cancers have a high probability of impairing sexual function. The psychological aspect of dealing with the cancer may also impact the individual's and thereby the couple's sexual function.

Many breast cancer patients experience negative sexual effects. Almost all treatments for what is termed as abdominal and pelvic malignancies, especially prostate cancer for men and gynecological cancers for women, usually impair sexual function vascularly (via blood vessels) and neurogenically (via nerves). Aggregating incidence statistics shows that about two-thirds of these patients, 6.5 million survivors in the United States, will have some impairment of their sexuality.

Psychological reactions overlay and exacerbate physical problems. Both patient and partner may experience distress, disruption and possibly depression.

> I think it's fair to say that every patient who is faced with a cancer diagnosis will have a profound emotional response or reaction to the news. It is particularly distressing in the early diagnostic phases when people are dealing with all kinds of uncertainties.
>
> Besides the fear of the unknown, there is the fear of body disfigurement, fear of no longer being able to carry on one's previously held roles. What is this going to mean in terms of my ability to be a husband, a lover, and a provider? Am I going to be able to maintain my position as breadwinner? Those fears start to shift as illness progresses (Chochinov & Schachter, 2002).

These comments of Dr. Harvey Max Chochinov and Sherry Schachter, coauthors of *The Psychology of Cancer*, reflect the dimension of the psychological issues that unsettle cancer patients.

Chochinov's list of cancer-related fears suggests that some or probably many cancer patients suffer a cancer stress disorder (CSD) analogous to a soldier's "post-traumatic stress disorder" (PTSD). Stress begins with the diagnosis. The patient may enter a traumatic mental state that fluctuates through the diagnosis, treatment, and post-treatment phases. After treatment, ongoing tests to determine cancer dormancy or biochemical recurrence are ongoing reminders and magnets for bouts of high anxiety.

In making the transition to the post-treatment stage, a couple's quality of life may be most severely impacted in sexual relations. The impact of treatment is obvious when there is a physical change. But patients always feel the change biologically and psychologically including, for some, the very real problem of not being able to achieve intercourse or climax, inability to be aroused, or having no desire. Analysis of incidence statistics for the different cancers indicates that about half of the 6.5 million patients may recover some sexual function. The other half, over 3 million people and their partners, will be those with permanent or long-term problems, who will have significant challenges trying to resume physical intimacy after cancer treatment. This is the group most in need of help.

Weijmar Schulz and colleagues (1990) concluded from their longitudinal study on psychosexual functioning after the treatment of cancer of the vulva that psychological and social variables are better determinants of the success for sexual rehabilitation than physical variables. According to these authors, psychosocial issues constitute the most promising focus for intervention.

Furthermore, by working with couples before and after cancer treatment over a two-year period, these researchers found that all women who were sexually active before the treatment had resumed their sexual activities within one year. Couples were assessed again at 6-month posttreatment and an increase in relational sexual dissatisfaction could be detected. Over the remaining observation period the women's satisfaction with sexual interaction with the partner was not found to be different from their pretreatment satisfaction and not different in the control group, in spite of the physical damage and persisting poor perception of genital symptoms of sexual arousal during lovemaking. Weijmar Schultz and colleagues concluded that satisfaction with the partner under these circumstances appears to be more an expression of satisfaction with the intimate aspects of the sexual relationship than of satisfaction with the physiologic arousal aspects of the sexual relationship" (Weijmar Schultz et al., 1990, p. 402).

Sexual rehabilitation does work. This is the premise of this chapter. Survivor couples can renew their physical intimacy after one or both partners have been treated for cancer. Appropriate short-term sex counseling may help them achieve a level of intimacy whereby they can derive pleasure and satisfaction. When couples go to a sexual therapist, they give him the job of director and conductor to help them work through their problem to get to a satisfactory level of intimacy.

SEXUAL REHABILITATION: DEFINITION AND CLARIFICATION

What makes sexual rehabilitation after cancer different from conventional sex therapy must be viewed from the perspectives of the therapist and client. Generally, therapists and couples must be cognizant of the problems a couple had prior to cancer as well as the psycho-social-biological-medical overlay of cancer and treatment. Many aspects of sexuality counseling are common regardless of the underlying problems. However, the plan for sexuality counseling must factor in the constraints imposed by the cancer treatments as well the way the couple copes with cancer and sexuality.

Sexual rehabilitation implies treatment to correct or overcome a sexual dysfunction in a way that supports the couple's need for physical intimacy. For the cancer couple, it cannot be assumed that they will be able to have sex the same way as before. It should also not be generally assumed that patients and couples had satisfactory intimacy and sex before one or both partners was diagnosed and treated for cancer.

The nature of the rehabilitation depends on the way cancer has impaired the couple's intimacy (e.g., prostate cancer treatment will usually affect the man's ability to have erections, and women with gynecological cancer may have pain during intercourse due to radiation or chemotherapy). These are significant physical problems. They will change almost every sexual pattern that a couple has established during their relationship. One of the key goals for rehabilitation therapy could be to help the couple find and appreciate that new ways could give them as much or more enjoyment than their previous habits. Sexual rehabilitation can help a couple renew their physical intimacy and may even improve their satisfaction when the problems and issues caused by cancer and its treatment overlay pre-cancer intimacy and sexuality problems.

Sexual rehabilitation after cancer treatment entails using a therapeutic modality that helps the client adjust to post-cancer life and adapt consistent with the new constraints and with the couple's desires. The therapist and couple must handle the effects of the disease and treatment: changes in the biological condition of the patient, the psychological effects on the partners, and the way they interact. The disease literally permeates all of the biological and psychological functions.

A couple requesting rehabilitation counseling presents the therapist with a complex situation that consists of six inter-related histories. One is the set of three histories (i.e., each partner's and the couple's) prior to the diagnosis and treatment of cancer. There is a second set of three histories after the diagnosis and treatment of cancer. Although this set by definition incorporates everything that went on before the cancer, the changes in the intimacy and sexual behavior occasioned by the diagnosis and the consequences of treatment are very significant. These histories are the basis for the rebuilding work that the therapist and the patients will do together. The therapist's objective is to bring the patient and partner to the point of restoring intimacy with the greatest satisfaction possible for both partners, regardless of intercourse capability.

THE SEX THERAPIST'S JOB

The sex therapist who works with cancer patients will find that the client's age, the desire for intimacy and sex, disease—cancer and co-morbidities, and preexisting intimacy and relationship problems all intersect. They will have to relate to the couple's world if they are to be successful in helping couples regain this part of their lives.

Therefore, therapists need to learn about the disease, treatment, and side effects to understand the complexity of the couple's cancer environment (i.e., the medical condition's biological/psychological/social aspects). To fully appreciate the full nature of the client's problem, the therapist should:

1. Know the cancer diagnosis, treatment and the prognosis. Knowing the stage of disease helps the therapist appreciate the patient's and partner's mental state.
2. Be familiar with treatment side effects.

3. Be informed regarding therapies to address the sexual issues—medications and aids, to guide clients in managing impediments to resuming physical intimacy (e.g., dealing with problems such as erectile dysfunction and vaginal lubrication).
4. Understand the clients' loving styles to aid partners to adjust to their limitations.

In a cancer patient, many normal physiological responses are altered. For example, a situation that would normally cause a person to get excited may have no such effects because the chemicals in the brain react differently as a result of chemotherapy (Schover, 2001a, 2001b). Or a man who is highly aroused may not get an erection because of the short- or long-term effects of treatment for prostate cancer.

One significant issue for many cancer patients is that the treatments suppress their capability for desire and arousal. Yet, desire and arousal are potentially accessible by understanding the dynamics of what can evoke them. For example, a man on hormone therapy for prostate cancer may never think of initiating sex, but may be able to react when his partner initiates it. This will only work if the partner feels free and comfortable to show her desire, so the therapist may need to focus on removing the partner's inhibition to initiate sex. Many breast cancer patients experience diminished desire and arousal from fear that they are less attractive and desirable (in addition to potential chemical depression analogous to the men on hormone therapy), and it may be critically important that the man express his desire and show her how attractive he finds her. The same applies to the partner in a same-sex relationship.

It may also be helpful to remember that, although the flow is generally thought to be desire, arousal, intercourse, orgasm, many women may be aroused by their partner before feeling desire or value the intimacy of the experience more than having an orgasm (for an overview of sexual response cycle models see volume 2, chapter 1, and the Appendix, volume 4). Focusing the couple more on the sensual pleasures and less on intercourse is likely to make the sexual experience much more satisfying for the woman and is an eye-opening experience to many men who never realized how much fun and satisfaction they can get from sensual sex. The sensual focus offers the opportunity for a deep emotional connection during the sex act.

Partners are often baffled by the changes taking place in the cancer patient. They may be used to an instantaneous response, or a reaction to a trigger ("when we kiss passionately, he gets an erection"), and suddenly those patterns do not apply any more. Some partners of men with erectile dysfunction think their spouses are having affairs or no longer find them desirable, as there is no erection. The men, frustrated and preoccupied with their reduced capability, have no idea what is going on inside their partners' heads, and suddenly there may be no sexual interaction at all, with devastating effects on both partners. A skilled counselor can get them back on track.

The therapist has to lead the couple down the road to understand the dynamics of lovemaking, work with the partners to relearn about each other's sexual response and rebuild the sexual relationship under the new constraints. Ideally, this will be a road where the partners rediscover each other and find new excitement. The change in sexual function may look like a door closing, yet rebuilding a couple's sex life offers the opportunity to get to a new and deeper level of sexual understanding between the partners and can greatly enrich a couple's relationship.

The therapist/counselor will find it necessary to instruct couples in the dynamics of lovemaking. For most of their lives, people often equate intercourse and sex. Outside of knowing how to have intercourse, many men do not know much about the woman's physiology. They may not know about vaginal lubrication or the effects of menopause and may not be sensitive when the woman suffers pain on intercourse. Some men are not aware how to stimulate and arouse a woman so that she is physically prepared for intercourse. Yet the preparation for intercourse is crucial for the satisfaction of both partners.

For men having erectile problems due to a broad range of problems, it is incumbent on the counselor to reorient them so they value the sensual part of sex. Many of these men have never given themselves the opportunity to enjoy and derive substantial pleasure from the art of loving. While using medications such as sildenafil (Viagra), tadalafil (Cialis), or vardenafil (Levitra), or aids like vacuum erection devices or penile injections may be an option, the couple should be introduced to the idea of fabulous erection-free sex. Similarly, in an environment where intercourse is painful for the man or woman, different options for sex should be explored.

Each couple will have to work through and evolve its own paradigm for seduction, desire and arousal. Many factors come into play from the couple's personalities to their sociocultural context to their patterns for resolving other problems. The therapist will need to understand "where the partners are coming from" and with this knowledge help the partners weave a therapeutic fabric that works for them.

The cancer couple looks to the sexuality counselor to hone in and define the problems, suggest ways to solve or alleviate friction even if the cause cannot be eliminated, and propose things the couple can do to reinvigorate the relationship. In the process of doing so, they label the counselor as an ombudsman—the impartial observer to resolve differences—although subjectively, many clients hope the therapist will take their side in dispute resolution.

The therapist's mission is to provide couples with a framework and methodology they can use as they encounter future problems as well as handle the current situation. In this therapeutic model, the therapist is a participant in an interactive dialogue as opposed to being in a passive listening mode with the client. The therapist would probe, suggest, generate ideas, and be an active participant in working toward solutions.

Short-term sex counseling can be an extremely effective tool for cancer patients. One study looked at the psychoadjustment of female patients with newly diagnosed gynecologic malignancies if they received in-hospital, individual counseling. The researchers concluded that counseling had a positive effect in boosting their return to normal and sexual functions during the first year after treatment. These results suggest that at a minimum, a subset of cancer patients may respond well to short term sexual counseling.

Implicitly, the counselors had the medical background, interacted dynamically with the patients and couples, and knew that they could do so only for a relatively short time. Counselors oriented to what we refer to as brief, introspective-integrative linked (BIILD) therapy can significantly improve the quality-of-life for many cancer couples.

MEDICAL CONDITION—CONTEXT

This section highlights some of the characteristics of common cancers that affect intimacy and sexuality. The therapist must be familiar with them and their effects to guide the couple to obtain satisfactory intimacy and sexuality. Even though the therapist will get information from the patient and partner, sometimes, the patients and partner may not be able to give the counselor the necessary information or may not be aware of the fact that many of the problems are related to cancer treatment.

Often, it is not the cancer itself but the required treatments that will harm sexual function. For example, pancreatic cancer is frequently associated with depression in excess of that imposed by other malignancies. Depression's effect on libido is well known, and this mood disorder should be a component of the differential diagnosis in all cancer patients. Uncontrolled pain also adversely affects sexuality and must be the focus of specific questioning.

Using the Bancroft model (Bancroft, 1989, p. 552) as a frame of reference, the possible effects of a clinical condition on a patient's sexuality may be categorized as follows:

   a. *Direct* physical effects of the cancer

   i. Specific interference with genital or other sexual responses due to pressure from tumor, including vascular impairment or neurological damage.

    ii. Nonspecific effects, such as pain, general malaise, fatigue, and lack of sexual desire, immobility with arthritis or spasticity making postural changes normally expected during sexual activity difficult or impossible.

  b. The *psychological* effects of the condition

    i. On the individual, such as feeling sexually unattractive, having loss of desire, or generally experiencing a loss of self-esteem as a result of the condition.

    ii. On the relationship (becoming dependent on partner, resulting in a child-parent rather than adult-adult relationship).

    iii. Concern about effects of sexual activity on the condition.

  c. Effects of *treatment* on sexual activity

    i. Drug effects. Chemotherapy has a wide range of side effects that affect sexual activity. It can cause lack of desire, neurologic changes, alopecia (hair loss) that alters body image, and mouth sores that make kissing or oral sex difficult or impossible. Hormone treatment may sharply reduce libido.

    ii. Effects of surgery and radiation, causing damage to genital structures or their neurological or vascular control, resulting in painful intercourse, erectile dysfunction, or vaginal collapse.

    iii. Psychological effects of treatment, such as surgery resulting in disfigurements.

The following table (Table 12.1) lists many cancers, and their treatments. Almost all the treatments directly affect the sexuality of the respective gender. Clinicians today have a fairly broad arsenal of medical options to treat these diseases. In many cases, the decision is left to the patient who may choose the treatment option based on a quality of life issue such as a concern with post-treatment sexuality. Most clinicians are solely concerned with the patient's survival regardless of sexual impact.

These are the major cancers where the treatments will directly affect a person's sexual capability. The primary means for treating these diseases may include one or more of the following: surgery, radiation, cryosurgery, and hormonal and chemotherapy. Watchful waiting (i.e., no treatment but monitoring the biological cancer markers for some period of time) is used primarily for older men with prostate cancer, and patients with chronic lymphocytic leukemia and some lymphomas.

Except for breast cancer, the other cancers presented are considered pelvic malignancies. Treatments directly affect the neural and vascular systems that are responsible for much of a person's sexual functions. A woman's sexual psychology may be impacted by breast cancer treatment. In addition, physical consequences of treatment frequently impose constraints on her participation for a few months after treatment.

The treatment for any pelvic malignancy in men is likely to result in erectile dysfunction. For example, prostate cancer treatment is likely to affect about 70 percent of the men sexually (Sexuality and Reproductive Issues, CancerWEB). The psychological impact is substantial when a man has to confront erectile dysfunction because this condition is bound up with their self-image of manliness.

Table 12.1
Major Cancers and Some Available Treatment Options

Disease	Surgery	Radiation	Chemotherapy	Other
Anal cancer	Wide excision for anal margin tumors. Radical therapy: Abdominoperineal resection removal of anus with permanent ostomy for anal tumors where anus cannot be preserved.	External beam or interstitial brachytherapy (seed implants). Radiation combined with chemotherapy to decrease local recurrence rate.	Chemo-radio therapy has become the standard of care for this disease.	
Bladder cancer	Transurethral resection. Cystectomy. Radical cystectomy.	External beam. Brachytherapy (interstitial) (seed implants).	Systemic chemotherapy (oral or infusion).	Intravesical immunotherapy.
Breast cancer	Lumpectomy. Mastectomy (with or without reconstruction). Sentinel node biopsy with or without subsequent axillary node dissection.	External beam. Brachytherapy (interstitial) (seed implants).	Systemic chemotherapy (oral or infusion if metastatic).	Monoclonal antibody. Hormonal (selective estrogen response modifiers, i.e. tamoxifen) or aromatase inhibitors.
Cervical cancer	Cervical removal. Hysterectomy.	External beam.	Systemic chemotherapy (oral or infusion).	Hormone (progestin). Cryotherapy (freezing).
Colorectal cancer (CRC)	Bowel resection (with or without reconstruction). Laparoscopic-assisted. Abdominoperineal resection for anal tumors or low rectal cancer where anus cannot be preserved. Colonoscopy—polyp removal. sessile scraping.	External beam. Brachytherapy (Needles, seeds, wires, catheters).	Systemic chemotherapy (oral and IV or IV, depending on stage). Chemo given first to shrink tumor to try to spare anus. Many chemotherapy drugs are used for colon cancer.	Cryotherapy (freezing). Chemotherapy may be accompanied by a monoclonal antibody.

(Continued)

Table 12.1
(Continued)

Disease	Surgery	Radiation	Chemotherapy	Other
Gynecological cancer, see also cervical cancer ovarian cancer uterine cancer vaginal cancer	Total pelvic exteneration.	External beam. Brachytherapy (intracavitary or interstitial) (seed implants).	Systemic chemotherapy (oral or infusion). Cytotoxic concerns.	Hormone (progestin). Intraperitoneal chemotherapy (only for ovarian).
Ovarian cancer	Total abdominal hysterectomy, with removal of ovary, tubes, and omentum (only for operable disease).	External beam. Brachytherapy (intracavitary or interstitial) (seed implants).	Cytotoxic chemotherapy used adjuvantly and palliatively.	Intraperitoneal chemotherapy.
Prostate cancer	Prostatectomy. Laparoscopic. Perineal. Retropubic.	External beam. Intensity modulated (IMRT). Neutron beam. Proton beam. Brachytherapy (intracavitary or interstitial seed implants).	Oral or IV. Hormonal therapy.	Cryotherapy. Watchful waiting (major use especially for advanced age or other severe illnesses).
Rectal cancer	See colorectal cancer			
Uterine cancer	Hysterectomy. Radical hysterectomy.	External beam. Brachytherapy (intracavitary or interstitial seed implants).		
Vaginal cancer	Partial or radical vulvectomy.	External beam for those undergoing less radical surgical procedures.		

Alterowitz, R., Alterowitz, B. © 2005.

Table 12.2
Glossary

Abdominoperineal resection—usually includes removal of anus with ostomy

Adjuvant—in addition to other therapy

Axillary node dissection—surgical removal of the axillary (armpit) *lymph nodes,* is usually performed on breast cancer patients during the course of a mastectomy

Brachytherapy—radiation therapy in which the source of the radiation is placed close to or implanted into the tissue to be treated (e.g., radioactive "seeds" implanted in the prostate gland for the treatment of prostate cancer). This allows specific tissues to be treated without broad area, external beam radiation, thus avoiding harming the surrounding normal tissue

Colonoscopy—use of an endoscope to examine the large intestine (colon) to look for to look for early signs of cancer in the colon and rectum.

Colostomy—establishment of an artificial opening through the skin into the colon

Cryotherapy—also called *cryosurgery, cryoablation,* or *targeted cryoablation therapy;* the application of extreme cold to destroy diseased tissue, including cancer cells

Cystectomy—removal of all or part of the bladder

Cystotomy—an incision into the bladder to drain urine from the bladder

Cystostomy—creation of an opening in the abdomen that allows a tube catheter to be inserted in order to drain urine from the bladder

Cytotoxic—detrimental to cells

Enervation—to weaken or destroy the strength or vitality of something (e.g., an organ)

External beam radiation—radiating an area of the body from an external source

Hysterectomy—removal of the uterus

Immunotherapy—a nonspecific term indicating treatment of a disease using one or more substances intended to stimulate the patient's immune system

Incontinence—often refers to inability to control the discharge of urine or feces

Intensity modulated radiation therapy—computer-calculated that permit delivering appropriate radiation dosage to the target and surrounding areas

Interstitial—relating to spaces within a tissue or organ

Intracavitary—within an organ or body cavity

Intraoperative—occurring during a surgical operation

Intraperitoneal—-the way medication is administered directly into the peritoneal cavity

Intravesical—inside the bladder

Intravesical immunotherapy—treating disease by administering antibodies inside the bladder

Laparoscopy—use of an endoscope to examine the abdominal cavity. (The endoscope is usually a very narrow cylinder containing a lens attached to a fiber optic cable.)

Lumpectomy—removal of a cancerous or noncancerous lesion from the breast without removing surrounding tissue

Mastectomy—removal of the breast

(Continued)

Table 12.2
(Continued)

Palliative care—reduce the severity of the symptoms without curing the underlying disease

Perineal—relating to the area between the thighs extending from the coccyx (tailbone) to the pubic bone

Polyp—a mass of tissue projecting from the surface and visible macroscopically (without use of magnifying devices); may be benign or malignant tumors, or the result of inflammation or degeneration of the affected tissue

Radical cystectomy—removal of the bladder, cervix, fallopian tubes, ovaries, uterus, and vaginal front wall

Radical hysterectomy—removal of all the female reproductive organs (including ovaries)

Radical vulvectomy—extensive surgical removal of the vagina and lymph nodes

Resection—removal of all or a significant part of an organ or bodily structure

Selective estrogen response—certain actions are initiated that have a primary effect on bone and cardiovascular tissue and less effect on endometrial, genital, and breast tissues

Sentinel node—removing the first node in the lymphatic chain that would receive drainage from a malignant tumor

Sessile—colon lesions having a broad base of attachment (i.e., not on a stalk)

Transurethral—through the urethra

Urethra—the tube which carries urine from the bladder to the outside of the body

Vesical—relating to the bladder

Source: The majority of the definitions were obtained from *Stedman Medical Dictionary for the Health Profession and Nursing,* Illustrated, Fifth Edition Baltimore: Lappincott Williams & Willems 2005.

As pointed out by Bancroft, the disease and the treatments can broadly impact the patient's sexuality. However, all the treatments do not have the same consequences, effects, or severity when they do occur. Other factors that come into play are the doctor's skills, the nature of the cancer, and the patient's age, general health, and coexistence of other diseases (e.g., cardiac), as well as their ability to cope with emotional issues involved.

To help the therapist, the following table (Table 12.3) lists some side effects of cancer treatments as they impact sexuality of men and women. Certainly, some treatment options lead to more severe problems than others. This table shows the major possible effects on each gender. Not every patient will experience these consequences and the degree of impact varies.

There is also a broad range of other effects that impact sexuality that are usually not thought about and are not reflected in the table. Breast cancer surgery often impacts a woman's sexuality physically such that she cannot have someone laying on top of her in the missionary position. Arm movement and strength is affected because of lymph node removal. She may have difficulty lifting things and her

Table 12.3
Sexual-Related Biological and Psychological Effects of Different Cancer Treatments

Disease	Women	Men
Anal cancer	Major effect on sexuality. Possible decreased clitoral stimulation and pain on intercourse. Surgery reduces fat pad cushioning area around vagina, anus, pelvis—may have increased pain with vaginal intercourse. If surgery to remove anus, many organs affected. Radiation also reduces vaginal lubrication.	Erectile dysfunction. Low or no libido. If surgery to remove anus, many organs affected and enervated.
Bladder cancer	Incontinence. Altered body image due to ostomy for urine collection. Chemotherapy also causes side effects (e.g., fatigue).	Incontinence.
Breast cancer	Body image. Hair loss. Early onset of menopause. Symptoms associated with hormonal therapy (weight gain, night sweats, vaginal dryness, etc). Reduced breast arousal after mastectomy (with or without reconstruction).	Body image.
Colon cancer	Pain. Cancer in upper colon may have little effect on sexuality. Psychological impact of colostomy. If lower rectum is operated on, there is less padding between vagina and sacrum, causing pain during intercourse. Diarrhea due to chemotherapy and surgery if significant part of colon is removed.	Psychological impact of colostomy. Possible erectile dysfunction. Diarrhea due to chemotherapy and surgery if significant part of colon is removed.
Gynecological cancers, including cervical, uterine, vaginal, and ovarian cancer therapy	Body image changes due to surgery. Hair loss from chemo. Lack of lubrication. Pain in pelvis and on intercourse. Loss of desire. Arousal difficulties. Orgasmic difficulties. Loss of clitoral stimulation.	

(Continued)

Table 12.3
(Continued)

Disease	Women	Men
Prostate cancer		Erectile dysfunction. Reduced level of orgasm. Retrograde ejaculation. Urinary dysfunction. Incontinence. Bowel dysfunction. Feminization (after hormone treatment): breast enlargement, nipple tenderness, hot flashes, weight gain, loss of upper body mass, man may feel he is less attractive. (Some people have greater estrogenic effect with combined androgen therapy.)
Other pelvic malignancies	Lubrication problems. Thinning of vaginal tissue. Vaginal collapse.	Erectile dysfunction.
All cancers	Chemotherapy may lead to loss or reduction of libido.	Chemotherapy may lead to loss or reduction of libido.

arm movements may be restricted. One woman asked her husband to sleep in another room because she was afraid that if he rolled over he could hurt her.

Treatment for female pelvic cancers may have sexual impacts in terms of pain, changes in vaginal anatomy, emotional distress, body image, sexual self concept, early onset of menopause and resulting problems. Moreover, there is often collateral damage in treating the cancer of one organ in that other "innocent" organs may be sacrificed (i.e., surgically removed or radiated because they are close to the diseased area). For example, a radical hysterectomy may be performed in treating some cancers of the cervix, ovaries and vaginal tissue so that all of the woman's reproductive organs are removed. Even the surgical treatment for bladder cancer may result in a radical hysterectomy. This involves removing the uterus, ovaries, fallopian tubes, cervix, front wall of the vagina as well as the bladder and the urethra.

Men's difficulties are usually discussed in the context of erectile dysfunction. However, the reality is that men may have difficulties in all areas of the sexual response cycle: lack of desire, failure to become aroused and to reach orgasm, and inability to achieve an erection. All treatments for pelvic malignancies will in most cases result in erectile dysfunction, ranging from partial impairment to complete impotence. Some men regain a level of potency over time as nerves recover from treatment trauma and regrow.

According to the Massachusetts Male Aging Study, 52 percent of men experience some level of impotence (Feldman, Goldstein, Hatzichristou, Krane, & McKinlay, 1994). The prevalence ranges from 40 percent of the men at age 40 to 70 percent of the men at age 70. Treatment for pelvic cancers worsens the man's situation when it comes to sexuality. Many men try to choose the treatment option that will help them best preserve their potency, especially when it comes to prostate cancer. Regardless of age, all treatments damage the nerves that are responsible for achieving an erection. Medications depress desire, interfere with arousal and over time cause some degree of erectile dysfunction.

The effects of systemic chemotherapy are also important to consider. Initially, patients must deal with the treatment-related adverse effects. These include, but are not limited to: nausea, vomiting, hair loss, and fatigue that are common with many regimens. In addition, many cancer therapies are immunosuppressive, requiring abstinence until white blood cell count recovery. Chemotherapy induced platelet decreases can make sexual activity dangerous as well until this cell line recovers. The negative sexual side effects of chemotherapy, especially hormonal therapy, decline soon after the therapy stops, whereas many effects of other treatments are long-term or permanent (Schover, 2001a).

Regardless of the treatment, the sexual and sensual selves of men and women are greatly impacted. The biological changes run the spectrum from significant etching on sexuality to less prominent side-effects that get in the way of physical intimacy. Even a broad overview of the many other side effects of treatment is beyond the scope of this chapter, but for sake of comprehending the magnitude, they can be reflected by the following highlights.

a. A woman will probably have physical problems if she has reconstructive trans-flap breast surgery. The flap is taken from the stomach and because muscles are cut, patients have difficulty sitting up. Until they heal and learn how to sit up because they need their stomach muscles to support themselves, there is usually no sexual activity.

b. A mastectomy removes one of a woman's most sensitive arousal areas. Surgery for a lumpectomy most likely will reduce a woman's breast sensitivity, but rarely eliminate it altogether. Although reconstructive surgery improves a woman's appearance, the reconstruction does not have the nerves and endings that can cause a woman to be aroused.

c. Women who have monthly saline injections as part of their reconstruction, may experience soreness and have severe discomfort under the arms. After the injection they go home, sit in a chair and must lift their arms over their head to get relief. The saline injection has a secondary and indirect side effect in that a woman often suffers from malaise and discomfort that reduces her desire for sex.

d. Lumpectomies (breast conservation procedures) are less radical and presumably have less impact. However, women who have this procedure often find they are numb in the area of the lumpectomy because some of the nerves are cut. Depending on breast size and size of the tumor, disfigurement causing altered body image may result. Most women who undergo lumpectomy (in lieu of mastectomy) require external beam radiation. This is generally associated with skin redness and discomfort that can make sexual activity intolerable during the period of, and for weeks after, treatment.

e. Most of the men and women who undergo hormone therapy lose their libido.

f. Women who have surgery for gynecological cancer also have nerves cut during the procedures such that sensitivity in the vaginal, clitoral, and cervical areas are reduced or eliminated. Nearby tissue may also be cut during the procedure. Women may experience vaginal pain (dyspareunia) during intercourse.

g. Chemotherapy often reduces the libido in men and women. Younger women may experience early menopause that can affect their responsiveness to sexually-related stimuli.

h. Surgery and radiation in the genital and pelvic areas create sexual difficulty for men and women. Surgery usually requires severing nerves essential to sexual stimulation in the course of removing diseased organs or controlling the spread of cancer. The nerves are dispersed throughout the abdominal cavity. The number of nerves that must be cut depends on the surgical procedure (e.g., laparoscopic or traditional abdominal surgery), the treatment objective, and whether the cancer is localized or whether it has spread to other organs, and competence of the surgeon.

For example, during a routine radical prostatectomy (surgery for prostate cancer), surgeons may attempt to spare the neurovascular bundles on each side of the prostate to preserve erectile capability but must still cut many of the smaller nerves thus reducing the man's potency. As a result, 70 percent of the men who undergo surgery have erectile dysfunction for some time or permanently (CancerWEB, National Cancer Institute). Radiation impacts potency gradually. At the four-year mark, surgery and radiation are equal in their effect on potency. After four years, 70 percent of patients are impacted. However, regardless of treatment modality, they do not affect a man's physical ability to have sex regardless of his erectile capability. Many men are capable of having partial penetration and orgasm and can engage in erection-free sex.

i. Then there are a number of "below-the-radar" radiation and chemotherapy problems that are experienced by patients but not often mentioned. These include:

Skin irritation.

Dry mouth because radiation decreases saliva production. This is generally preventable with newer techniques such as intensity-modulated radiation therapy (IMRT) that can be restricted to the target area.

Mouth sores that make kissing or oral sex impossible.

Severe fatigue, although patients may just mention being tired.

Low platelet counts that might make intercourse dangerous.

Diarrhea and constipation that would make lovemaking difficult.

Headaches—from mild to severe.

> Severe urinary or bowel incontinence, which is not a frequent side effect, is devastating to a couple's sex life. Urinary stress incontinence is a more frequent consequence that can be managed to minimize its impact on a couple's sex life.

Cancer treatment-related effects arise from many biomedical directions to impede the pursuit of sexuality. That said, sexual pleasures can still be had although some of the steps to achieve them may be different than previously. With the help of a knowledgeable and innovative counselor, cancer couples can be successful in rebuilding their sexual intimacy.

PATIENT & PARTNER, "THE COUPLE ENVIRONMENT"

The Cancer Couple's Emotional Climate: Stunned, Confused, Overwhelmed, Angry, Depressed

Four groups of people have to cope with cancer disease: male patients, female patients, male partners, and female partners. The patient and partner often react differently to the consequences of the cancer treatment. And it is well-known that men and women deal with issues in different ways.

The cancer diagnosis stuns, as if the patient or partner were hit in the head by the cancer two-by-four, or kicked in the stomach. For many people denial comes first, only to be followed by the stunning realization: "I have cancer." "My partner has cancer."

After the diagnosis and some explanations, the doctor frequently makes the patient responsible for deciding on the treatment option, especially if the situation is not life-threatening and there are several options with similar medical outcomes. The challenge of this settles in when patients try to cope with the enormous and often overwhelming volume of information. Since most patients have minimal or no medical background, the information is difficult to understand. Most patients come out of this confused state by telling the doctor that they will go with his or her recommendation.

The "Why me?" effect comes into the equation some time after the patient leaves the doctor's office after diagnosis. That's when the word *cancer* hits the patient. Anger usually surfaces after the treatment when they realize the side effects and other consequences they were not told about.

On top of the consequences of the diagnosis, patients feel a lack of preparedness for dealing with the side effects when they confront the everyday tasks in resuming life. For a time, treatment and the near-term follow-up consumed the patient's attention. Then, when things slow down and they try to resume their normal activities, the physical and psychological side effects cause additional problems. Patients may feel deceived and betrayed by the medical establishment. Besides treatment causing an impairment of sexual function, they may also have an elevated risk of developing osteoporosis, congestive heart failure and other heart problems, strokes and blood clots. In some cases, chemotherapy may cause leukemia or bladder cancer. Yet there is no post-treatment cancer plan. They feel let down, lost, and neglected (Hewitt, Greenfield, & Stovall, 2006).

Contributing to this feeling is the lack of information. A common complaint is that "my doctor didn't tell me." Patients expect their doctors to tell them about everything regarding resuming their life without having to ask for it. Unfortunately, oncologists frequently focus only on the immediate issue of removing the cancer and many patients are reluctant or unable to ask for any information when it is not forthcoming because they are intimidated by the white coat syndrome or by some doctor's arrogance or overbearing attitude.

Even if many questions are answered, the notable exception concerns sexuality. Often when patients and partners ask about the effects of treatment on their sexuality, doctors do not discuss the sexual implications of the recommended treatment or treatment options. Unfortunately, many clinicians who do respond either minimize the therapy effects on sexuality, discount the questions as being irrelevant or suggest postponing the discussion until after the treatment.

Returning to life's routine after the disruption by the need for medical tests, doctor visits, and one or more courses of treatment is difficult alone. When overlaid by uncertainty and no answers for the many questions that arise, patients are unsettled to put it mildly. Some people expected only a temporary disruption, and thought their routine would return to normal after treatment. However, treatment complications and medication side effects keep the situation in flux and increase the distress and anxiety levels. Think about resuming sexual activities under these circumstances!

Temporary or long-term depression can be present in almost 40 percent of the population, especially in the older group. Depression hits many cancer diagnosed patients and many of their partners. When the medical condition or treatment present barriers to intimacy, partners may become depressed. When men question their manhood because of impotence or incontinence, they retreat from interaction with people close to them. Women with breast cancer often anticipate rejection because of poor body image and question their attractiveness. Both major and minor depression can last for more than a few weeks and lead to impairment of many daily functions. With this in mind, it is helpful to take a closer look at couples in the post-treatment period.

Post-Treatment Pictures of Patients and Partners

A Breast Cancer Survivor

The daughter told the therapist her mother had both breasts removed at age 48 due to breast cancer. To this day the mother "has never 'recovered' emotionally from the 'loss.' She didn't want reconstructive surgery. She was divorced and has never remarried. Her 'femininity' was totally wrapped up in her body-image as a woman. She always took pride in the way she looked and how she dressed . . . and suddenly, everything she *was* was taken away from her by the surgery."

A Prostate Cancer Patient

Sometimes I sit and ponder, too . . . I'm 54 years old. I'm thankful for so much. But I'm sad, too for what I've lost. I don't feel like a man anymore.

A Gynecological Cancer Patient

A year and a half after we got married, I was diagnosed. I was early stage and had the radiation therapy the doctor suggested. He said I would be fine after the five weeks of radiation. Then we found that my vagina collapsed. I had a lot of pain and couldn't sometimes bear to go to the bathroom. Certainly, I could not have intercourse. My husband was very understanding. Then my vagina closed up. I'm amazed, my husband even wants to touch me and kiss me.

The gamut of emotions from being upbeat to depressed may evolve at any time during diagnosis and treatment, and afterwards emotions go up and down in reaction to events. Patients may exhibit seemingly contradictive behaviors.

One woman who generally tended to complain about almost anything, was surprisingly upbeat after she was diagnosed with breast cancer, had a mastectomy and chemo. Her family expected substantial complaining along the lines "why did this happen to me?" and "what did I do to deserve this?" She continued to complain that things unrelated to the cancer were not good for her and that no one, especially those close to her, could do things right. However, as regards her cancer, everything was matter of fact. Was it denial or successful coping?

Patients usually demonstrate different emotions and feelings than do their partners. Partners' set of broad emotions may include empathizing with the other person, wanting to help the patient, feeling uncomfortable and just not sure what to say. Some want to avoid discussion because they may identify with the condition, dreading the thought that it could happen to them. Many partners feel a loss of control over their life and their most important relationship.

Emotions are driven by many factors. For the patients some of the principal ones are the threat–to-life; the conflict with the sense of self that occurs when the person's sexuality is at risk, real or imagined; the patient's personality, well being, and gender. The partner's primary emotions are usually related to the fear of losing the loved one, and also reflect the couple's level of emotional involvement with each other, the partner's degree of dependency on the patient, as well as personality, well being, and gender.

Men are more often angry. Where impotence is concerned, as in the treatment for prostate cancer, men get confronted with the questions: "Am I still a man? What does it mean to be a man? Many men with pronounced erectile dysfunction feel "I am no longer a man."

Men with prostate cancer have three things to be angry about: inability to have an erection firm enough for intercourse (even if they do, their erections are usually not as hard as they were previously), lack of ejaculate (also referred to as dry ejaculations), and a shorter penis. Men tend to be focused on the size of their penis, notwithstanding that women's sexual pleasure does not depend on large/long penises.

Men who have advanced disease and are placed on anti-androgen therapy, also referred to as hormone therapy, will usually lose all desire and often cannot be aroused or find it difficult to do so. Consequently, they are also impotent.

Breast cancer is the major disease that affects sexuality for more than one-third of all women with cancers. No matter whether it is a mastectomy or a lumpectomy, the removal of a breast or the scar blemish of a lumpectomy, the body image may be that of the imperfect woman. Although breast cancer treatment does not prevent intimacy and intercourse, surgery can impose the questions "Am I still a woman?" and "Will I still be desired?" on the mind. One woman would not go on dates for fear she would be rejected when the man saw her breast. The therapist asked if she ever thought of wearing a camisole or a bandanna across her breast. She said no. She was persuaded to go on a date. Afterwards she reported that she wore a camisole and everything went well.

Many patients are anxious before treatment due to uncertainty about the extent and severity of the disease and whether the therapy will cure them. After diagnosis, almost all cancer patients function against a backdrop of *anxiety: this persistent feeling of dread and apprehension impinges on all*. Once cancer is in the picture, the worry faucet is turned on. After treatment, anxiety is a constant companion. Many patients are encouraged to look forward to resuming the life they led prior to the diagnosis. But they experience anxiety when they dwell on whether they will be able to carry on their duties, fulfill their responsibilities and do things they enjoy. Overall, there are so many changes in their lives will they be able to handle them? The discordant notes cancer introduces in a couple's relationship adds more anxiety.

Most anxiety is not overt (i.e., not readily seen or detected in conversation or the person's appearance). Nevertheless, it may become a constant state of tension not only for the patient but the partner as well. Both of them may have an ever-present fear that the cancer will recur or progress, the uncertainty of how the disease will be dealt with, the impact on the family, and so forth. A partner expresses her concern in one e-mail:

And every time in those two years if Joe had a headache or some body ache that appeared out of the blue, I would cringe with fear that the cancer was spreading.

Anxiety hangs over fundamental questions concerning intimacy. Breast cancer patients ask themselves "Will my partner still desire me (with one breast gone)? After prostate cancer treatment causing impotence, men wonder "Will my partner still want me (when I can't have an erection)?" Apprehension accompanies the cancer patients into the bedroom.

Unresolved open *conflict* generates anxiety as to when the next confrontation will occur and what will be the outcome. One woman describes her situation

> Sometimes there is one person in the relationship who "pushes the envelope" and insists on the communication, openness and confrontation of issues and problems.

Although communication is a healthy way to approach the situation, when the envelope being pushed concerns sex/physical intimacy, the *self-esteem* of each partner is involved. The woman is concerned with her being desirable. The man is concerned with his manliness based on his ability to "perform." Partner disagreement on any aspect of resuming sexual activity can implicitly mean conflict, will cause upset at the moment, and set the stage for anxiety on all aspects of intimacy. Yet, as discussed later, it is often essential to recovering intimacy that one of the partners initiates communication about the topic of sex.

A patient's self-esteem problems following treatment may cause the person to withdraw from any physical contact. Some couples stop touching and even talking intimately when their sex life is affected by cancer treatment and they have not learned to communicate about it. This is often devastating to the partner, as in the following example:

> I'm desperate. I don't know what to do. I am up at this hour of night, because I have been rejected again by my husband. God, I wish I had a man that just wanted to be with me. I miss being touched, cuddled, and held. We have no intimacy. Touching one another is out of the question because he is afraid that I will want sex if we have any contact. There is a wall between us and I don't know what to do. I am to the point of filing for a divorce because I feel inadequate. What should I do?

In other couples, the opposite may be true. The lack of sexual interaction may be welcome. This situation became apparent when sildenafil (Viagra) was introduced. As the first easy-to-take medication to help men obtain quick erections, one might think that every adult would be happy, especially older couples. This was not the case in many marriages. Many women complained that things were going along okay and they were glad their men could no longer perform and did not bother them for sex. The availability of this new drug would cause their male partners to pester them for sex just when both had gotten used to living together without any sexual interaction. A representative comment from women was that things were okay. "We were getting along and I thought we were finished with sex. And now he is going to want sex again."

The Viagra response points to a fundamental misconception. Although there are many studies that point to couples wanting and having sex throughout their lives, quite often a couple had no sex before the cancer diagnosis. It may be that the sex life patients would like to recover may be closer to that which existed at the onset of their relationship or may only have been dreamt of and is not what actually existed before treatment. Consequently, their "benchmark" for measuring the extent of recovery may have no basis in reality. This may be one reason why a high percentage of men who have been successfully treated for erectile dysfunction, discontinue their treatment.

A fundamental requirement for sex therapy is that the therapist must obtain as correct a picture of the intimacy that existed before cancer and each partner's motivation for resuming sexual activity. And then seek to answer the question whether therapy can help the couple bridge the gap between expectation and reality.

Emotions Experienced by Cancer Couples and Their Causes

As indicated in the foregoing, the cancer situations cause patients and partners to experience a broad array of emotions throughout the cancer course. These feelings may hamper their recovery after treatment and adjustment to post-cancer life as well as hinder their attempts to renew their intimacy. Sometimes the sex life is completely erased because the emotions are swirling around and not dealt with.

Their feelings may be expressed either verbally or behaviorally or both. Therapists will notice that there is substantial shifting, replacement and recycling of emotions. The following table (Table 12.4) provides an overview to the patient's and partner's emotional landscape. It highlights one inescapable fact: partners express emotions similar to patients and there may be widely different perceptions and mismatched expectations. Although this is the case for many couples, cancer now gives them additional psychological and biological obstacles to deal with. For those couples who come from a dysfunctional intimacy pre-cancer, incompatibility may become aggravated. Couples desiring to make their loving work, may not know how to get it back on track.

Patient and Partner Actions

Actions of the patients and partners during the course of cancer can lead to or worsen emotional estrangement between them. Quite often they coalesce

Table 12.4
Emotions Experienced by Cancer Couples and Their Causes

Emotion	Cancer Patient	Partner
Anger (When guilt cannot be expressed it can surface as anger.)	Toward the outside world. "What did I do to deserve this?" "I tried to do the right things for my body and this had to happen." Guilt often gets expressed as anger because some people feel anger is a more acceptable social emotion.	"Why will the cancer patient not discuss the situation, not listen to reason, not express intimacy by touching . . ."
Anxiety (related to concerns about health implications, incompatible desires)	Cancer recurrence, he/she can't fulfill partner's demand.	Worried about partner's health and survival; unable to get partner to talk; does not know how partner feels.
Apathy	No sex because of real or perceived inability to "perform."	No sex because of real or perceived inability to "perform." "I don't want to make demands of him/her."
Denial (Comes, goes, and may return. When MD diagnoses the disease, the patient is in shock and denies.)	"They can't mean me." "It's not me they're talking about." Often occurs during the time of diagnosis. May suppress it or come out of denial and then accept the situation. Then a bad lab result may push the patient into denial again.	Confused: does not know why partner does not take the situation seriously. Or Denial: "This can't be happening to us."
Depression	Disease changes life: treatment is costly, and routines and plans are disrupted. Lower quality of life.	Worried about partner's survival. Quality of life is lower. Paying for treatment may be a financial burden.
Discouragement	Given a raw deal; has to deal with cancer. Becomes pronounced when treatment goes badly.	Same as for patient.
Distressed	Feeling powerless and sad.	May feel distressed and guilty because he/she could not protect the loved one.
Frustration	"Why doesn't my partner understand what I am going through?" "Nothing's going right." "He wants me to feel sexual. But I don't."	"I can't get him to open up." "I have needs also, and she or he shuts me out." "I want to help and he/she won't let me."

(Continued)

Table 12.4
(Continued)

Emotion	Cancer Patient	Partner
Guilt	"I'm causing all this worry for my partner and family."	"I was not able to protect the person I love from this terrible disease." "I would just like to go on with my life, but I'll feel guilty about that."
Lack of desire (may be caused by chemo-therapy)	Hormone treatment. Poor body image. Feeling unattractive or not sexual. Poor relationship history.	Poor relationship history.
Lack of trust (medical establishment, breaking trust)	"My doctor did not tell me about the conse-quenced/side effects of the treatment/medication. He/She did not discuss what happens to sexuality after treatment." "My body has let me down." Not feeling safe in the relationship.	Similar to patient.
Pessimism	"Nothing ever goes right for me." "He won't like me if he sees I have only one breast."	"Nothing goes right for me."
Rejected (or anticipating rejection)	"He can't stand me because I have only one breast." "The lumpectomy scar will turn him off." "She won't want me because I can't come up."	"If I touch him, he'll run away because he can't fol-low through." "I think my wife/husband is having an affair because we have not made love in months.
Self-pity	Why did it happen to me?	"Everything is about the cancer. Everyone focuses on the patient. Nobody asks how I feel."
Stress	Life is disrupted. Time spent for treatment.	Life is disrupted. Sex life evaporated.

Table 12.5
Patient and Partner Negative Actions

Action	Cancer Patient	Partner
Alienation	Negative feelings result in alienating behavior that further reinforces negative feelings.	Partner feels isolated, shut out, and rejected. Partner may have negative feelings about self. "You don't have to feel paranoid."
Avoidance (Both partners may take this action.)	Refuses to communicate and interact. Does not know how to start talking.	No intimate interaction. Does not know how to start talking. Tiptoes around the issues.
Conflict	Conflict predating the cancer. Sometimes the patient has the burden of getting the partner to be supportive and intimate. This can lead to conflict.	Conflict predating the cancer. Pushing the patient to talk and to cooperate. Can lead to conflict.
Rejection (active or passive)	Rejects intimacy; rejects interactions with others. May find reasons to criticize and reject partner in order to avoid intimacy.	In some cases, the partner rejects interactions with the patient.
Repression (automatic restraint of drives and urges; a means for dealing with anxiety)	Dealing with irreconcilable desires.	Wants to encourage patient to talk and engage in even simple intimacy but does not. May be related to interpretation of role in the marriage.
Suppression (willful restraint of drives and urges)	Patient suppresses the need to talk with partner and/or touch and be touched. "This is my problem to solve."	Partner concerned about upsetting patient does not bring up important issues (e.g., intimacy, patient's feelings and needs, personal needs, family issues).
Withdrawal	Partial or total withdrawal due to feelings of inadequacy e.g., body image, feeling less of a man/woman.	Concern regarding making the patient feel inadequate or fear of rejection by the patient.

Alterowitz, R., Alterowitz, B. © 2005.

into emotional boulders manifested by destructive actions such as rejection. When carried on for some time, they may lead to irreconcilable difficulties. By dwelling on non-constructive emotions, a partner may create more divisive scenarios, sometimes leading to irreconcilable difficulties. Ultimately, this disconnect increases sexual dysfunction.

As the situation continues, one or both partners will require even greater support to pull him or her out of the emotional tailspin. One or both of them may need pharmacological support to arrest the emotional illness before corrective measures can be taken.

The preceeding table (Table 12.5) was prepared to offer insight into behavioral expressions of emotions. It is not intended to be all-inclusive but merely to highlight some of the frequently observed actions, their manifestations, and the consequences.

Positive Action: Communications

The actions and behaviors described above are destructive to the interaction between the partners and can even lead to a death spiral for the relationship. The starting point for an upward spiral is clearly that one of the partners opens the door to communication. Any couple seeking sex therapy has already taken an important step in that direction. It is the counselor's task to reinforce the positive potential of the communication and use this as the basis for rebuilding the physical intimacy of the couple.

Communication is also the key for single cancer patients who are embarking on a new relationship. An extreme negative case is the new wife who found out on her wedding night that her husband was impotent—she was not pleased. She didn't have a problem with the erectile dysfunction and figured they could overcome that (she was right). But she wished that he had told her in advance. Similarly, a woman who tells a new partner beforehand that she lost a breast or has a "dimple" in her chest from a lumpectomy has a greater chance for a normal and positive reaction the first time they make love. Surprises that can possibly change a partner's receptivity to lovemaking are best taken care of in advance. A counselor can work with a single person to prepare them for the conversation. "First tell, then show" works a lot better than "show and then tell" where sexual function or body changes are concerned.

TREATMENT PROTOCOL

Sexual rehabilitation of the cancer couple is complex. Even without cancer and its treatment, Joel Kovel in *A Complete Guide to Therapy* writes "sex is at once the most easily disturbed of functions and the one whose disturbances are the most easily put aside" (Kovel, 1976, p. 203). When cancer is involved, it is often the last aspect of recovery to be addressed, if it gets addressed at all.

The nature of the sexual connection between partners is a mirror that reflects the state of the relationship. For partners who do not have the desired physical bond, their quality of life is less satisfactory. As noted previously, the sexual side of intimacy is sometimes impacted directly by the disease, or more often by the biological and psychological consequences of cancer treatment. They can carry over into social interaction, thus presenting the therapist with a bio-psycho-social-medical case. Quite often, therapy must be implemented in a medical context (i.e., in a collaborative arrangement with the medical care provider).

At this point, it may help to look at the subtlety of the "rehabilitation objective." Revamping (i.e., to reconstruct or renovate) probably better conveys the objective of the therapy whereas rehabilitation could be interpreted as restoring to a former state. After cancer treatment, the former state cannot be recovered if there is a permanent effect such as total impotence or other biological cause for sexual dysfunction.

Many couples have commented that their renovated sexuality is better, more satisfying than what they had prior to the cancer diagnosis. This can happen if they open themselves up to each other and to new ideas. The change forced by the consequences of cancer treatment can be used positively to reinvigorate and revitalize the sexual relationship.

Treatment Protocol Model

The proposed protocol model is a brief-term, focused, interactive approach that is directed exclusively at the objective of sexual rehabilitation. Collateral issues may need to be dealt with if they underlie or contribute to the sexual difficulties. In one case, the male partner felt his spouse continually criticized him in their daily life. He acknowledged that he was sensitive because he was often told that he did something wrong during his younger years. His partner said that she was "bitchy" and "critical" partly because she let her first husband get away with doing very little. Their "criticism conflicts" played themselves out in the kitchen when he would load the dishwasher. Both partners started out declaring "that's the way it is." The therapy needed to move the partners toward understanding themselves so that different behavior patterns could be implemented in order to achieve the desired physical intimacy.

Dealing with their respective behaviors was necessary because good communication is essential for intimacy. Moreover, disagreements during the day will preclude or impact quality physical intimacy.

Brief-term, focused, interactive therapy (B-FIT) helps clients to experience feelings, reflect on their observations, and consider using constructive approaches to resolve difficult situations. The client will then be moving away from resolving problems through detachment, defensiveness, and destructive behavior.

B-FIT therapy means the client and therapist work toward achieving their objectives in a shorter period than conventional therapy. They inherently agree to collaborate on defining the problem and channeling the client towards positive solution options for sexual intimacy.

Protocol components may be defined as follows:

Brief term

Research has shown that even as few as four weeks can aid in improving a couple's sex life after prostate cancer. The research reported in the December 2005 issue of *Cancer* magazine showed that a group of patients who had undergone short-term sexual counseling were functioning better sexually three months after completing the therapy than the control group. Elsewhere in this chapter, it is noted that vulva cancer patients also functioned better after counseling.

Several factors increase the likelihood of accomplishing the objective in a short term. The client couple or individual:

a. Self-selects for the therapy.
b. Is positively disposed to the therapy.
c. Has sexual problems and concerns and believes assistance is needed.
d. Sets a realistic objective.
e. Has a positive outlook that the therapy will help.

Focused

The sex counseling must be limited to the key issues concerning the sexual relationship. Discussions during the sessions may bring to the surface and highlight many significant issues concerning past relationships of the client as well as the current one, previous sexually related difficulties, how they grew up, and so forth. Although worthy of examination and meaningful, pursuing the many threads that arise can mean going down long roads. The clients can feel that they will never get to the issue at hand. Therefore only immediately relevant issues should be explored as part of B-FIT therapy.

Interactive

During sessions, the therapist serves as an instructor, mediator, and participant in discussions addressing the concerns of the clients. The clients, in turn, direct their comments to both the therapist and to each other. Under the guidance of the therapist the clients improve their ability to examine their thought processes, feelings, interpretation of events and resultant behavior. This orientation should aid the clients in dealing more effectively with the current problem as well as being able to deal optimally with future situations. As one psychiatrist puts it, "Ideally, therapists look for their patients to get to the point of knowing what they feel and feeling what they know." This is what the therapist should be consciously working toward during the sessions.

The interactive component is intended to help the client translate intent into appropriate action. The ideal outcome of therapy is for the client to change their behavior by applying the improved understanding that introspection gives them. Implicitly, that means a change in reasoning. Over time, it is expected that the client will go through an iterative process of finding more ways to achieve his objectives and integrate appropriate actions into his daily pattern.

Directed, purposeful achievement of the objective in the short-term insists on a high level of interaction between the therapist and client. The therapist listens to the client's (or couple's) presentation of symptoms and possible problem statement, asks questions and prompts the client to discuss the situation, and works jointly with the client to arrive at a concrete statement of the problem(s). For clarification, the therapist might reframe the problem statement. Then over a period of time, the counselor may reorient the client through discussion, solicitation of views and comments, and exercises to resolve issues and problems.

Treatment Protocol

The treatment protocol consists of the B-FIT model described above and the following additional factors:

a. Qualifying clients for compatibility with the therapist and therapeutic approach.
b. Client history.
c. Considering the challenges created by the resumption of sexual relations resuming sex after a long interruption is tough.
d. Using therapeutic modules specific to cancer couples in addition to conventional units of therapy.
e. Homework assignments (e.g., sharing fantasies, sensate focus exercises, scheduling talk and touch time).

Qualifying the Patient/Client Couple for Therapy

To maximize the chance of success, counselors/therapists need to ensure that they have the necessary expertise, and that they are compatible with the client. They also need to ensure concord on objectives and collaboration (i.e., will the client take an active role in the therapy)?

The prospects for improvement depend on the "fit" between the therapist, the therapy, and the client(s). The therapeutic approach must be suitable for the client and the situation—no therapy works for everyone. Equally important, can the therapist and client mutually agree on the objective, the idea of change, motivation, and approach?

The Therapist-Client "Fit"

The appropriate therapy with the wrong therapist still means the therapeutic relationship will not work. In the course of counseling, the therapist and client develop a social relationship that becomes the medium by which the therapist delivers direction, is constructive, and guides the client. Defects in the relationship can impede the message being heard, correctly understood, and lessen client motivation to implement beneficial measures.

"Fit" is absolutely critical for an effective and successful therapeutic relationship. It speaks to whether two or more people have interaction characteristics in common that reflect whether they are well-matched. This match is essential for any joint endeavor. "Fit" includes personalities, how the people express themselves, mannerisms, how they think, and sometimes even how they dress.

The provider cannot be absolutely sure beforehand that he and the client will be compatible for effective delivery of therapy. However, indicators that the therapist can consider concern the client's:

a. Behavior and appearance.
b. Cultural background.
c. Manner of expression, affect and mood.
d. Speech content.
e. Cognitive function (attention and concentration, memory, intelligence).
f. Introspective ability.

The "Agreement": Setting the Stage with the Patient

One criterion for gauging therapist-client compatibility is whether they can easily come to agreement on the goals and process of the therapy.

An effective therapeutic situation is more likely when the therapist and client have established a contractual-like situation. After a few sessions, they can summarize the client's key problem areas. The "contract" helps the therapist and client ascertain the latter's motivation and broader question whether the client couple is appropriate for sex therapy, especially the dynamic short-term course.

Much in the same way, a salesperson "qualifies" a customer to increase the probability of "making a sale," a therapist should try to assess the likelihood of success for a couple seeking sex therapy. A therapist may want to use the following list of client characteristics as a check list. In fact, the therapist may want to review this with the client so they can agree on related issues. We have found that sex therapy is only likely to be more successful for clients with the following characteristics.

Objective—the therapist and partners help set the therapy objective and are committed to achieve it.

Motivation—both partners must be involved and motivated to seek therapy and work together to implement changes. Their desire for a satisfactory outcome must be high on the priority scale. Getting their sexual relations back on track requires both partners to be at the bargaining table working on their issues.

Mutual trust—the partners are committed to each other and trust the therapist.

Interaction—the partners must be actively involved and interact with each other and with the therapist to realize the highest possible level of success.

Willingness to embrace change—The partners must be willing and actively involved in exploring different techniques and approaches.

In general, good candidates for sex therapy are at least of average intelligence, with the capacity to understand their psychological orientation, have good self-esteem, and are able to articulate their problems and feelings. Moreover, they are committed to each other and their joint objective.

Client History

Good health care and appropriate treatment determinations demand that providers obtain a client history. The breadth and level of detail may vary among providers and for different types of cases and healthcare purposes.

The initial two to four meetings provide the foundation and context for the therapist-client dynamics and the architectural plan for the therapy. This is also the time when the therapist establishes and defines the nature of the rapport.

The intake history should include the following:

a. Client's complaint and objective
b. Background—history of the partners and their relationship

  1. How the partners met
  2. How the relationship proceeded
  3. How their relationship changed over the years they've been together
  4. How much time do they spend together and what are the activities do they share?
  5. What kind of work or activities does each partner do?

c. Medical history of both partners

  Diseases diagnosed and when (e.g., heart disease, diabetes, depression may affect sexual function)
  Medical procedures and date performed
  Medications past and current (Many medication affect sexual function, e.g., beta blockers for hypertension, medications for depression. Others, especially the potency pills, are contraindicated for cardiac disease patients on nitrates.)
  How has the relationship and sexual interaction changed after cancer diagnosis and treatment?

d. Status of the current sexual problem

  How did it start and when?
  What treatment has been sought, if any?
  How well did it work?

During the initial sessions the therapist should observe the partner dynamics and look for signs that indicate the nature of the couple's relationship. Do they sit near each other? Do they address each other and look for confirmation when they say something or do they avoid looking at each other? What is their body language? These observations will fill in much of the undiscussed dynamics.

Resuming Sex After an Interruption Is Tough

Treatment for almost all pelvic cancers, will force a couple to interrupt their lovemaking for some period, anywhere from a month to several years. Resuming sex after any sustained interruption, demands that the partners prepare for resumption. They need to think through their feelings, desires, physical and emotional capability, and changes that may be necessary. When medical considerations were responsible for interrupting normal sexual activity, the partners must consider their feelings toward the intervention and the loss. At the end of this internal inquiry, they must set their expectations

In his thought-provoking article, *When an Erection Alone Is Not Enough,* Dr. Stanley Althof (2002) sets forth a framework of six questions that a couple must answer before a prostate cancer couple resumes sex. All couples who have not had sex for some time need to understand the cause for the cessation, their impact, and their reasons for restarting their sexual relationship.

In modifying Althof's framework so they are applicable to a broader segment of cancer patients and couples and help the therapist create a context to orient the therapy, the questions could be:

1. What is the quality of the couple's non-sexual relationship?
2. How long has it been since the couple has not had sex? And what were the reasons for stopping?
3. Are both partners physically and emotionally ready to resume lovemaking?
4. Do the partners have compatible love styles? If different and a partner has different/unconventional arousal patterns, how does the other partner feel about it?
5. Do the partners need and wish to use medications and/or devices? How do they feel about it and how should it be integrated into the lovemaking?

The first question is the key point for assessing a couple's readiness to resume lovemaking and the probability of achieving satisfaction. The longer a relationship exists, the more likely it is to settle into a lovemaking routine. Generally, routine depresses desire and obviates arousal. In a couple's early years, infatuation and a focus on the physical tend to drive the sexual part. Over time, bonding physically is driven by the good feeling the partners have for each other. If there is substantial, conflict, the emotional turmoil cannot be swept aside to permit them to enjoy physical interaction.

Unless the partners have continuously worked on energizing their relationship and sexual interest in each other, their quality of lovemaking will have drifted from high-intensity excitement that existed at the beginning to a somewhat, dull, boring union—even before the cancer diagnosis and treatment. The key question, what have the partners done to maintain the relationship's vitality, viability and freshness, clearly applies even more when cancer adds to the complexity. Physical as well as emotional attraction is in large part a function of their efforts.

So What's a Therapist to Do with a Cancer Couple?

A therapist should provide a safe, secure, and nonjudgmental environment, guidance, support and assistance. They aid patients in revising nonconstructive thinking, helping them achieve thought-behavior congruence, and encourage them to initiate satisfying activities. Fundamentally their work and the therapy concern the sexual flow: desire, arousal, play, and/or climax. The therapist accomplishes this:

a. While working within constraints.
b. By helping partners to communicate.
c. By informing couples about therapies—medications and aids that are available, if desired by the couple
d. By telling them about different techniques to help couples reawaken the arousal sensitivities and sexual play leading to climax

Therapy Modules

Many major components of standard sex therapy are equally applicable for a cancer couple. However, there are additional complexities, and sex therapy after cancer requires the therapist to also discuss information concerning the disease, treatment and sexual behavior modification. All of these are combined to help couples reestablish patterns that will continue to work for them in their new situation and revamp others that would not help them accomplish their ends.

When dealing with a couple affected by cancer, a therapist can:

- Help couples to be accepting of the changes the disease has forced on them.
- Position their situation as being an opportunity to reinvigorate their sex life and even improve the sexual satisfaction compared to the pre-cancer situation.
- Motivate patients and partners to use the cancer-induced changes positively in the post-cancer sexual situation and work with their new constraints.
- Clear away thought process obstacles such as myths that interfere with achieving sexual satisfaction.

Accepting and Working with Change: Cancer Means Change; Therapy Means Change

There are a few key modules that are required for most couples dealing with the effects of cancer. Very often, clients rebuff a therapist's ideas because they involve making some change. Generally, people resist change. They are rooted where they stand concerning ideas, activities, and ways of doing things—even if they no longer have the capability of doing them the same way as before. Getting the client even to accept something intellectually as being valid may be a difficult first step. These vernier adjustments in the client's attitude are often major accomplishments. Even after that is achieved, behavior change is not automatic. Client fixations are rarely modified in major steps.

Cancer has already forced the client to change in major ways such as an altered daily schedule with office visits to doctors, treatments, perhaps different eating schedules, changing the foods they eat and possibly some of their activities. To address their sex problems, the clients must alter sexual habits and often, also the relationship.

The therapist has a valuable tool by leveraging the change introduced by the cancer diagnosis and treatment. So while there may be new and different constraints, the partners also have been released from their commitment to past practices, conditions, and loving styles. They were forced to change. They need to think about and try new approaches if they want to resume their love life. The therapist can help them decide to make improvements.

But bringing about change demands the counselor clearly understands the client. The therapist determines what needs to happen and guides the client toward the agreed-on objective. The therapist must convey the concepts in words and a framework understandable by the patient. This is one reason why compatibility in speech is important.

Sex Is an 11-Letter Word: Communicate

Probably the most difficult task for a couple is changing the communication pattern. Long-term habits, such as being uptight, are not likely to be improved. Type A personalities are not likely to become open and transparent. Herein lies the therapist's greatest challenge. Intimacy suffers when the partners are reticent and suppress talking about things that the other person does not like to discuss. Sexual problems are frequently on the list of topics to avoid.

Male cancer patients habitually want to resolve the problem by themselves because they have "always taken care of things." An often used excuse is that they do not want to saddle the partner with concerns. Most partners' emotional response is to feel shut out, isolated and alone at a time when they need to feel connected to the man they love. A man confronts an identity crisis when he has erectile dysfunction: is he a man? What about his manliness, capability to perform, ability to please his partner? If the couple avoids talking about sex, these issues will never be satisfactorily addressed. The therapist needs to facilitate an ease of communication so that the thorny issues can be discussed and dealt with on a timely basis.

Women also may refrain from discussing sensitive topics with their partners fearing rejection or the possibility of driving their partner into mental seclusion. Often, their partners convey their thoughts by looks and actions. One woman treated for breast cancer said her husband looked at her after she came home and immediately turned his head away. One husband went on a business trip to California, the day his wife returned from the hospital. Their partner's responses may express disappointment, rejection, and in some cases abandonment.

The therapist can create a "talk climate" during the therapy sessions that ultimately gets carried back to the couple's home. "Communications" really means contact of any and all types including looking, touching, and talking. Part of becoming comfortable with each other may be achieved by looking at the treated area. This is especially true regarding breast surgery. Getting both partners to look at the scars as part of their "homework" can help. One woman had her husband apply cream on the scar after she returned from the hospital. With her guidance as to the amount of pressure he should apply, he learned what she could tolerate and where she was sensitive so that their lovemaking was never affected.

Setting the Stage for Loving: Creating a Positive Loving Environment and Getting Reacquainted

Experimenting with new approaches is easier if the partners give each other love and affection all day long, but many couples in long-term relationships have fallen into a rut. As a result, the partners become less sensitive to the needs of each other. The simple caring gestures of the day are forgotten.

The counselor can help them get back on track by creating a loving environment which is essential for having and restoring substantive intimacy and sex. This intimacy requires that partners do many little things for and with each other. Boston therapist Mira Kirshenbaum, author of the book, *The Weekend Marriage-Love in a Time Starved World*, talks about a clinical research study that showed "the people who were successful . . . were doing little things consistently . . . The key is in concentrating on each other and having positive experiences the way they did when they were first in love" (Kirschenbaum was interviewed by Rebecca Adams of the *Washington Post*).

The therapist can remind and suggest to them things that can do for each other constantly and consistently. They could include:

- Putting their arms around each other occasionally
- Touching and kissing each other
- Taking walks and doing things that they enjoy together
- Taking a shower together

- Putting lotion on each other's body after showering combines touching, caring, and sensuality
- Retelling each other (or other people) how they fell in love, to remind them why they are together and what makes their relationship special

These things may not be considered sexual, but they can initiate and maintain a couple's physical sensual connection. In this key module, the therapist can guide the client to creating a loving environment so the partners can think of each other positively. By reducing the daily friction the partners will have fewer unfavorable factors distracting them from sexual activity.

Increasing Desire and Arousal: Getting Reacquainted and Using the Power of Anticipation

After cancer, body sensitivity changes, and the way people respond to various aspects of lovemaking may also change. This is an opportunity for partners to get to know each other all over again sexually, to explore each other's likes and dislikes and rediscover each other's anatomy. The partners need to test and find out what turns them on and how they react. Things that felt good previously may not feel that way any longer. Different or new areas may now have heightened sensitivity. The only way to find out is for them to touch each other and have the partner provide feedback. The partners may need to be creative to restore some of the pleasures they used to have. Sensate focus is an extremely useful tool for getting reacquainted.

Arousal is a special challenge for most men who are undergoing hormone treatment or had their testicles removed to treat prostate cancer. Many of them will not initiate sex. However, the man often can be responsive if their partner initiates sex. One woman put on clothes that used to turn her husband on. Even though it took a little longer for him to get aroused, it worked. Some hormone patients also report success from using a vibrator or having their partner using the vibrator on them.

Desire and subsequent arousal occurs when there is a high degree of anticipation. The partners can create a mood for anticipation so they get into loving with advance excitement. They can do things hours before getting together such as:

- Writing a love note and invite their lover to a romantic tryst that day.
- Telephone the partner for a romantic dinner.
- Dressing up for each other.
- Arranging to "chance on each other" at a museum, a store, coffee-hour at a Starbucks or other such place.
- Going to a store and try on different clothes and then go home.

And before and during loving, desire and arousal can be increased by:

- Being playful.
- Touching each other all over, and/or massage.
- Many couples find it helpful to watch erotic videos. (An 84-year-old woman who came to a cancer intimacy workshop brought her collection of books and videos that she and her 87-year-old partner use to get excited.)

Dealing with Sex Flow

Desire, foreplay and arousal, intercourse, and orgasm—most people do not think explicitly about the sexual flow or sequence. Yet when there are difficulties in the flow as a couple has practiced it, they need to understand how to achieve the same satisfaction. Desire may not be automatic, but it can be stimulated. And sometimes arousal must be initiated by one partner with desire following from the other partner.

The therapist must help the client understand that although the cancer treatments may have introduced some obstacles and in fact prevent some activities, a different approach can be used. The therapist can introduce the concept of intercourse-free sex and if both partners are interested, there may be medications and aids.

The most important consideration is for clients to appreciate that sex can be as great as they want it to be, even if it will be different than before. Clients are likely to feel frustrated that some of the things they did previously are no longer possible, or do not provide satisfaction. Cancer treatment may have imposed changes on the way couples can interact sexually. The partners may not be able to do their foreplay in the way they used to do, they may not be able to have intercourse, and they may not have the same feelings from some of their sexual acts. Still, they can give each other sexual pleasure and satisfaction. So the first major task is to help couples accommodate to their current capability. But that means they may need to understand the discrete components of the sexual flow.

Sex and Intercourse

In the book, *Father Joe*, the protagonist, Father Joe, says, "Sex is a wonderful gift, a physical way to express the most powerful force in all existence—love. Sex is a brilliant idea of God's, I think. Almost like a sacrament" (Hendra, 2005, p. 118).

But as each person is different in so many ways—culture, religion, gender, age, and other factors—bringing two people together as a couple means that the way they think about, practice and experience sex will be unlike another couple. Therefore, the therapist at best can merely point them in a direction and provide guidance and suggestions to get them to a satisfactory sexual relationship. For many that will mean an orgasm, and some will not be able to separate that from intercourse in their mind. Separating the two is one task for the therapist since some couples may not be able to have intercourse. For couples affected by erectile dysfunction, the first step is to help them understand that the neurological paths for erection and orgasm are different, so a man can have an orgasm without an erection—and that neither orgasm nor erection are possible without arousal, The therapist may need to explain that a woman does not need penetration in order to have an orgasm.

Three major myths must be dispelled at the outset as a means of revising the client's sexual mind-set.

- Sex does not come with the precondition of intercourse. Couples can have sex and orgasms with and without penetration.

- Intimacy and sex are not the same. Intimacy can define a relationship between partners without the presumption of physical contact. Intimacy should be viewed as the umbrella for a fulfilling emotional relationship.

- There is no one way to have sex. The couple may like the pattern it has established over the years. But that pattern may no longer be feasible. Adapting and implementing changes can facilitate the resumption of sexual activity. Moreover, changes to lovemaking can be cause for anticipation and arousal, thus heightening the partners' respective pleasures.

With the foregoing context in mind, a couple can transform their sexual environment by making the following key changes:

- Change the *place* for making love—it does not always have to take place in the bedroom.

- Change the *way* and the *places* they *touch* each other. Sensate focus can be a very helpful tool here.

- Change the *pace*—slow down, undress each other, change from a strong style to delicate to vice-versa.

- Change the *time* to make love. This is especially important for older couples. They need to move up the sex timetable—do it in the morning or in the afternoon, or at least early in the evening.

- Change their loving *style*. Over time they have probably developed a style or a way to go about making love. Doing the same thing all the time means that they can get comfortable, but the partner does not get the same kick out of it. So now there is an opportunity to change. For example, become expert at clitoral stimulation, using any means that feels comfortable to the couple—finger, tongue, vibrator, or an erect or completely flaccid penis.

- Change positions. Sometimes as in the breast cancer reconstruction, sexual positions previously enjoyed by a couple may cause discomfort and even pain.

The partners may need to test whether positions they've been accustomed to place a strain or weight on a sensitive place. Even pressing on a scar can cause pain.

For men with erectile dysfunction, using gravity to enhance blood flow may help retain some engorgement of the penis, if in the missionary position or where the man is standing at the side of the bed.

- Change lovemaking.

In addition, couples are encouraged to share and build on some of the *fantasies* the partners have had. Fantasies are constructive in helping couples revive their sex life. The fundamental condition is that both parties have to agree on acting them out. By setting an environment of trust and openness, the counselor can create a threat-free atmosphere such that safe and exciting fantasies can be implemented.

Fantasies that involve staging seduction scenes, dressing in a certain way and undressing, and trying new positions, may be especially arousing if the couple has not done them previously. Other useful fantasies may consist of being sensuously touched, naked caressing, having sex in different locations, oral sex, and having one partner masturbate the other. The therapist can help the partners talk about fantasies and help them work out how a situation could be played out to everyone's satisfaction.

Men with erectile dysfunction may have some penile engorgement even though it may not be sufficient for intercourse. With sufficient foreplay and vaginal relaxation, the *penis may be stuffed into the vagina.* Both partners may be able to climax

Alternatively, the female partner may *rub the flaccid penis against the clitoris* in the manner of a vibrator. Women may achieve greater stimulation due to the softness of the penile tissue (which is less abrasive than that of a vibrator) and its warmth.

Engaging in sex when one partner is recovering from treatment can be difficult. Couples can find it helpful to *focus on different areas.* For example, women recovering from breast cancer may find that oral sex will focus sex on the genital area and take the pressure off the breast area and allows the breast to heal. Sensate focus and, if desired, anal stimulation, may shift attention from the penis and intercourse.

Sex toys are novelties for the baby boomer and older generations. The topic has to be introduced sensitively, so that neither member of the couple feels awkward in either accepting or rejecting the idea. It often helps to have samples of the products available for the partners in an emotionally safe and secure environment (i.e., without embarrassment or feeling under pressure).

Therapies: Medications and Aids

Many medications and aids are available to support treatment for the client with sexual dysfunction. The therapist may weave their consideration into the dialogue with the client to address a specific problem if this is of interest to both partners.

Medications and aids may be suggested with the mutual understanding that only a medical professional can ascertain and prescribe the medication and aids most appropriate for the patient. Many medications for sexual problems have side effects that may conflict with medications for other conditions.

Although the sex therapist is often not in a position to prescribe a particular medication or aid, the therapist can prepare the client by setting the appropriate level of expectations. They need to tell the prospective user:

> The medications do not work on all patients. When they do work, they may not work equally well each time.
> They have side effects. Couples need to be aware of what they are and prepared to respond should they occur.
> Many medications (especially the oral medications for erectile dysfunction) must not be taken by people with certain medical conditions or with other medications.
> Most medications for erectile dysfunction only work or when the man is aroused. When the relationship is conflict ridden, they are not likely to work.

For men with erectile dysfunction, an array of therapies and medications have been developed to improve the probability of achieving an erection. These include oral pills, injections, intra-urethral suppositories, and vacuum erection devices (pumps). Companies are developing lotions and gels to aid men in obtaining an erection as well as an inhalation medication. (see volume 4, chapter 3)

For women, lubricants like KY Jelly and Astroglide have been available for years. In 2000, the first clitoral therapy device, a vacuum pump, was approved by the FDA (Eros Device). A number of chemicals have also been found to increase clitoral stimulation and are being explored for future products. Some products currently being used to improve men's erectile capability also show promise in aiding women's sexual response.

Although the medications and aids do offer the prospect of benefits, these are not certain to confer on every person who uses them. They do introduce new factors in the sexual equation that the patients and partners should be aware of. Since these products were developed for people with sexual problems at large, they may have side effects that preclude their use by cancer patients. For example, many men cannot take testosterone because it can increase the probability of prostate cancer recurrence, and hormone injections for women may be likewise contraindicated. All medications and nonprescription approaches must be reviewed by the appropriate health care professional.

Volume 4 in this series has three chapters that discussed details of the therapies: medications and aids available and in development. These include the following:

Volume 4, Chapter 3—Pharmacological Treatment of Male Erectile Dysfunction, provides an extensive review of the pharmacology, clinical trials and side effects of pharmaceutical products that deal with erectile dysfunction.

Volume 4, Chapter 4—Devices Used for the Treatment of Sexual Dysfunctions in Men, covers the broad range of vacuum constriction devices, external penile splints, penile implants, and vibrators.

Volume 4, Chapter 6—Therapy Update for Women, discusses the pharmacophysiology of female sexual disorders, with a special focus on hypoactive sexual desire and arousal.

NOTE

1. Therapist/counselor hereinafter may be referred to as either counselor or therapist.

REFERENCES

Adams, R. (2005). Interview of Myra Kirschenbaum. *Washington Post*, Health Section, May 17, 2005.

Althof, S.E. (2002) When an erection alone is not enough: Biopsychological obstacles to lovemaking. *Journal of Impotence Research, 14*(Suppl. 1), S99–S104.

Bancroft, J. (1989). *Human sexuality and its problems* (2nd ed.). New York: Churchill Livingstone.

CancerWEB. National Cancer Institute.(n.d.). *The prevalence and types of sexual dysfunction in people with cancer*. Sexuality and Reproductive Issues. Retrieved September 10, 2006, from http://cancerweb.ncl.ac.uk/cancernet/310207.html.

Chochinov, H.M., & Schachter, S., (2002). *The psychology of cancer*. Lymphoma Focus. Retrieved May 23, 2006, from http://www.lymphomafocus.org/focus_article.asp?b=lymphoma&f=lymphoma_issues&c=cancer_psychology&pg=1.

Feldman, H.A., Goldstein, I., Hatzichristou, D.G., Krane, R.J., & McKinlay J. B. (1994). Impotence and its medical and psychosocial correlates: Results of the Massachusetts Male Aging Study. *Journal of Urology, 151*(1), 54–61.

Hendra, T. (2005). *Father Joe: The man who saved my soul*. New York: Random House.

Hewitt, M., Greenfield, S., & Stovall, E. (Eds.) (2006). *From cancer patient to cancer survivor: Lost in transition*. Washington, D.C.: National Academies Press.

Kirschenbaum, M. (2005). *The weekend marriage: Abundant love in a time-starved world*. New York: Harmony.

Kovel, J. (1976). *A complete guide to therapy*. New York: Pantheon Books.

Schover, L. (2001a). *Sexuality and cancer for the man who has cancer*. Atlanta: American Cancer Society.

Schover, L. (2001b). *Sexuality and cancer for the woman who has cancer*. Atlanta: American Cancer Society.

Weijmar Schultz, W. C., van de Wiel, H. B., Bouma, J., Janssens, J., & Littlewood, J. (1990). Psychosexual functioning after the treatment of cancer of the vulva. A longitudinal study. *Cancer, 66*(2), 402–407.

Additional Resources

Books

Aftel, M., & Lakoff, R.T. (1985). *When Talk Is Not Cheap.* New York: Warner Books.

Alterowitz, B., & Alterowitz, R. (2004). *Intimacy with Impotence: The Couple's Guide to Better Sex After Prostate Disease.* Cambridge, MA: Da Capo Books

Anand, M. (1989). *The Art of Sexual Ecstasy.* Los Angeles: Jeremy P. Tarcher, Inc.

Angier, N. (1999). *Woman.* New York: Houghton Mifflin.

Bostwick, D.G., Crawford, E.D., Higano, C.S., & Roach, M. (2005). *Complete Guide to Prostate Cancer.* Atlanta, GA: American Cancer Society.

Diamond, J. (1997). *Why is Sex Fun?* New York: Basic Books.

Engel, B. (1999). *Sensual Sex.* Berkeley, CA: Hunter House Publishers

George, S.C., & Caine, K.C. (1998) *A Lifetime of Sex.* Rodale.

Heffernan, M., & Quinn, M. (2003). *The Gynaecological Cancer Guide.* Melbourne, Australia: Michelle Anderson Publishing.

Hewitt, M., Herdman, R., & Holland, J. (Eds.) (2004). *Meeting Psychosocial Needs of Women with Breast Cancer.* Washington, D.C.: National Academies Press.

Hughes, J.M. (1989). *Reshaping the Psychoanalytic Domain.* Berkeley and Los Angeles: University of California Press.

Inkeles, G., & Todris, M. (1972). *The Art of Sensual Massage.* New York: Simon & Schuster.

Kolb, L.C. (1968). *Noyes' Modern Clinical Psychiatry.* Seventh Edition Philadelphia: W.B. Saunders.

Leiblum, S., & Sachs, J. (2002). *Getting the Sex You Want.* Lincoln, NE: ASJA Press.

Levine, S.B., Althof, S.E., & Risen, C.B. (2003). *Handbook of Clinical Sexuality for Mental Health Professionals.* New York: Brunner-Routledge.

Love, S.M. (2000). *Dr. Susan Love's Breast Book,* Third Edition. Cambridge, MA: Da Capo Press.

Marks, S. (1999). *Prostate & Cancer.* Cambridge, MA: Fisher Books.

McCarthy, P., & Loren, J.A. (1997) *Breast Cancer? Let Me Check My Schedule!* Boulder CO: Westview Press.

Schnarch, D. (1997). *Passionate Marriage.* New York: Henry Holt and Company.

Schwartz, R., & Olds, J. (2000). *Marriage in Motion.* Cambridge, MA: Perseus Publishing.

Spark, R.F. (2000). *Sexual Health for Men.* Cambridge, MA: Perseus Publishing, 2000

Strum, S.B., & Pogliano, D. *A* (2005) *Primer on Prostate Cancer.* Hollywood, Florida: The Life Extension Foundation.

Toronto, E.L.K., Ainslie, G., Donovan, M., Kelly, M., Kieffer, C.C., & McWilliams, N. (Eds.)(2005). *Psychoanalytic Reflections on a Gender-free Case.* New York: Routledge.

Truax, C.B., & Carkhuff, R.R.(1972). *Toward Effective Counseling an Psychotherapy: Training and Practice.* Chicago & New York: Aldine-Atherton.

Articles/Abstracts

Ameda, K., Kakizaki, H., Koyanagi, T., Hirakawa, K., Kusumi, T., & Hosokawa, M. (2005). The long-term voiding function and sexual function after pelvic nerve-sparing radical surgery for rectal cancer. *International Journal of Urology, 12*(3), 256–263.

Canada, A. L., Neese, L. E., Sui, D., & Schover, L. (2005). Pilot intervention to enhance sexual rehabilitation for couples after treatment for localized prostate carcinoma. *Cancer, 104*(12), 2689–2700.

Carmack Taylor, C., Basen-Engquist, K., Shinn, E. H., Bodurka, D. C. (2004). Predictors of sexual functioning in ovarian cancer patients. *Journal of Clinical Oncology, 22*(5), 881–889.

Donahue, V. C, & Knapp, R. C. (1977). Sexual rehabilitation of gynecologic cancer patients. *Obstetrics & Gynecology, 49,* 118–121.

Gallo-Silver, L. (2000). The sexual rehabilitation of persons with cancer. *Cancer Practice, 8*(1), 10–15.

Goldstein, I. (2000). Female sexual arousal disorder: new insights. *International Journal of Impotence Research, 1* (Suppl. 4), S152–S157.

Latini, D. M., Elkin, E. P., Cooperberg, M. R., Sadetsky, N,, Duchane, J., Carroll, P. R. (2006). Differences in clinical characteristics and disease-free survival for Latino, African American, and non-Latino white men with localized prostate cancer: data from CaPSHURE. *Cancer, 106*(4), 789–795.

McKee, A. L., Jr., & Schover, L. R. (2001). Sexuality rehabilitation. *Cancer, 92*(Suppl. 4), 1008–1012.

Schover, L. R. (2005). Sexuality and fertility after cancer. *Hematology* 2005:523–527.

Schroder, M., Mell, L. K., Hurteau, J. A., Collins, Y. C., Rotmensch, J., Waggoner, S. E., et al. (2005). Clitoral therapy device for treatment of sexual dysfunction in irradiated cervical cancer patients. *International Journal of Radiation Oncology*Biology* Physics, 61*(4), 1078–1086.

Thomas, D. F., (Host), Rosenberg, K., & Filewich, R.J., (Participants). (2003). Conquering performance anxiety [Webcast]. October 12, 2003, http://sexhealth.healthology.com.

Chapter Thirteen

ACCESS TO PLEASURE: ON-RAMP TO SPECIFIC INFORMATION ON DISABILITY, ILLNESS, AND CHANGES THROUGHOUT THE LIFE SPAN

Mitchell S. Tepper and Annette Fuglsang Owens

All too often, sexual health is overlooked or ignored in the health care system (Tepper, 1992). The most common reasons for not providing sexual health care services from a provider's perspective include anxiety with regard to discussing sexuality with patients, inadequate training, lack of appropriate curriculum, and the health provider's belief that it is someone else's responsibility (Ducharme & Gill, 1990; Krueger 1991; Novak & Mitchell, 1988). Discomfort and resistance to talking about sexual issues with people who have disabilities, chronic conditions, and who are elderly is reinforced by societal attitudes that do not embrace the sexuality of those who are not young and healthy. Instead of routinely assessing patients' sexual health needs, many health professionals will wait for the patient to bring up a concern.

From the patient's or client's perspective, research shows that both men and women fear discussing sexual problems with their doctors because of concerns that physicians would be embarrassed with the topic (Partnership for Women's Health at Columbia, 1999). A telephone survey of 500 Americans over age 25 found that 68% of those polled worry that their physicians would be uncomfortable discussing sexual issues, with 75% of women expressing such concerns compared to 61% of men. Survey respondents also believe that sexual problems have an impact on a number of medical issues, including depression (91%), emotional stress (93%), poor self-image (88%) and extramarital affairs and marriage breakups (91%). Historically, men and women who interact with the health care system have sexual concerns but felt they had nowhere to turn for help.

Silence about sexual health-related issues has made access to sexual health care from traditional sources difficult, resulting in unnecessary suffering for many. This is especially true for the three discrete populations that are the focus of this chapter, namely (a) people with disabilities, (b) people with chronic conditions, and (c) people who are in their later years. As noted, these groups have been traditionally sexually disenfranchised. Misconceptions about sexuality as they relate to these populations often add to the generally negative societal attitudes toward sexuality.

Now patients can turn to the Internet for help. The Internet has begun to bridge the sexual communication gap between provider and consumer. It offers a novel medium providing direct, private, and anonymous access to information about sexual health. The concept of sexual health includes treatment of underlying medical conditions that interfere with sexual and reproductive functions as well as freedom from fear, shame, guilt, false beliefs, and other psychological and social factors inhibiting sexual response and impairing sexual relationships.

In this chapter we will give a brief overview of previous research about sexuality and disability, chronic illness, and aging; provide demographic information on Internet use among the groups focused on; examine how people with disabilities, chronic conditions, and age after midlife have begun to utilize the Internet to gain access to sexual health information; and provide suggestions as to how the therapist can incorporate this phenomenon into his or her practice. We will discuss this in general terms and give examples of existing Web sites.

BRIEF HISTORICAL OVERVIEW

A rapidly growing novel focus on sexual health in the late '60s and early '70s brought along several publications on sexuality in conjunction with physical disability and chronic conditions (Anderson & Cole, 1975; Diamond, 1974; Krieger, 1977). Pioneering studies on individuals with spinal cord injuries in the '50s and early '60s laid some of the foundations for this work (Zeitlin et al., 1957; Tsuji et al., 1961). As reviewed by Kaplan (1990), some studies on sexuality and aging date back even further (Kinsey et al., 1948, 1953; Masters & Johnson, 1966, 1970; Palmore, 1970, 1974).

When reviewing past literature it is striking how little progress has been made. Society's regard of physically disabled people as nonsexual beings is largely unchanged (Mona & Gardos, 2001). It is still widely believed that a physically disabled person is either unable to engage in sexual activity or does not have a need for sexual expression (Anderson & Cole, 1975). Sex primarily appears to be reserved for the young, healthy, and fertile population.

Why have attempts to abolish these myths and to educate the general public about the rich sexual experiences and potential of people of age and with disabilities or chronic conditions failed? One simple explanation may be that the information has yet to reach a wider audience. While articles can be found in academic journals, and movement is underway within the disability community, within populations of specific chronic conditions, and among retired people, the mainstream media has not given much attention to this matter. Media portrayals of the sexuality of people with disabilities is sensationalized and still exaggerates the tragedy of lost sexuality after a devastating injury instead of producing plots that include people with disabilities as sexy and capable of healthy sexual relationships.

The Internet may prove a superior medium for dissemination of information on sexual health that heretofore has been relegated to academic journals and segregated identity movements. By providing access to information about sexual health to a broader population, including older people, people with disabilities, and people with chronic conditions, it may finally become obvious that sexual expression does continue after midlife and that it presents an important part of life for people with chronic illness and disability.

PEOPLE WITH DISABILITIES, CHRONIC CONDITIONS, AND NATURAL CHANGES WITH AGING AND THEIR USE OF THE INTERNET

Adult Internet users with disabilities, chronic illnesses, and natural changes associated with growing older comprise a large and very broad demographic group. The U.S. Department of Justice, in its deliberations on the Americans with Disabilities Act, estimates that 20% of the American population has a disability that impairs a major life function. Within this group, an estimated 21.6% have Internet access (U.S. Department of Commerce, 2000). With 196 million adults in the United States in 2000 (U.S. census projection for persons over 20 years old, U.S. Census Bureau, 1996), these percentages give a figure of 39.2 million adults with disabilities, of whom 8.5 million have Internet access. Of course the Internet is not limited to the United States, so the global number of people with disabilities is much larger.

Within this broad demographic group there are segments defined by specific disabilities and/or chronic conditions. These include spinal cord injury, multiple sclerosis, cerebral palsy, cancer, diabetes, arthritis, developmental disabilities, psychiatric disabilities, HIV/AIDS, and learning disabilities to name just a few. The Internet offers opportunities for continuous tailoring of Web site content to specific needs and conditions.

The Internet provides individuals with chronic illness, disability, and/or age-related concerns access to pleasure by making professional information available to them. It also allows individuals to emerge from isolation and to establish contacts with others in similar situations, thereby providing each other understanding support (Cooper, McLoughlin, & Campbell, 2000).

Overlapping the disability and chronic condition populations is the aging population. A significant group that might be considered under this categorization is the baby boomer population. Over time, most individuals will develop some disabling conditions with possible repercussions on their sexual health. With the baby boomers moving into their older years, this population is growing much faster than that of the general population. While 22% of adults in the U.S. reported a disability in 1999, this figure increased to 50% for adults 65 years of age and older (Centers for Disease Control and Prevention, 2001).

The baby boomer population includes people born between the late 1940s and the early 1960s. Thus, today most boomers are nearly or already over 40. Boomers have transformed every stage of life they have reached. Retirement and old age are likely to be changed as well. Boomers brought the sexual revolution as soon as they reached adulthood. Never inclined to accept limitations, boomers are not likely to settle for less satisfactory sex lives just because they get older. Thus they are likely to be eager consumers of any product or service that helps them meet these needs.

The level of interest by boomers is likely to increase as they move into the older age groups, and as their Internet access and sophistication increases. U.S. population projections show an increase in the population over age 40 from 116 million to 137 million over 10 years (U.S. Census Bureau, 1996). During this same time, Internet access is projected to increase from 56% in 1999 to 90% in 2009, and the over 40 population with Internet access is estimated to nearly double over a period of five years, from 65 million in 1999 to 115 million in 2004. More than 1 billion people are estimated to have Internet access by year 2005 (eTForecasts, 2001), and a recent study by NetValue, a global leader in tracking and interpreting online behavior, shows that the number of retired people going online in the U.S. jumped by 28.1 percent in December 2000, to a total of 8.6 million unique visitors. This surge has the online retired population now representing 10.2% of the overall Internet population (NetValue, 2001).

THE INTERNET AS A USEFUL TOOL FOR THE DESCRIBED POPULATIONS

The driving force for the Internet with respect to sexual expression consists of three key factors: access, affordability, and anonymity. Cooper (1998) has termed these factors the "Triple-A engine" of the Internet, which makes the Internet a unique forum for accessing information about sexuality, pursuing specific sexual interests, and establishing sexual contacts. No other more conventional medium such as books, magazines, TV, or video has a similar promise as the Internet (Cooper, Boies, Maheu, & Greenfield, 1999).

For the populations discussed in this chapter, accessibility is of major importance and carries special meaning. People with disabilities, chronic conditions, and who are retired regularly face architectural and attitudinal barriers to sexual health. As will be described in the following, people with disabilities, chronic conditions, or advanced aging may now access information about their specific needs and concerns through the Internet. Chat rooms, forum boards, instant messaging, and "ask the expert" columns are all mediums that have helped the sexual lives of these populations, as they do for all others.

The populations discussed in our chapter can use the Internet as a very positive tool. These sexually disenfranchised populations can benefit from the access, affordability, anonymity, and the virtual communities that develop around common sexual questions, concerns, and shared experiences. The Internet enables previously isolated individuals to become part of such virtual communities where they may find empathy, support, and a sense of community and belonging (Cooper et al., 1999). This, in return, may have positive psychological effects on the individual. As a flip side, increased Internet use may expose some of these individuals to the dangers of the Internet.

The following case example demonstrates how the Internet helped a quadriplegic man to overcome a long-term fear of having sex. His adolescent sexual inhibition became compounded by a spinal cord injury acquired at age 20. Online communication served as a bridge to establishing and pursuing a successful offline sexual relationship for the first time in his life, 17 years after his accident.

Bruce (an alias) is a 37-year-old quadriplegic, who acquired a cervical (c4/5) spinal cord injury from a diving accident. He is college educated, interested in journalism, and lives in an addition to his parents' house with 24-hour personal care assistants (PCA) who help with activities of daily living. Bruce's pre-injury sex life consisted of one occasion of heavy petting as a teenager. His injury left him with no sensation below his upper chest and with only limited function in one arm. He has reflex erections in response to touch but does not experience orgasm or ejaculation. He received no sexual education or counseling during his rehabilitation.

For years after his accident Bruce was in unrequited love with his former best friend. Bruce contacted Dr. Tepper's Web site (www.sexualhealth.com) with the following comments:

> The lust I had for her and others, while never directly expressed, tortured me and drove me to selfish, hostile behavior that hurt very kind friends ... I have little desire to attempt physical sex, and lots of reservations. I fear I might be more of a spectator

than a participant. When prone, I have no arm/hand function, no sensation below my upper chest, and penetration is not feasible. All that works is my mouth. I know these problems aren't insurmountable for everyone, but it would be great to hear about any similarly (dys)functioning guys or women who have succeeded at an ongoing relationship.

In subsequent postings, Bruce expressed doubt that he would ever have a physical relationship. He relayed that he had several wonderfully close platonic women friends but was unable to appreciate some of them because of unexpressed sexual desires. In his own words:

I lusted for them, feeling guilty and frustrated. It's not just society that emphasizes sex; it's biological urges too, especially with my massive libido. When one friend offered to listen to my repressed feelings about sexuality, presto! Everything changed! Discussing sexuality with women cured my unrequited lust, and freed me to find a great sex-oriented relationship online. I am very fulfilled now, just curious about crips like me who manage successful long-term relationships.

Bruce coined the term "hands free whoopee" to describe sexual excitement and fulfillment through mental activity and without involvement of physical stimulation of sex organs. He was now able to describe fantasies to partners verbally over the phone and by email exchanges. He later wrote:

My experience with written sex doesn't seem typical of "cybersex." I feel that my circumstances are fairly unusual—lack of privacy, lack of in-person confidence, love of and talent for writing, hyper-horniness, and most of all luck in finding a couple of women whose needs matched mine. These relationships were also not typical of cybersex because they included a dimension of love. I have felt guilty and ashamed of my libido for years; so have my disabled lovers, and we cured each other—sort of a self-help sex therapy. Maybe there are more lonely, isolated and horny disabled folks than I think, but a great majority of people online either have in-person sex lives or very much want them.

Reservations and fear contributing to little desire to attempt physical sex are predictable outcomes of disability when sexual education is lacking during rehabilitation and there are few role models to learn from (Tepper, 1996; Tepper dissertation, 2001). The Internet had given Bruce an outlet for his sexual expression and a source of brief professional counseling. His relationships based on written online communications combined with a greater vision of his possibilities provided by Dr. Tepper gave him the confidence to overcome his reluctance about sex. Eventually, a chance for a physical love relationship developed, and in the following, Bruce describes a physical encounter with Wendy (an alias), an acquaintance he had met online:

Writer that I am, I'm not sure I can find the words to convey how wonderful Wendy's visit was. It can't be true that waiting till age 37 was worth it! And yet if

I had it to do over again, I really don't think I could bring myself to choose a life that doesn't include every blissful second of our 16 hours in heaven. In the realm of physical love, I have been massively deprived of quantity but extraordinarily blessed with quality. It's almost as if those two extremes are inversely proportional! Wendy's visit provided so much incentive! Not just the obvious kind; she makes me feel so confident in areas unrelated to sex and love, too . . . But probably our greatest discovery wasn't primarily sexual. As she stood next to the chair, I realized that I could get my good arm around her and hug her quite strongly. I can hold her, Mitch! She LOVED it! I loved it! Until we get a lot more extended time together (which probably will happen, though not for several months), a lot of the brief time we have is bound to go to holding each other. Then we'll break out the toys!

Wendy eventually relocated with her teenage daughter to be closer to Bruce with the intentions of eventually getting married.

SCIENTIFIC STUDIES

While there are some early studies outlining the demographics of cybersex users of the Internet (Cooper, Delmonico, & Burg 2000; Cooper, Scherer, Boies, & Gordon, 1999) and a new study that seeks to understand user profiles in online sexual activity (Cooper, Morahan-Martin, Mathy, & Maheu, 2002), we are unaware of any published studies that quantify the number of people utilizing the Internet to gain access specifically to information about sexual health. Data from our own Web site offering general information about sexual health is briefly summarized below. Parts of this analysis have been previously communicated (Tepper & Owens, 2000).

Nearly 600 questions presented over a 4-month period in 2000/2001 to a team of over forty sexual health experts at www.SexualHealth.com, were analyzed. About 75% of inquisitors were from within the U.S., while most other continents were represented to lesser degrees. Men and women represented equal groups, and a few individuals listed their gender as transgender or intersex. Visitors' ages ranged from teenagers to individuals over 59 years with the mode in age range from 20 to 29 years.

Not surprisingly, women mostly asked about low sexual desire, sexual pain, and orgasm, while men's top concerns were about masturbation, erections, and questions about ejaculation, including premature and delayed ejaculation.

Roughly 20% of the questions were requests for basic information about items such as anatomy (3%), physiology (10%), medication effects (2%), sexual positions (1%), and terminology (2%). The remaining 80% of questions were requests for specific information, including topics such as sexual problems related to age, chronic conditions, and disability.

From this small sample, we conclude that whether otherwise healthy or challenged by chronic illness, age, or disabilities, online users are willing to use the Internet as a medium for seeking general advice and specific information about sexual concerns (Tepper & Owens, 2000). As a consequence, the Internet is a viable option for health professionals to provide information to a wide audience. Our analysis further reveals the broad range of sexual issues people have been struggling with, some heretofore in silence, and reflects the dire need for more and better sexual education and counseling.

DIFFERENT WAYS OF UTILIZING THE POWER OF THE INTERNET TO GAIN ACCESS TO PLEASURE

In the following we have summarized different ways for clients and clinicians to utilize the Internet for specific purposes. The listed categories not only apply to sexual health information but in general to many other areas of interest as well.

Specific Information

The Internet makes access to pleasure possible by making general and disability and/or illness specific sexual health information easily available. Heretofore, this type of information was relegated to obscure journals targeted toward academics and was not accessible to consumers. Clarifying myth-information and finding accurate information is the first step toward sexual enlightenment.

Affordable, Anonymous Access

The Triple-A engine (Cooper, 1998) allows Internet users easy access to credentialed health professionals who can inform and offer advice regarding sexual health and sexual problems one-to-one and in groups. There is a shortage of well-trained sexual health professionals with expertise in the intersection of sexuality and disability and illness. The Internet offers those with experience to make themselves known, and it provides users affordable, anonymous access to these health professionals.

Peer Support

Access to pleasure is also made possible by providing forums and chats for objective discussions of sexual matters among peers and facilitating interpersonal contacts. Potential pitfalls of using the Internet are noted elsewhere in this book. Also, if someone learns to rely too much on computer mediated relating (CMR; Cooper et al., 1999) as a way of fulfilling their sexual needs, there may be too little motivation to pursue in-person relationships. However, for disabled, chronically ill, as well as more mature Internet users, it is sometimes difficult to meet sexual partners in general, and online sexual contacts may be welcome additions to their lives.

e-Learning

The Internet increases opportunities for training and continuing education of health service personnel with respect to sexual health. Equipped with superior knowledge, these individuals will be better prepared and more likely to address sexual health related concerns with their patients. The major sexuality organizations provide listservs for members where difficult cases can be discussed in a professional forum and information and announcements may be posted on bulletin boards. Other educational resources are online seminars and courses. The field of eLearning is rapidly growing and will revolutionize the ways in which professionals will be able to receive continuing education.

e-Commerce

The Internet makes access to pleasure possible by making sexual health related products easily available for purchase (Fisher & Barak, 2000). Clients may be more comfortable buying sex related products online. Retail stores for such products tend to be located in major metropolitan areas and only a minority of potential customers has direct physical access to these stores.

Links and Contacts

Finally, computer links to the disability community and information about other online as well as offline resources make up a sexual health network, which allows clients and clinicians to effectively navigate the broad field of sexual health. For people with disabilities, this network of sexual health information provides a true onramp to pleasure.

HOW CLINICIANS CAN UTILIZE THE INTERNET TO BETTER SERVE THEIR CLIENTS

In addition to taking advantage of the above mentioned ways to keep informed and up-to-date, clinicians should become familiar with the best sites in their specific area of interest and use them to complement their therapies (The Network for Family Life Education, 2001). Therapists and other health professionals may want to provide patients with a list of regularly updated, high quality sites and help them navigate "the mean streets" by demonstrating how to avoid exploitive or pornographic sites (Gotlib & Fagan, 1997). Due to a rapidly changing market, it is advisable to periodically use the major search engines for newly developed sites. The Sexuality Information and Education Council of the

United States (SIECUS) provides regularly updated lists of Internet sources at SIECUS.org. The American Association of Sexuality Educators, Counselors, and Therapists (AASECT) has a Web site, AASECT.org, with current information and links. Many organizations with a specific focus, such as the American Heart Association, the National Multiple Sclerosis Society, or the American Diabetes Association, specifically address sexual health topics on their Web sites. University or hospital based sites and sites that have been approved by Health On the Net or Truste are likely to be reliable sources as well.

Clinicians also may find the Internet a useful tool for informing themselves in areas in which their clients are well versed, thereby gaining greater understanding of the patient perspective. They should find out what sites their clients are visiting and what types of support, chat, or news groups they frequent. Clinicians may then be able to assist their clients to better use these resources. Health professionals even may aid with specific tasks, such as helping their patients to write personal ads and assisting them in registering for community classes promoting computer skills and literacy. We recommend having informational brochures about such services readily available in the office. Clinicians may find useful information on these sites, or they may take online continuing education courses, or join a professional listserv within their particular area of interest. At present, several organizations such as the American Association of Sexuality Educators, Counselors, and Therapists (AASECT), the Female Sexual Function Forum (FSFF)[1] and the International Society for Sexual and Impotence Research (ISSIR)[2] have listservs that offer professionals a forum and network for discussing difficult cases. This is one particular area of communication between clinicians that is likely to expand considerably in the future.

TELEHEALTH: IMPLICATIONS AND SPECIAL CONSIDERATIONS

The use of the Internet for telehealth applications provides a unique medium for distributing basic sexual health information, education, and specific advice to a growing population. The Telemedicine Report to Congress of January 1997 (U.S. Department of Commerce) defines telemedicine as the use of electronic communication and information technologies to provide or support clinical care at a distance. Telehealth is a broader concept that includes clinical care in addition to the related areas of health professional education, consumer health education, public health, research, and administration of health services. The World Wide Web has the potential of reaching users in remote and rural settings, where medical care and mental health assistance are not readily available. However, ethical considerations and concerns need to be carefully evaluated before telehealth is more fully adopted and utilized along with traditional healthcare models (U.S. Department of Congress: National Telecommunications and Information Administration in consultation with the U.S. Department of Health and Human Services, 1997).

Some of these ethical issues have been addressed previously (Cooper et al. 1999) and within this book (references to selective chapters in the book). In the following, we will summarize special considerations and issues of concern to health professionals who work with disabled and/or chronically ill clients, or with individuals who are in their upper years. Many of these issues are covered more fully in The Telemedicine Report to the Congress (1997).

Licensure Requirements

Licensure requirements for health professionals vary between geographical regions. Licensure and malpractice concerns arise when a licensed health professional works across state lines or provides services on a multi-state basis, as it is highly likely using the Internet. The major issue is which state has the power to regulate or discipline a provider who "enters" a state to practice via telehealth technology and in which state or jurisdiction will the provider answer a telehealth malpractice claim.

Anonymity

One of the driving factors of the Internet and part of the Triple-A engine, anonymity, carries several negative implications for telehealth. The fact that Internet users have the option to remain anonymous may impact and limit the relationship between the sexual health professional and the client. The professional has no guarantee that the information provided is accurate. As a consequence, thorough exchange of information and in-depth therapy is often limited. However, basic guidance and, if necessary, encouragement to seek out health care providers within the client's local area can usually be given. Thereby, someone who has previously relied on self-help may be moved to consult a trained local provider.

Another consequence of anonymity is that the physical location of the person seeking assistance is often unknown. Possible legal implications of this fact are manifold. Consider a client acknowledging pedophilic tendencies or someone who confirms being sexually abusive to a child or to a partner. How can the telehealth professional take the necessary steps to protect potential or actual victims if the physical location of those individuals cannot be revealed without involving major, ethically debatable efforts of tracing?

Privacy, Confidentiality, and Security

Privacy, confidentiality, and security issues unique to telemedicine, especially mental health records on conditions that carry a social stigma such as

HIV, are other areas of concern, as are the verification of credentials by the consumer and verification of the consumer's identity by the provider. The Telemedicine Report to the Congress (U.S. Department of Congress: National Telecommunications and Information Administration in consultation with the US Department of Health and Human Services, 1997) notes that unlike standard medical record documentation, in which the health professional has discretion to selectively record his or her findings, most interactive telemedicine consultations are recorded in toto. This record usually is maintained as part of the documentation of the consultation. As a result, practitioners have less discretion to remove information that they might otherwise not record. Another concern is that the patient may not be able to "see" who else is viewing the session along with the clinicians on the other end of the long distance consultation. Health Internet Ethics (HI Ethics) has defined ethical standards regarding privacy, confidentiality, credibility, reliability, and security at http://hiethics.com. Another Web site, National Board for Certified Counselors (NBCC) Standards for the Ethical Practice of WebCounseling at http://www.nbcc.org/ethics/wcstandards.htm, recommends certain codes of conduct with respect to online counseling.

Treatment Concerns

Several implications relate to treatment concerns. Sex therapy has an enormous potential for client resistances and failures to complete assignments given by the therapist. Providing supportive counseling may be possible but trying to elicit significant behavioral changes may prove more challenging, especially in the sexual areas. Only ongoing evaluation will determine how effective "full-fledged" sex therapy can be online and how well it will deal with clients with very complex issues. Furthermore, many clients with disability, illness, or changes with age have at least some biological etiology to their sexual dysfunctions and may need to undergo physical exams and treatments. Lastly, there is some concern about the ability to obtain an appropriate assessment without visual cues like facial expressions and body language. However, since visually impaired individuals are not barred from doing therapy, this challenge may be overcome if telehealth providers begin to develop and rely on different cues germane to the Internet. Also, there is the option of setting up cameras on both ends that becomes more viable with the proliferation of broadband access.

Billing for the service may be difficult if the client remains anonymous or does not have an internationally accepted credit card. Reimbursement for services by third parties, managed-care, Medicare, and Medicaid is a concern for long-term growth of telemedicine and telehealth.

Finally, the Telemedicine Report to the Congress (1997) highlights the need for evaluating certain telemedicine projects. The questions of whether patients and providers can accept telemedicine-enabled care, and whether outcomes associated with the use of telemedicine are acceptable can only be answered in the future and after pilot programs have been established and evaluated.

These general implications on telehealth all apply to the specific populations discussed in this chapter. As the Internet and telehealth evolves, access to disability, chronic condition, and aging specific information, education, counseling, and support will be expanded and even more accessible and user-friendly.

CONCLUSIONS

We hope to have given clinicians an overview of past and present efforts to provide sexual health information to those who are physically challenged by disability or chronic conditions and by normal and expected changes throughout the lifespan. We also have attempted to provide health professionals with specific tools to help them and their patients take the right exit from a potentially disturbing cybersex maze. We believe that as health care providers use the Internet to improve their clinical skills and expertise, the general sexual climate and interaction with their patients will benefit. Finally, looking into the future as ethical guidelines with respect to telehealth are being developed, we invite clinicians to consider making their expertise available to future eCounseling services, thereby reaching out to a much broader group of clients.

The title of this chapter, "Access to Pleasure," reflects a positive approach to human sexuality based on the right to sexual information and the right to pleasure. The concept of sexual health includes treatment of underlying medical conditions that interfere with sexual and reproductive functions and freedom from fear, shame, guilt, false beliefs, and other psychological factors inhibiting sexual response and impairing sexual relationships. People with disabilities, chronic conditions, and people who do not generally fit the dominant culture's depiction of sexy no longer have to suffocate in a veil of sexual silence. The Internet as an onramp to specific information and related resources for heretofore sexually disenfranchised populations is one of the most positive aspects of the World Wide Web.

NOTES

This chapter was reprinted from Tepper, M.S., & Owens, A.F. "Access to Pleasure: Onramp to Specific Information on Disability, Illness, and Changes Throughout the Lifespan." In *Sex and the Internet,* ed. Al Cooper. New York: Brunner-Routledge, 2002, pp. 71–86. Reproduced with permission of Routledge/Taylor & Francis Group, LLC.

1. This organization has been renamed The International Society for the Study of Women's Sexual Health (ISSWSH).

2. This organization has been renamed International Society for Sexual Medicine (ISSM).

REFERENCES

Anderson, T.P., & Cole, T.M. (1975). *Sexual counseling of the physically disabled. Postgraduate Medicine, 58*(1), 117–123.

Barak, A., & King, S.A. (2000). The two faces of the Internet: Introduction to the special issue on the Internet and sexuality. *Cyberpsychology & Behavior, 3*(4), 517–520.

Centers for Disease Control and Prevention (February 23, 2001). Prevalence of Disabilities and Associated Health Conditions among Adults—United States, 1999. *Morbidity and Mortality Weekly Report 50*(7);120–125 Retrieved September 10, 2006, from http://www.cdc.gov/mmwr/preview/mmwrhtml/mm5007a3.htm.

Cooper, A. (1998). *Sexuality and the Internet: Surfing into the new millennium. Cyberpsychology and Behavior, 1,* 181–187.

Cooper, A., Boies, S., Maheu, M., & Greenfield, D. (1999). *Sexuality and the Internet: The next sexual revolution.* In F. Muscarella and L. Szuchman (Eds.), *The psychological science of sexuality: A research based approach,* (pp. 519–545). New York: Wiley Press.

Cooper, A., Delmonico, D.L., & Burg, R. (2000). Cybersex users, abusers, and compulsives: New findings and implications. *Sexual Addiction & Compulsivity, 7,* 5–29.

Cooper, A., McLoughlin, I.P., & Campbell, K.M. (2000). Sexuality in cyberspace: Update for the 21st century. *Cyberpsychology & Behavior, 3*(4), 521–536.

Cooper, A., Morahan-Martin, J., Mathy, R., & Maheu, M. (2002). Toward an increased understanding of user demographics in online sexual activities. *Journal of Sex and Marital Therapy, 28,* 105–129.

Cooper, A., Scherer, C., Boies, S. C., & Gordon, B. (1999). Sexuality on the Internet: From sexual exploration to pathological expression. *Professional Psychology: Research and Practice, 30*(2), 154–164.

Diamond, M. (1974). Sexuality and the handicapped. *Rehabilitation Literature, 35,* 34–40.

Ducharme, S., & Gill, K.M. (1990). Sexual values, training, and professional roles. *Journal of Head Trauma Rehabilitation, 5*(2), 38–45.

eTForecasts. (2001, February 6). *Internet users will surpass 1 billion in 2005* [Press Release]. Published online at http://www.etforecasts.com/pr/pr201.htm.

Fisher, W. A., & Barak, A. (2000). Online sex shops: Phenomenological, psychological, and ideological perspectives on Internet sexuality. *Cyberpsychology & Behavior, 3*(4), 575–589.

Gotlib, D. A., & Fagan, P. (1997). Mean streets of cyberspace: Sex education resources on the Internet's World Wide Web. *Journal of Sex Education and Therapy, 22*(1), 79–83.

Kaplan, H. S. (1990). Sex, intimacy, and the aging process. *Journal of the American Academy of Psychoanalysis, 18*(2); 185–205.

Kinsey, A. C., Pomeroy, W. B., & Martin, C. E. (1948). *Sexual behavior in the human male.* Philadelphia, PA: W. B. Saunders.

Kinsey, A. C., Pomeroy, W. B., & Martin, C. E. (1953). *Sexual behavior in the human female.* Philadelphia, PA: W. B. Saunders.

Korn, K. (1998). Computer comments: Disability information on the Internet. *Journal of the American Academy of Nurse Practitioners, 10*(9), 413–414.

Krieger, S. M. (1977). Sexuality and disability. *ARN J., 2* (1), 8–10, 12–14.

Krueger, M.M. (1991). The omnipresent need: Professional training for sexuality education teachers. *SIECUS Report, 19*(4), 1–11.

Masters, W. B., & Johnson, V. E. (1966). *The human sexual response.* Boston: Little, Brown & Co.

Masters, W. B., & Johnson, V. E. (1970). *Human sexual inadequacy.* Boston: Little, Brown & Co.

Mona, L.R., & Gardos, P.S. (2001). Disabled sexual partners. In L.T. Szuchman & F. Muscarella (Eds.), *Psychological Perspectives on Human Sexuality* (pp. 309–354). New York: John Wiley & Sons.

NetValue. (2001, January 29). *NetValue study on: Retirees' behavior online "retired and wired."* Retrieved from http://us.netvalue.com/presse/index_frame.htm?fichier = cp0024. htm.

Novak, P.P., & Mitchell, M.M. (1988). Professional involvement in sexuality counseling for patients with spinal cord injuries. *American Journal of Occupational Therapy, 42*(2), 105–112.

Palmore, E. (Ed.). (1970). *Normal aging.* Durham, NC: Duke University Press.

Palmore, E. (Ed.). (1974). *Normal aging II.* Durham, NC: Duke University Press.

Partnership for Women's Health at Columbia. (1999). *Adult Attitudes Towards Sexual Problems. National Survey of American Adults Aged 25 and Older.* Prepared for Gender and Human Sexuality: A Continuing Medical Education Conference presented by the Partnership for Women's Health at Columbia. Survey conducted by telephone by Bennett, Petts & Blumenthal, 1010 Wisconsin Avenue NW Suite 208, Washington, DC 20007, March 25–31, 1999.

Tepper, M.S. (1992). Sexual education in spinal cord injury rehabilitation: Current trends and recommendations. *Sexuality and Disability, 10,* 15–31.

Tepper, M. S. (1996). Hands-free whoopee. *New Mobility,* 88–89.

Tepper, M. S. (2001). *Lived experiences that impede or facilitate sexual pleasure and orgasm in people with spinal cord injury.* Unpublished doctoral dissertation. University of Pennsylvania, Philadelphia.

Tepper, M.S. (2000, May). *Telemedicine and telehealth: Implications for sex counseling and therapy.* Paper presented at the American Association of Sex Educators, Counselors and Therapists Annual Meeting, Sexuality and the Millennium: Integrating Tradition, Technique and Technology, Atlanta, GA.

Tepper, M. S., & Owens, A. F. (2000, October). Women's questions about sexual health using the Internet as a medium for information and advice [Abstract]. For the Female Sexual Function Forum, New Perspectives in the Management of Female Dysfunction, Boston University School of Medicine.

The Network for Family Life Education. (2001, Winter). *Family Life Matters,* no. 42, 4–5.

Tsuji, I., Nakajima, F., Morimoto, J., et al. (1961). The sexual function in patients with spinal cord injury. *Urologia Internationalis, 12,* 270–280.

U.S. Census Bureau (1996, February). *Current Population Reports. P25–1130 Population Projection of the United States by Age, Sex, Race, and Hispanic Origin: 1995 to 2050* (pp. 1–131). Retrieved from http://www.census.gov/prod/1/pop/p25–1130/.

U.S. Department of Commerce (in consultation with the U.S. Department of Health and Human Services). (1997). The Telemedicine Report to Congress, January 1997. Retrieved January 11, 2000, from http://www.ntia.doc.gov/reports/telemed/index.htm.

U.S. Department of Commerce (2000, October). *Falling Through the Net: Toward Digital Inclusion. A report on Americans' Access to Technology Tools.* Economics and Statistics Administration; National Telecommunication and Information Administration (pp. 1–120). Retrieved from http://www.esa.doc.gov/fttn00.pdf.

Zeitlin, A. B., Cottrell, T. L., & Lloyd, F.A. (1957). Sexology of the paraplegic male. *Fertility and Sterility, 8,* 337–344.

Chapter Fourteen

IATROGENIC CAUSES OF FEMALE SEXUAL DISORDERS

Elizabeth A. Baron-Kuhn and Robert Taylor Segraves

When students graduate from medical school, part of the ceremony has traditionally included the Hippocratic oath. This of course states the ideal of causing no harm to the patient. As medicine has become so much more technologically based, the potential to inadvertently cause harm has increased markedly. Today, we have many therapies that are truly effective, but often, these treatments have a greater possibility of side effects. The doctor treating his patients really is still committed to doing no harm, but today, may not even be aware of all the potential side effects. The concept that therapies may cause sexual side effects is relatively new, and sadly, it is still often an uncomfortable thing to ask patients about. Hopefully, this chapter will provide some insight into the impact that our therapies can have on female patients' quality of life.

This chapter will focus on the iatrogenic causes of female sexual disorders (negative effects of therapy that inadvertently occur during the treatment of a medical condition), and for the purposes of this chapter, the actual existence of female sexual disorders will be assumed. Because of the current political debate concerning whether female sexual disorders are real or are created by the pharmaceutical industry, we will use a patient-driven model. For our purposes in this chapter, any patient complaint of a detrimental change in sexual function occurring after a medical or surgical therapy will be considered iatrogenically caused female sexual dysfunction. We will follow the currently accepted classification developed at the First International Consensus Conference on Definitions of Women's Sexual Dysfunction in 1998: Disorders of arousal, desire, and orgasm, and pain disorders (Basson et al., 2000; see the appendix in this volume). The term *sexual disorders* for women is preferred rather than *sexual dysfunctions*. This terminology was recommended at the World Association for Sexual Health World Congress held in Montreal in 2005 (see the appendix of this volume).

Further, this chapter will be organized by medical and surgical treatments rather than by disorder type, as many of our current disease treatments can cause disruption of more than one aspect of sexual function. For the purposes of this chapter, we will also assume that all the patients, prior to a "therapeutic instrumentation," had acceptable sexual function as assessed by the patient and that no intervening relationship issues are involved. Although, when evaluating a patient, one would certainly assess all aspects of the patient's complaint.

MEDICATIONS THAT CAN CAUSE SEXUAL SIDE EFFECTS

For the female patient with chronic medical problems, pharmacological intervention is often prescribed. In the male patient, it is usually obvious if a drug causes sexual issues, as erectile dysfunction is an easily identifiable physical sign. For the female patient, a change in arousal status can be harder to discern, and hence, sexual side effects in women are not as often reported. But, the sexual response in women occurs due to central and peripheral nervous system and vascular system responses that are similar to the response in men. Therefore, some generalizations will be made, since the physiology of women's sexual response is not as well understood as that of men. And often the complaint will be vague, such as dryness or discomfort, rather than lack of arousal.

Oral Contraceptives

Probably the most prescribed group of medications in younger women is the oral contraceptive pill. All of these use ethinyl estradiol as the estrogen component, and use various progestins in combination with the estrogen. It is the progestin component that gives each pill its unique characteristics. All of the progestins except for one are derivatives of testosterone, and in general, these progestins behave similarly to one of the two female sex steroid hormones: estrogen or progesterone. Often, the oral contraceptive chosen is deliberately picked in order to take advantage of the characteristics of the progestin. For example, to prevent breakthrough bleeding (intermenstrual bleeding during the time of the cycle which is usually without bleeding) strong progestins are used, such as norgestrol. Similarly, to decrease premenstrual symptoms, a more estrogen-like progestin may be used, such as diethnodiol diacetate, or the progestin that is a derivative of the antihypertensive drug aldactone: drospironone.

If a patient complains of sexual side effects after being placed on oral contraceptives, often a change in progestin can help. I (E. Baron-Kuhn) have managed patients on oral contraceptives for over 20 years, and wish I could say that a change to a stronger progestin always helps, but occasionally a change to a more estrogen-like progestin makes the difference. A new study suggests that oral contraceptives cause female sexual disorder by inducing an increase in sex hormone binding globulin (SHBG), a carrier protein for testosterone. If SHBG is increased, then active, unbound testosterone is decreased. This study found that even six months after discontinuing the oral contraceptive, the SHBG was still twice as high as for nonusers (Panzer et al., 2006). There are many problems with this study, the main one being that all the study subjects had sexual health complaints. Further, no patients without sexual health complaints were studied. As always, when studying only a group of subjects with a specific issue, it is difficult to generalize to the normal population, but this study does create interesting questions for future study. The most basic question being whether the oral contraceptive pills increase SHBG in normal women. A cohort of patients on the oral contraceptive who do not have any sexual complaints (this is called a control group) need to be tested for levels of SHBG to see if the levels are the same or different than in the study group. If the control patients have similar levels of SHBG, then they will likely have similar levels of free testosterone. This then would raise the question of whether the SHBG levels are even related to sexual dysfunction. If testosterone levels are related to sexual function in women, then the levels would of course be different. Again, this is an area that has not been elucidated in women (Davis, Davison, Donath, & Bell, 2005).

Currently, all the oral contraceptives, as well as the patch and the vaginal ring, contain a constant dose of estrogen each treatment day of the cycle, with the exception of one brand, Estrostep. Most hormonal contraceptives have a constant dose of progestin also, but a significant group of oral contraceptives use a changing dose of progestin during the cycle. In some, the progestin increases during the month, stepwise, and in others, it increases midcycle and then decreases again (this group is called the triphasic oral contraceptives.)

There is one oral contraceptive pill in which the estrogen component changes (Estrostep). It is a novel approach that is not necessarily useful for bleeding or mood issues. However, it is worth considering for the patient who wishes hormonal contraception, but for whom the other types of oral contraceptives are causing sexual side effects. (In a normal fertile cycle, the estrogen levels increase and then decrease throughout the month, and perhaps mimicking this pattern could help specific patient types.) I have used it successfully for this purpose in a few patients.

Other Medications (Antihypertensives, Antifungals, Anticonvulsants, etc.)

Other medications used in gynecology that can cause sexual problems include therapies for endometriosis. Danazol is an attenuated androgen that is active orally. It produces both a hypoestrogenic (low level of estrogen) and a hyperandrogenic (high level of androgen) effect on sex steroid sensitive organs. And, although it causes the androgenous side effects of hirsuitism, acne, and occasionally deepening of the voice, it can cause decreased desire. Its hypoestrogenic effects can also cause decreases in arousal. The gonadotropin releasing hormone (GnRH) agonists block the hypothalamic—pituitary—gonadal axis, which causes a medically induced menopause. With a lack of circulating sex steroid hormones, it is not surprising that complaints of lack of desire and arousal, as well as pain are common. Depo-Provera is used for both endometriosis and contraception. It can also cause decreased libido (mechanism unknown).

Ketoconazole is an antifungal that is used to treat yeast infections. This medication can cause decreased desire, also. Fortunately, this drug is rarely used for extended periods of treatment. But, because of the frequency of yeast infections in women, it is an often-prescribed medication.

Hypertension is of course treated in order to prevent cerebral-vascular accidents (strokes) and myocardial infarctions (heart attacks.) Beta-blockers are very effective agents, which act on the sympathetic nervous system (adrenergic) and directly on the vascular system. While being effective at decreasing blood pressure, those same mechanisms of action can cause disorders of arousal and orgasm by direct effects. Alpha-blockers can cause similar side effects, but the mechanism of action is uncertain. Diuretics can cause desire, arousal, and orgasmic disorders also; however, the mechanism of action is again unclear (Thomas, 2003).

The National Heart, Lung, and Blood Institute and The Office of Rare Diseases at the National Institute of Health, and the Executive Summary, Third Report of The National Cholesterol Education Program: Expert Panel on Detection, Evaluation, and Treatment of Hugh Blood Cholesterol in Adults recommends not only treating high blood pressure, but also treating elevated cholesterol. While of course a diet and exercise program is the first line therapy, and it is known to have beneficial sexual effects, all too often, patients need lipid-lowering agents. These drugs are known to have effects on arousal and orgasm. The mechanism of this action is not known. Digoxin, the cardiac anti arrhythmia drug, can cause arousal disorders, due to its sex hormone-like structure (Thomas, 2003).

The anticonvulsants carbamazepine, phenytoin, phenobarbital, and primidone are used to treat epilepsy and related disorders. These drugs affect the P-450 pathway (which is the enzyme system in the liver that breaks down toxins and drugs), and they cause an increase in the metabolism of androgens. This causes a decrease in circulating androgens and thereby causes nonspecific sexual dysfunction (Thomas, 2003).

Gastrointestinal disorders are sometimes treated with medications that can cause sexual difficulties. Gastro esophageal reflux disease, severe heartburn, and irritable bowel disease sometimes need to be treated long term. Histamine H2-receptor blockers can cause decreased libido by affecting the hypothalamic—pituitary—gonadal axis (increasing prolactin). It can sometimes also interfere with arousal (possibly by a local effect on histamine receptors). Metoclopramide has several gastrointestinal uses, and it also can decrease libido (as a dopamine-receptor antagonist) (Trimmer, 1981).

The antihistamine group is used for treating allergies, often seasonally. As discussed for H2-blockers, this class also causes disorders of arousal and this is likely for the same reasons (local effects).

Chronic pain patients that are treated with long-term narcotics may find difficulties with orgasm. The mechanism can be either via a central or peripheral nervous system effect.

Antidepressants and Other Centrally Acting Drugs

There is considerable evidence that many commonly prescribed psychiatric drugs adversely affect female sexual dysfunction. Most classes of antidepressant drugs may cause anorgasmia and decreased libido. Wyatt et al. (1971) were the first to report orgasmic difficulty with monoamine oxidase inhibitors. Numerous other clinicians subsequently made similar case reports (Lesko, Stotland, & Segraves, 1982; Moss, 1983; Pohl, 1983). Couper-Smartt and Rodman (1973) were the first to report orgasmic delay on imipramine, a tricyclic antidepressant. Subsequently, clinicians reported anorgasmia in individuals on other tricyclic antidepressants (Souvner, 1983). A double-blind, placebo-controlled study by Harrison and colleagues (Harrison et al., 1985) established that orgasmic delay was associated both with phenelzine (a monoamine oxidase inhibitor) and imipramine (a tricyclic antidepressant). A double-blind placebo controlled study also found a high rate of orgasm delay with clomipramine, a serotonergic tricyclic antidepressant (Monteiro, Noshirvani, Marks, & Lelliott, 1987). Clinical case reports suggest that desipramine, a tricyclic antidepressant with predominantly adrenergic activity, may have much lower rates of orgasm delay than more serotonergic tricyclic antidepressants (Segraves, 1995).

Fluoxetine was the first selective serotonin reuptake inhibitor (SSRI) introduced into the United States, in 1987. This was followed by the introduction of other SSRIs (e.g., sertraline, paroxetine, fluvoxamine, citalopram, and s-citalopram). Premarketing clinical trials underestimated the incidence of sexual dysfunction for all of these drugs. For example, the *Physicians' Desk Reference* (1990) did not mention orgasm delay as possible side effect of fluoxetine.

However, clinicians began reporting that fluoxetine and other SSRIs had a high incidence of sexual dysfunction in both sexes (Rosen, Lane, & Menza, 1999). The reason that premarketing trials underestimated the incidence of SSRI-induced female sexual dysfunction is probably related to the observation that many patients experiencing drug-induced sexual dysfunction do not report this unless directly asked (Montejo-Gonzalez et al., 1997). Studies using direct inquiry have found that the SSRIs, with the possible exception of fluvoxamine, have approximately a 30 percent incidence of drug-induced sexual dysfunction. The most common side effect is anorgasmia. Many patients also complain of decreased libido (Croft, Settle, Houser, Batey, Donahue, & Ascher, 1999). It is probable that paraxetine has a higher incidence of sexual dysfunction than the other SSRIs (Rosen et al., 1999).

A number of clinical investigators have examined the sexual side effect profile of antidepressants affecting multiple neurotransmitters. Double-blind studies have shown that bupropion, an antidepressant with both dopamine and norepinephine reuptake inhibition, has fewer sexual side effects than sertraline (Segraves et al., 2000) or fluoxetine (Coleman et al., 2001). There is also evidence that this drug may facilitate several aspects of sexual responsiveness (Segraves et al., 2004). Double-blind controlled studies indicate that nefazodone has a lower incidence of sexual side effects than sertraline (Ferguson et al., 2001) and that duloxetine has a lower incidence of sexual side effects than paraxetine (Delgado et al., 2005). Duloxetine and nefazodone are both serotonin and norepinephrine reuptake inhibitors. There is some evidence that mirtazapine and venlafaxine may have lower rates of sexual side effects than SSRIs, but the evidence is inconsistent (Clayton et al., 2002; Montejo-Gonzalez et al., 2001). Both drugs have serotonergic and adrenergic activity. Since sexual dysfunction is less common in serotonergic drugs with 5-HT 2 antagonism, it has been hypothesized that the sexual side effects of serotonergic drugs are mediated by 5-HT 2 receptors (Segraves, 2002). Most of the data concerning possible sexual side effects of mood stabilizers consists of case reports. Part of the difficulty of interpreting data in this area is that mania is associated with increased sexual activity (Goodwin & Jamison, 1990). Thus, a complaint of decreased libido could be an effect of mood stabilization as opposed to a drug side effect. Case reports of decreased libido on lithium have been reported in both sexes (Segraves, 2003). Anticonvulsants are frequently employed as mood stabilizers. There have been case reports of anorgasmia with gabapentin (Drabkin & Calhoun, 2003; Grant & Oh, 2002). Valproate has been reported to be associated with decreased libido in female patients (Schneck et al., 2002). Lamotrigine has been reported to increase libido and other measures of sexuality in female epileptics (Gil-Nagel et al., 2006). Carbamazepine can induce changes in sex hormones and thus might be expected to adversely affect libido (Herzog & Fowler, 2005; Rattya et al., 2001; Verrotti, Green, Latini, & Chiarelli, 2005).

One double-blind controlled study demonstrated that diazepam can cause anorgasmia in women (Riley & Riley, 1986). Some assume that this is true for other benzodiazepines although this is unproven.

Most of the evidence concerning antipsychotic drugs consists of case reports and clinical series. Anorgasmia and decreased libido appears to have been a common side effect with the traditional antipsychotics such as thioridazine (Segraves, 2006). Sexual side effects also appear to be quite common with risperidone, a drug associated with prolactin elevation (Dickson, Seeman, & Corenblum, 2000). Of the atypical antipsychotics, it appears that olanzapine and quetapine may have very low rates of sexual dysfunction (Bobes, Garcia-Portilla, & Rejas, 2003). It is unclear whether ziprasidone and aripriprazole have sexual dysfunction as a major side effect.

It should be mentioned that for any medication, sexual side effects should be considered by the prescribing physician; however, if no complaints are voiced by the patient, it may wrongly be assumed that there are no negative side effects. Therefore, both the physician and the patient should be encouraged to discuss these issues. The patient should be reassured that in most instances a different drug can be tried, which usually will provide the desired therapeutic effect with fewer sexual side effects. For example, as mentioned, bupropion is an antidepressant which often has fewer sexual side effects. Additionally, there is an over the counter product, Zestra, which in a small study, was shown to improve sexual satisfaction in women with all types of sexual dysfunction, including patients experiencing negative effects from antidepressants (Ferguson et al., 2003).

Diabetes Mellitus Management

Diabetes is a chronic disease which adversely affects the vascular and peripheral nervous system. This is most commonly recognized in the need for cautious treatment of a diabetic's feet. Any small injury can cause severe infection which will not be initially perceived as painful because of poor nerve function and due to poor circulation will not heal well. These same vascular and neural defects occur in the female genital tract. Therefore, a lack of aggressive diabetic management can result in inadvertent sexual disorders and should be considered as possibilities in the diabetic patient (Esposito et al., 2005; Muniyappa, Norton, Dunn, & Banerji, 2005).

As previously noted, a decrease in sensation is associated with disorders of desire, arousal, and orgasm (Connell, 2005). Although, there are currently no definitive treatments, practitioners can optimize function by general support and individualized treatments: estrogens or androgens if not contraindicated, counseling, and oil based treatments (perhaps Zestra, which can improve nerve stimulation may end up being useful). The practitioner should be careful to advise against any lubricants containing any known skin irritants. A skin test on the patient's forearm may save some grief. Unfortunately, the phosphodiesterase-5 inhibitors are not likely to work for this group of women for the same reason that they are not very useful in men: they do nothing for sensation in these patients with neuropathies.

Of course, the most common long-term complication of diabetes is kidney failure. The patient on dialysis has a unique situation with multiple possible causes for sexual dysfunction. Usually these patients have many other illnesses and either the illness or its treatment can cause side effects. Dialysis itself alters the levels of sex steroid hormones and can cause decreases in desire and arousal and orgasm from this direct effect. The older and sicker the patient, the more significant these problems (Peng et al., 2005).

Chemotherapy and Other Forms of Cancer Treatment

The cancer therapies are truly the class for which balancing risk versus benefit is a grave challenge. It would seem to the cancer specialist that prolonging life is a simple choice, but lately, more patients are questioning side effects. The chapter on cancer and sexuality has a very nice discussion of this topic. We do not wish to be repetitive, but would like to expand on one particular aspect of chemotherapy.

Chemotherapy can destroy ovarian function. It does so because of its mechanism of action. It targets rapidly growing cells (by interfering in different phases of the cell growth cycle). The follicles of the ovary are of course rapidly growing due to their task of producing mature oocytes (eggs) for release each month. The destruction of follicles causes not only infertility/sterility but it also results in the cessation of hormonal function. The patient is put through a medical menopause.

It is a well accepted fact in gynecology that the abrupt cessation of menstrual hormones caused by the surgical removal of the ovaries results in a far more severe climacteric. The patient who undergoes a surgical menopause is more often in need of estrogen replacement because of severe hot flashes and troubling vaginal dryness.

The patient that undergoes a medical menopause should be expected to have a similar experience. As chemotherapy is destroying the tumor cells, the health practitioner should remember that it is also changing patients' sexual function. We should be grateful for our successful cures, but also mindful of the life changes we have caused our patients.

Following a successful course of chemotherapy, the physician should help provide support for the long-term quality of the patient's life. Hot flashes and vaginal dryness are most effectively treated with estrogen replacement. The skillful physician will choose a dose appropriate to the patients' age (consider an oral contraceptive because of its higher estrogen dose for the adolescent, and 20 and 30 year old) (Mishell, Stenchever, Droegemueller, & Herbst, 1997).

Some of the cancer survivors will have been treated for a tumor that is estrogen sensitive. In this patient population, estrogen is relatively contraindicated (meaning not to be given except under special circumstances with much counseling given).

The patient who should not receive estrogen can have hot flashes treated by clonidine; the SSRIs; or perhaps an herbal remedy, such as black cohosh. However, none of these therapies will help with vaginal dryness. Topical vaginal estrogen treatment could be considered; however, it must be remembered that some of the vaginal estrogen will be absorbed systemically. Alternatives to vaginal estrogen include topically applied vitamin E, olive oil, and oils high in GLA (gammalinoleic acid, one of the essential fatty acids) such as borage oil. Another option is a new product called Zestra, which in a small study showed improvement in desire and arousal in women with FSD due to many different causes (Ferguson et al., 2003). Zestra holds promise because it is topical and nonhormonal, and it appears to be effective regardless of the cause of FSD.

Certain cancers are treated most effectively with radiation therapy. Radiation not only kills tumor cells, but can also help make local recurrences less likely because of destruction of blood vessels and lymphatic channels near the tumor. It is worth noting that other types of normal tissue are also in the radiation field.

In the case of pelvic tumors (gynecologic, gastrointestinal, neuromuscular, or metastatic ones), the radiation field often includes both the internal and external female genitalia. The vascularity as well as the nerve tissue is often compromised. Sensation can be decreased, and the arousal response of vascular engorgement can be decreased. The autonomic nervous system and the orgasmic response can also be compromised. Radiation can cause poor long-term sexual function (DiSaia & Creasman, 1993; Thompson, 1992).

With such global destruction of these tissues, what can be done to mitigate the dysfunction that is caused? Some of the newer philosophy in the treatment of prostate cancer includes ongoing support of erectile function with small nightly doses of phosphodiesterase-5 inhibitors such as sildenafil (Viagra). In the female patient, perhaps nightly use of a vibrator would be beneficial, but this is currently unstudied. Certainly, the vaginal mucosa must be protected during coitus with either silicone or oil based lubricants, or in the worst case even a zinc-oxide based ointment.

A 42-year-old patient presented to my office for a Pap smear. Her last Pap smear being at the start of prenatal care for her only child who was now 8 years old. She had not had a postpartum examination. Cervical cancer was diagnosed after this visit, and evaluation by the gynecologic oncologist showed that she required radiation therapy. She received whole pelvis irradiation (no areas of the pelvis were shielded). Following therapy she was considered clinically cured. However, on return visit for a routine annual exam, she was not as pleased as expected about being cured because she was no longer able to have satisfying sexual relations. The only suggestion that the gynecology oncologist had was to use dilators and "have more sex." Because the radiation had destroyed nerves and blood vessels, sex was painful as well as unsatisfying. A novel suggestion was made: topical use of Zestra to encourage healing and promote better sensation. The patient did apply a small amount twice daily on most days for eight weeks and by self-report had become 30 percent improved, a better relief than the patient had gotten from dilators. The patient was lost to further follow-up because of a move out of the area.

The surgical treatment of pelvic cancers would seem by comparison to be less detrimental to the patients' sexual function because it is a localized treatment and it does not seemingly damage surrounding tissues. Unfortunately, this does not seem to be the case. Because cancer is not usually confined to one organ, and further, it can invade lymphatic vessels, which infiltrate all tissues of the body, the surgery for cancer is often extensive. Blood vessels, and more often, nerves can be compromised. In fact, between 10 and 75 percent of female patients treated with either radiation or surgery had poor sexual functioning after treatment (Amano, Takemae, Sakai, Sugasse, & Kondou, 2005; Corney, Crowther, Everett, Howells, & Shepard,1993; Freeman, 1992).

Cervical Cancer

The surgical treatment of cervical cancer is a radical hysterectomy. The name implies that rather than staying as close to the uterus as possible, the surgeon must dissect tissue as far from the uterus as possible. Usually this dissection will include as much tissue as possible on each side of the pelvis. The great vessels to the legs, the nerves to the bladder, rectum, and external genitalia, as well as the ureters, all pass through this area. Because the dissection is so extensive it is easy to understand how not only sexual function, but also bowel and bladder function can be negatively affected (Amano et al., 2005; Freeman, 1992; Stead, 2004).

The complaints of sexual problems following radical hysterectomy are so common that similar to the nerve sparing prostatectomy, a nerve sparing radical hysterectomy has been devised (Barton, Butler-Manuel, & Buttery, 2002; Hockel, Horn, Hentschel, Hockel, & Naumanns, 2003; Raspagliesi et al., 2004). The procedure is still being perfected as the need to remove lymphatic tissue while attempting to preserve nerve tissue presents an anatomic challenge. However, when the surgery is eventually performed, it will also have to provide excellent cure rates in order to be an acceptable choice.

The surgical treatment of ovarian cancer is more varied because the goal is to remove as much tumor as possible with a cancer that spreads over all interabdominal organs. Not only is a clean dissection of the pelvic nerves often not possible, but colostomy can sometimes be necessary due to rectal involvement of the tumor. Because the rectum is lying immediately behind the vagina, the nerves and blood supply often cannot be separated and preserved.

The removal of the ovaries can also cause hormonal problems regarding sexual function. As mentioned earlier, this can exacerbate vaginal dryness, as well as decrease desire and arousal (Stead, 2004).

An 18-year-old college student was sent by her student health service physician for evaluation of an abdomino-pelvic mass. This had been found during evaluation of a cough. Unfortunately, the mass was found to be a malignant germ cell tumor and required surgical removal of the uterus, cervix, both tubes and ovaries, and lymph nodes. She needed radiation, also. After treatment, the gynecologic oncologist gave her a very low (menopausal) dose of estrogen. Following her treatment, she dropped out of school, moved away, and joined the art scene. Eventually, she met a wonderful man. He made her return to my office (E. Baron-Kuhn) to discuss her lack of desire, as well as decreased arousal and overall decreased sexual response. She was no longer on any hormones and also was having hot flashes and a generalized lack of well being. Placing this patient on age-appropriate hormonal therapy was indicated, and the oral contraceptive pill was started with very good results. The patient was surprised at how much better she felt in all areas of her life.

Vulvar Cancer

The last gynecologic cancer to discuss is vulvar cancer. The treatment for this is always surgical, but may sometimes also include radiation therapy. The surgical treatment consists of excision of the tumor and often the whole external genitalia are removed (the labia major and minora) as well as the clitoris and groin lymph nodes. The anatomy of the clitoris is such that muscle fibers extend into the labia as well as under the pubic bone along the urethra (O'Connell & Delancey, 2005). This decrease in sensation can cause any type of sexual dysfunction (Connell et al., 2005). Most patients report a decrease in sexual satisfaction, but surprisingly, some patients still report having orgasms (DiSaia & Creasman, 1993). The ability of some patients to still have orgasms is likely related to the presence of clitoral fibers intravaginally or to the use of G spot or cervical stimulation.

The other pelvic malignancy that is surgically treated is rectal cancer. This, of course, also involves surgical resection of tissue that lies directly behind the vagina. As mentioned earlier on a purely anatomic basis, this disrupts nerves and blood vessels. But, the sexual effects are wider than that: body image can be damaged if a colostomy is needed, and urinary and fecal incontinence can be problematic. These problems can be compounded by radiation therapy when utilized (Fischer et al., 2005; Henderson et al., 2005).

OBSTETRICAL CAUSES OF FEMALE SEXUAL DISORDERS

This topic is already covered nicely in the chapters on pregnancy and sex, and sexual pain disorders; however, a couple of other points deserve discussion. Obstetrical deliveries have, for centuries, been natural, spontaneous, and normal. Today, in many developed countries, the expectations of an extraordinarily perfect result have caused an increase in obstetrical interventions. We shall not debate whether this has actually improved outcomes, but we should recognize the impact these interventions can have on our patients.

For many years, episiotomies were routinely performed. Today, the trends have turned away from this, and in most labor and delivery suites today, episiotomy is no longer a routine procedure. As a resident, I (E. Baron-Kuhn) was exposed to an obstetrician who asked all of his patients how they would like their episiotomy repaired: "tighter, looser, or the same." It seemed a curious question, and thankfully, I met a unit secretary that same year who emphatically told me that she had asked for a "tighter" repair and forever regretted the discomfort she had caused herself. This is a good lesson for all. We as health care providers should be careful to repair obstetrical lacerations, including episiotomies, as anatomically correctly as possible. I have also seen extensive obstetrical lacerations that were allowed to heal spontaneously and, because of improper healing, caused sexual problems. (For example, part of the left labia minora healed down into the perineal body of one patient). We should always try to promote meticulous wound healing.

Another issue that should be mentioned is the matter and mode of delivery. Prolonged pushing and the use of vacuum extraction or forceps can cause nerve and muscle damage, which can result in long term pelvic floor problems. Muscle laxity and decreased arousal and orgasmic sensation can be consequences. Nerve damage can result in poor arousal response also.

The issue of how to best deliver pregnant patients in order to cause the least amount of pelvic floor damage is currently greatly debated. The annual American College of Obstetricians and Gynecologists meeting recently held a two-day seminar discussing these issues and the best approaches to repairing obstetrical damage without causing further sexual disorders. Currently, there is no consensus as to best practices in obstetrical deliveries, so the concept of

---

For example, a 22-year-old patient came to my (E. Baron-Kuhn) office one year post partum. She stated that since the birth of her daughter, she had had problems with sexual intercourse. She stated that her uterus would protrude through her introitus (opening of the vagina) for two days after making love. She also stated that it was much more difficult for her to have an orgasm since the birth. Further history revealed that this patient had been allowed to push for six hours. It was decided after six hours to perform a caesarian section.

Physical examination of this patient revealed marked pelvic floor laxity, and examination of sensation of her external genitalia revealed *no* sensation of the labia minora bilaterally and decreased sensation of the clitoral hood.

Because of such poor pelvic muscle strength, this patient is undergoing aggressive physical therapy, including pelvic weights and she may be started on electrical muscle stimulation. Every possible effort will be made to not do any surgical repair. In an attempt to improve sensation, a novel therapy is being tried: this patient is using Zestra (Ferguson et al., 2003) nightly, applied externally and on the G spot in an attempt to encourage better innervation of the external genitalia.

The pelvic laxity was still present but slightly improved (at 10 weeks of therapy), and the patient stated that the Zestra is helping with arousal, although examination at 10 weeks still showed poor sensation. By four months, examination showed not only improved muscle tone but a slight increase in sensation (to vibration).

---

causing no harm should be our best guide. And we as health care providers should not use the highly stressful time of birth as an opportunity to improve things surgically that were not in need of our intervention in the first place.

SURGERY-INDUCED SEXUAL DISORDERS

Most drugs can be discontinued or changed if the patients' side effects are severe enough, but some disorders cannot be well treated medically. For the female patient, the vast majority of these problems are gynecological (endometriosis, severe bleeding, pain, or relaxation of the support tissues of the pelvis leading to prolapse of those organs into or beyond the vagina, and often urinary or fecal incontinence). The major procedure for these types of problems is surgical.

A considerable debate is ongoing regarding the need for hysterectomies, the proper percentage of hysterectomies, the best route for hysterectomies, and the best type of hysterectomy. As the majority of hysterectomies in the United States are performed for benign reasons, the debate is crucial, and the final conclusions will be important for the care of our patients. Fortunately, as of 2006, the questions are being seriously discussed.

Most abdominal hysterectomies are performed for abnormal bleeding, due to either fibroids or adenomyosis. Most studies currently measuring quality of life in patients who have had a hysterectomy for bleeding show an improvement in all measures of quality of life. This includes sexual function (Carlson, Miller, & Fowler, 1994; Davies & Doyle, 2002; Kuppermann, Varner, Summitt, Hearman, & Ireland, 2004; Rhodes, Kjerulff, Langenberg, & Guzinski, 1999; Thakar, 2004). However, even though most of these studies showed satisfaction with the procedure, most also showed a small percentage of women who had poorer sexual function postoperatively. The current hypothesis for a negative impact include both the possibility of nerve disruption (Lowenstein et al., 2005) or vascular impairment (Meston, 2004).

A further consideration regarding abdominal hysterectomy is whether to leave the cervix intact (supracervical hysterectomy) or to perform a total hysterectomy (remove the cervix and the uterus). Reports are conflicting as to whether the supracervical hysterectomy leads to better post operative sexual function (Kuppermann, Summitt, Varner, McNeiley, & Goodman-Gruen, 2005). Current research suggests that the reason for the lack of a difference in sexual response after total versus supracervical hysterectomy is that for most women clitoral stimulation is dominant in the sexual response cycle (Flory, 2005). However, with no definite agreement on this point, the gynecologist should consider asking each patient about her perceived most "erogenous" zone.

Indeed, asking a patient where they perceive the most pleasurable stimulation—the clitoris, the cervix, or the G spot—would have prevented the following situation.

In addition to asking about whether the patient prefers to keep her cervix, the gynecologist should reconsider the routine removal of the ovaries. In the 1980s, it was routine to remove them in all patients aged 40 and older. By the

A 49-year-old white female patient presented to my (E. Baron-Kuhn) office with a complaint of lack of sexual arousal since her vaginal hysterectomy, two years prior. The patient had undergone a vaginal hysterectomy for cervical dysplasia. During the office evaluation, it was noted that the patient had normal sensation of the entire external genitalia. Unfortunately, a pelvic examination revealed that the patient had had an anterior colporrhaphy (bladder suspension), which caused scarring over her G spot. Additional questioning revealed that the patient prior to surgery had always gotten the most pleasure from stimulation of her G spot. Sadly, the patient had not had any urinary incontinence symptoms and did not need any bladder surgery. Hopefully, over time, she will be able to successfully focus on clitoral stimulation.

1990s, gynecologists had moved the age parameter back to 45 years. However, surgical removal of the ovaries results in worse hot flashes and vaginal dryness and the potential for a decrease in desire. Leaving the ovaries also appears to result in an increased life span (Parker, Broder, Liu, & Shoupe, 2005). Because of less negative impact on sexual function and a real gain in life span, the routine removal of the ovaries should be seriously reconsidered.

By discussing vaginal surgery last, it is not meant to imply that this is any less important of a procedure. Vaginal surgery is performed to correct defects in the support of the pelvic organs: the uterus, the bladder, and the rectum. Any or all of these organs can protrude to varying degrees because of factors such as age, damage to the supporting tissues due to child birth, or simply gravity. The prolapse of these organs is actually a type of hernia through the floor of the pelvis.

By thinking of this problem as a hernia, it can be more easily understood. The surgical approach to correction of the defect is to reattach supportive structures just as in an abdominal hernia repair (Shull & Bachofen, 1999). Unfortunately, the support of the pelvis is mostly muscular tissue with very little tissue of any real strength. This results in attempts to increase the thickness of tissues by forcing tissue that is next to the vagina to be pulled either above or below the vagina in the midline, which can cause constriction of the vagina and pain (Kahn & Stanton, 1997). Sadly, even in the best surgical hands, many of these attempts fail (Vassallo & Karram, 2003).

For many of these women with pelvic organ prolapse, sexual function is poor to begin with (Navi, Jeronis, Morgan, & Arya, 2005). In fact, one vaginal surgery textbook warns the surgeon not to try to improve the "marriage relationship" by performing vaginal surgery (Nichols & Randall, 1983). This is also emphasized in an operative gynecology textbook with the warning that significant dysparunia can be caused by vaginal surgery (Thompson, 1992).

The ideal vaginal surgical technique has not been developed yet. Ideally, it would both correct defects long term as well as not cause sexual dysfunction. So, at this time, it is best to remember that although many women become or remain sexually active postoperatively, a significant number consider sexual activity less satisfactory after surgery (Lemack & Zimmern, 2000; Poad & Arnold, 1994; Weber, Walters, & Piedmonte, 2000).

While we await much improved surgical techniques, we as physicians should at least discuss these issues with our patients. As an 80-year-old woman with a large bladder prolapse states: "I still have sex. I'm old, not dead!" We should never assume that our patients are not sexually active, even if they are widowed and living in a nursing home.

REFERENCES

Amano, T., Takemae, K., Sakai, H., Sugasse, M., & Kondou, K. (2005). Analysis of mailed questionnaire for female sexual dysfunction after intra-pelvic surgery. *Nippon Hinyokika Gakkai Zasshi, 96*(3), 453–461.

Barton, D.P.J., Butler-Manuel, S. A., & Buttery L.D.K. (2002). A nerve-sparing radical hysterectomy: Guidelines and feasibility in Western patients. *International Journal of Gynecologic Cancer, 12*, 319–321.

Basson, R., Berman, J., Burnett, A., Derogatis, L., Ferguson, D., Fourcroy, J., Goldstein, I., Graziottin, A., Heiman, J., Laan, E., Leiblum, S., Padma-Nathan, H., Rosen, R., Segraves, K., Segraves, R.T., Shabsigh, R., Sipski, M., Wagner, G., Whipple, B. (2000). Report of the International Consensus Development Conference on female sexual dysfunction: Definitions and classifications. *Journal of Urology, 163*, 888–893.

Bobes, J., Garcia-Portilla, M., & Rejas, J. (2003). Frequency of sexual dysfunction and other reproductive side effects in patients with schizophrenia treated with ripseridone, ola-nazapine, quetiapine, or haloperidol. *Journal of Sex and Marital Therapy, 29*, 125–147.

Carlson, K., Miller, B., & Fowler, F., Jr.(1994). The Maine women's health study: 2. Out-comes of nonsurgical management of leionyomas, abnormal bleeding, and chronic pelvic pain. *Obstetrics and Gynecology 83*, 566–572.

Clayton, A., Pradko, J., Montano, C., Leadbetter, R., Bolden-Watson, C., Bass, K., Donahue, R., Jamerson, B., & Metz, A. (2002). Prevalence of sexual dysfunction among newer antidepressants. *Journal of Clinical Psychiatry, 63*, 357–366.

Coleman, C., King, B., Bolden-Watson, C., Book, M., Segraves, R., Richard, N., Ascher, J., Batey, S., Jamerson, B., & Metz, A. (2001) A placebo-controlled comparison of the effects on sexual functioning of bupropion sustained release and fluoxetine. *Clinical Therapeutics, 23*, 1040–1058.

Connell, K., Guess, M., La Combe, J., Wang, A., Powers, K., Lazarou, G., & Mikkail, M. (2005) Evaluation of the role of pudendal nerve integrity in female sexual function using non-invasive techniques. *American Journal of Obstetrics and Gynecology, 192*, 1712–1717.

Corney, R. H., Crowther, M. E., Everett, H., Howells, A., & Shepard, J.H. (1993). Psy-chosexual dysfunction in women with gynecological cancer following radical pelvic surgery. *British Journal of Obstetrics and Gynaecology, 100*(1), 73–78.

Couper-Smartt, J., & Rodman, R. (1973). A technique for surveying side effects of tricyclic drugs with reference to reported sexual side effects. *Journal of International Medical Research, 1,* 469–772.

Croft, H., Settle, E., Houser, T., Batey, S., Donahue, R., & Ascher, J. (1999). A placebo-controlled comparison of the antidepressant efficacy and effects on sexual functioning of sustained-release bupropion and sertraline. *Clinical Therapeutics 21,* 643–658.

Davies, J., & Doyle, P. M. (2002). Quality of life studies in unselected gynecological outpatients and in-patients before and after hysterectomy. *Journal of Obstetrics and Gynecology, 22,* 523–526.

Davis, S., Davison, S., Donath, S., Bell, R. (2005). Circulating androgen levels and self-reported sexual function in women. *Journal of the American Medical Association, 294,* 91–96.

Delgado, P., Branman, S., Mallinckrodt, C., Tran, P., McNamara, R., Wang, F., Watkins, J., & Detke, M. (2005). Sexual functioning assessed in 4 double-blind placebo and paroxetine controlled trials of dulexetine for major depressive disorder. *Journal of Clinical Psychiatry, 66,* 686–692.

Dickson, R. A., Seeman, M. V., & Corenblum, B. (2000). Hormonal side effects in women: typical versus atypical antipsychotic treatment. *The Journal of Clinical Psychiatry, 61*(suppl. 3), 10–15.

DiSaia, P., & Creasman, W. (1993). *Clinical Gynecologic Oncology* (4th ed.). St. Louis, MO: Mosby-Year Book.

Drabkin, R. B., & Calhoun, L. (2003). Anorgasmia and withdrawal syndrome in a woman on gabapentin. *Canadian Journal of Psychiatry, 48,* 125–126.

Esposito, K., Ciotola, M., Marfella, R., Di Tommaso, D., Cobellis, H., Giugliamo, D. (2005). The metabolic syndrome; A cause of sexual dysfunction in women. *International Journal of Impotence Research, 17*(3), 224–226.

Ferguson, D. M., Singh, G. S., Steidle, C. P., Alexander, S., Weihmiller, M., & Crosby, M. G. (2003). Randomized, placebo-controlled, double blind, crossover design trial of the efficacy and safety of Zestra for Women in women with and without female sexual arousal disorder. *Journal of Sex and Marital Therapy, 29,* 33–44.

Ferguson, J., Shrivastava, R., Stahl, S., Hartford, J., Borian, F., Leni, J., Mc Quade, R., & Jody, D. (2001). Reemergence of sexual dysfunction in patients with major depressive disorder; a double blind comparison of nefazodone and sertraline. *Journal of Clinical Psychiatry, 62,* 24–29.

Fischer, F., Mirow, L., Gondeck, C., Schwandner, O., Brusch, H. P., & Farke, S. (2005). Influence of postoperative radio-chemotherapy for rectal cancer on quality of life. *Zeitschrift für Gastroenterologie, 43*(11), 1213–1218.

Flory, N., Bissonette, F., & Binik, Y. M. (2005). Psychosocial effects of hysterectomy: literature review. *Journal of Psychosomatic Research, 59,* 117–129.

Freeman, M. (1992). Te Linde's Operative Gynecology (7th ed.). Philadelphia, PA: J.B. Lippencott.

Gil-Nagel, A., Lopez-Munoz, F., Serratosa, J. M., Moncada, I., Garcia-Garcia, P. & Alamo, C. (2006). Effect of lamotrigine on sexual function in patients with epilepsy. *Seizure, 15(3),* 142–149.

Goodwin, F., & Jamison, K. (1990). *Manic-depressive illness.* New York: Oxford University Press.

Grant, A. C., & Oh, H. (2002). Gabapentin-induced anorgasmia in women. *American Journal of Psychiatry, 159,* 1247.

Harrison, W., Stewart, J., Ehrhardt, A., Rabkin, J., McGrath, P., Liebowitz, M., & Quitkin, F. A. (1985). Controlled study of the effects of antidepressants on sexual function. *Psychopharmacology Bulletin, 21,* 85–88.

Henderson, S. K., O'Connor, B. L., Liu, M., Asano, T., Cohen, Z., Swallow, C. J., Macrae, H. M., Gryfe, R., & McLeod, R. S. (2005). Prevalence of male and female sexual dysfunction is high following surgery for rectal cancer. *Annals of Surgery, 242*(2), 212–223.

Herzog, A. G., & Fowler, K. M. (2005). Sexual hormones and epilepsy: Threat and opportunity. *Current Opinion in Neurology, 18,* 167–172.

Hockel, M., Horn, L. C., Hentschel, B., Hockel, S., & Naumanns, G. (2003). Total mesometrial resection: High resolution nerve-sparing radical hysterectomy based on developmentally defined surgical anatomy. *International Journal of Gynecologic Cancer, 13,* 791–803.

Kahn M, Stanton S.(1997). Posterior Colporrhaphy: Its Effects on Bowel and Sexual Function. *British Journal of Obstetrics and Gynaecology.* 104, 82–86.

Kuppermann, M., Summitt, R., Varner, R. E., McNeiley, S. G., & Goodman-Gruen, D. (2005). Sexual functioning after total compared with supracervical hysterectomy: A randomized trial. *Obstetrics and Gynecology, 105,* 1309–1318.

Kuppermann, M., Varner, R. E., Summitt, R., Hearman, L., & Ireland, C. (2004). Effect of hysterectomy as medical treatment on health-related quality of life and sexual functioning. *Journal of the American Medical Association, 291,* 1447–1455.

Lemack, G. E., & Zimmern, P. E. (2000). Sexual function after vaginal surgery for stress incontinence: Results of a mailed questionnaire. *Urology, 56*(2) 22–227.

Lesko, L., Stotland, N., & Segraves, R. (1982). Three cases of female anorgasmia associated with MAOIs. *American Journal of Psychiatry, 1389,* 1353–1354.

Lowenstein, L., Yarnitsky, D., Gruenwald, I., Deutsch, M., Sprecher, E., Gedalia, U., & Vardi, Y. (2005). Does hysterectomy affect genital sensation? *European Journal of Obstetrics, Gynecology, and Reproductive Biology, 119*(2), 242–245.

Meston, C. (2004). The effects of hysterectomy on sexual arousal in women with a history of benign uterine fibroids. *Archives of Sexual Behavior, 33*(1), 31–42.

Mishell, D., Stenchever, M., Droegemueller, W., & Herbst, A. (1997). Comprehensive Gynecology (3rd ed.). St. Louis, MO: Mosby-Year Book.

Monteiro, W., Noshirvani, H., Marks, I., & Lelliott, P. (1987). Anorgasmia from clomipramine in obsessive-compulsive disorder: A controlled trial. *British Journal of Psychiatry, 151,* 107–112.

Montejo-Gonzalez, A., Llorca, G., Izquierdo, J., Ledesma, A., Bousono, M., Carrasco, J., Ciudad, J., Daniel, E., de la Cndara, J., Derecho, J., Franco, M., Gomez, M., Macias, J., Martin, T., Perez, V., Sanchez, J., & Vicens, E. (1997). SSRI-induced sexual dysfunction: Fluoxetine, paroxetine, sertraline, and fluvoxamine in a prospective, Multicenter and descriptive clinical study of 344 patients. *Journal of Sex and Marital Therapy, 23,* 176–194.

Moss, H. (1983). More cases of anorgasmia after MAOI treatment. *American Journal of Psychiatry, 140,* 266.

Muniyappa, R., Norton, M., Dunn, M. E., Banerji, M. A. (2005). Diabetes and female sexual dysfunction: Moving beyond "benign neglect," *Current Diabetes Report, 5*(3), 230–236.

Navi, J., Jeronis, S., Morgan, M., & Arya, L. (2005). Sexual function in women with pelvic organ prolapse compared to women without pelvic organ prolapse. *Journal of Urology, 173,* 1669–1672.

Nichols, D., & Randall, C. (1983). Vaginal surgery (2nd. ed.) Baltimore, MD: Williams and Wilkins.

O'Connell, H., & Delancey, J. (2005). Clitoral anatomy in nulliparous healthy, premenopausal volunteers using unenhanced magnetic resonance imaging. *Journal of Urology, 173,* 2060–2063.

Panzer, C., Wise, S., , Fantini, G., Kang, D. , Munarriz, R., Guay, A., & Goldstein, I. (2006). *Journal of Sexual Medicine, 3,* 104–113.

Parker, W., Broder, M., Liu, Z.,& Shoupe, D. (2005). Ovarian conservation of the time of hysterectomy for benign disease. *Obstetrics and Gynecology, 106,* 219–226.

Peng, Y. S., Chiang, C. K., Kao, T. W., Hung, K. Y., Lu, C. S., Chiang, S. S., Yang, C. S., Huang, Y. C., Wu, K. D., Wu, M. S., Lien, Y. R., Yang, C. C., Tsai, D. M., Chen, P. Y., Liao, C. S., Tsai, T. J., Chen, W. Y. (2005). Sexual dysfunction in female hemodialysis patients A multicenter study. *Kidney International, 68*(2), 760–765.

Poad, D., & Arnold, E. P. (1994). Sexual function after pelvic surgery in women. *Australian and New Zealand Journal of Obstetrics and Gynecology, 34*(4), 471–474.

Pohl, R. (1983). Anorgasmia caused by MAOIs. *American Journal of Psychiatry, 140,* 510.

Physicians' Desk Reference. (1990). *Physicians' desk reference.* Oradell, NJ: Medical Economics.

Raspagliesi, F., Ditto, A., Fontanelli, R., Solima, E., Hanozet, F., Zanaboni, F., & Kusamura, S. (2004). Nerve-sparing radical hysterectomy: A surgical technique for preserving the autonomic hypogastric nerve. *Gynecologic Oncology, 93,* 307–314.

Rattya, J., Turkka, J., Pakarinen, A. J., Knip, M., Kotila, M. A., Lukkarinen, O., Myllyla, V. V., Isojarvi, J. I. (2001). Reproductive effects of valproate, carbamazepine, and oxcarbamezpine in men with epilepsy. *Neurology, 56,* 31–36.

Rhodes, J., Kjerulff, K., Langenberg, P., & Guzinski, G. (1999). Hysterectomy and sexual functioning. *Journal of the American Medical Association, 282,* 1934–1941.

Riley, A. & Riley, E. (1986). The effect of single dose diazepam on sexual response induced by masturbation. *Sexual and Marital Therapy (UK), 1,* 49–53.

Rosen, R., Lane, R., Menza, M. (1999). Effects of SSRIs on sexual function: A critical review. *Journal of Clinical Psychopharmacology, 19,* 67–85.

Schneck, C., Thomas, M., & Gunderson, D. (2002). Sexual side effects of valproate. *Journal of Clinical Psychopharmcology, 22,* 532–534.

Segraves, R. (1995). Antidepressant-induced orgasm disorder. *Journal of Sex & Marital Therapy, 121,* 192–201.

Segraves, R. (2002). Female sexual dysfunction: psychiatric aspects. *Canadian Journal of Psychiatry, 47,* 419–425.

Segraves, R. (2003). Recognizing and reversing sexual side effects of drugs. In S. Levine, C. Risen, & S. Althof (Eds.). *Handbook of clinical sexuality for mental health professionals* (pp. 377–392). New York: Brunner-Routledge..

Segraves, R. (2006). The role of the psychiatrist. In I. Goldstein, C. Meston, S. Davis, & A. Traish (Eds.). *Women's sexual function and dysfunction* (pp. 701–705). New York: Taylor & Francis.

Segraves, R., Kavoussi, R., Hughes, A., Batey, S., Johnston, J., Donahue, R., & Ascher, J. (2000). Evaluation of sexual functioning in depressed outpatients: A double-blind comparison of sustained-release bupropion and sertraline. *Journal of Clinical Psychopharmacology, 20,* 122–128.

Segraves, R. T., Clayton, A., Croft, H., Wolf, A., Warncok, J., & Segraves, K. (2004). Buporopion for the treatment of hypoactive sexual desire disorder in premenopausal women. *Journal of Clinical Psychopharmacology, 24,* 339–342.

Shull, B., & Bachofen, C. (1999). *Urogynecology and reconstructure pelvic surgery* (2nd ed.) M. Walters, & M. Karram (Eds.). St. Louis, MO: Mosby.

Souvner, R. (1983). Anorgasmia associated with imipramine but not desipramine: A case report. *Journal of Clinical Psychiatry, 44,* 345–346.

Stead, M. (2004). Sexual function after treatment for gynecological malignancy. *Current Opinion in Oncology, 16,* 492–495.

Thakar, R., (2004). Dispelling the myth—Does hysterectomy cause pelvic organ dysfunction? *British Journal of Obstetrics and Gynaecology: An International Journal of Obstetrics and Gynaecology, 111*(Suppl. 1), 20–23.

Thomas, D .R. (2003). Medications and sexual function. *Clinical Geriatric Medicine., 19,* 553–562.

Thompson, J. (1992). TeLinde's operative gynecology (7th ed.). Philadelphia, PA: J.B. Lippencott.

Trimmer, E. (1981). Iatrogenic sex problems. *British Medical Journal, 283,* 953–955.

Vassallo, B., & Karram, M. (2003, September). Management of iatrogenic vaginal constriction. *American College of Obstetricians and Gynecologists. 101*(3), 512–520.

Verrotti, A., Green, R., Latini, G. & Chiarelli, F. (2005). Endocrine and metabolic changes in epileptic patients receiving valproic acid. *Journal of Pediatric Endocrinology and Metabolism, 5,* 423–430.

Weber, A., Walters, M., & Piedmonte, M. (2000). Sexual function and vaginal anatomy in women before and after surgery for pelvic organ prolapse and urinary incontinence. *American Journal of Obstetrics and Gynecology, 182,* 1610–1615.

Wyatt, R., Fram, D., Buchbinder, R., & Snyder, F. (1971). Treatment of intractable narcolepsy with a monoamine-oxidase inhibitor. *New England Journal of Medicine, 285,* 987–991.

Chapter Fifteen

CURRENT CONTROVERSIES IN SEXUAL HEALTH: SEXUAL ADDICTION AND COMPULSION

INTRODUCTION

Mitchell S. Tepper and Annette Fuglsang Owens

People can become addicted to chemicals such as alcohol, nicotine, or heroin; but can someone be addicted to love, sex, masturbation, or pornography? Dr. Patrick Carnes defines addiction as "a pathological relationship with a mood-altering experience or thing that causes damage to the individual or others."[1]

By those criteria, sexual arousal or orgasm could be addictive. Sexual addiction, however, as both Carnes and Dr. Eli Coleman point out in the essays that follow is not recognized as a mental disorder in the *Diagnostic and Statistical Manual of Mental Disorders* of the American Psychiatric Association. Coleman refers to the phenomenon as compulsive sexual behavior until more research is available to determine more suitable terminology. Whether someone calls it sexual addiction or compulsive sexual behavior, if sexual thoughts or actions are causing significant distress or problems, experts agree that it is time to get help.

Both men and women can be affected. Nearly 9 percent of respondents in a study conducted by Dr. Al Cooper, editor of *Sex and the Internet: A guidebook for clinicians,* showed signs of online sexual compulsivity. Cooper describes the Internet as a "triple-A engine" of access, affordability, and anonymity (see chapter 13 in this volume). Depressed or irritable feelings from a bad day may prompt someone who is addicted to go online to escape negative emotions.

The study found women more likely to visit chat rooms, while men visited pornography sites.

Often, people with difficulty controlling their sexual behavior will deny and ignore the problem, especially if the sexual behavior is being used to cope with stress. Partners or spouses may be the first to spot the trouble and can encourage the person to seek professional help. Treatment may include talk therapy and medical treatment for underlying problems, such as depression or obsessive compulsive disorder.

In this chapter, we will present opinions by two leading figures in their respective fields, Dr. Eli Coleman and Dr. Patrick Carnes. Although Coleman and Carnes approach problematic sexual behaviors from different fields of study, which have historically been highly critical of each other's theoretical orientations, both experts realize there is much research to be done before anyone can claim they know the definitive answers, and both agree there is benefit to be gained from being open to different perspectives. We hope that the reader will gain a broader understanding of the complexity of what sexual compulsion or addiction entails.

The final chapter of this volume, by Dr. Richard Leedes, will delve deeper into theories that may explain psychological processes underlying sexually addictive tendencies.

COMPULSIVE SEXUAL BEHAVIOR: WHAT TO CALL IT, HOW TO TREAT IT?

Eli Coleman

Like most behaviors, sex can be taken to extremes. It can become excessive, impulsive, obsessive, compulsive, driven, and distressing. Some people suffer with these behavioral problems to the point that it interferes with their daily lives.

Unfortunately, clinical sexologists appear unable to reach consensus on what to call or how to treat such sexual behavior. Terms used to describe this phenomenon include *hypersexuality, erotomania, nymphomania, satyriasis,* and, most recently, *sexual addiction* and *compulsive sexual behavior.* The terminology often implies different values, attitudes, and theoretical orientations, and we remain in a quagmire about classification, causes, and treatment.

Debate over Cause

Disagreement exists as to whether compulsive sexual behavior is an addiction, a psychosexual developmental disorder, an impulse control disorder, a mood disorder, or an obsessive compulsive disorder.

Patrick Carnes popularized the concept of compulsive sexual behavior as an addiction. He believes that people become addicted to sex in the same way they become addicted to alcohol or drugs. Although this theory has become popular in recent years, it remains quite controversial and many other theories exist.

Robert Barth and Bill Kinder have agued that compulsive sexual behavior is an impulse control disorder.[2] Others have argued that it is a variation of an obsessive compulsive disorder.[3] A relatively new hypothesis put forth by John Bancroft and Erick Janssen explains sexual disorders as dysregulations of our excitatory and inhibitory mechanisms.[4]

The more psycho-dynamically oriented theorists have described this syndrome as a psychosexual disorder.[5] Heinz Kohut views it as a disorder of the self and an intimacy disorder.[6] Sexologist John Money conceptualizes it as lovemap pathology—a developmental and psychosexual disorder resulting from deprivation in, or punishment for, normal sexual rehearsals in infancy and childhood and/or from childhood trauma or abuse that would impair love and love bonding.[7] Money implicates cultural factors as well for potentially creating schisms between "love" and "lust" that result in the development of psychosexual disorders.[8]

While I have seen compulsive sexual behavior as an example of an "intimacy dysfunction" stemming from childhood abuse and trauma and highly restrictive attitudes about sexuality, I now view the behavior as having a multitude of causes and presentations.[9]

In my work and throughout this article, I use the term *compulsive sexual behavior (CSB)* to describe this syndrome. I chose this term in an attempt to find language that would describe the clinical phenomenon but leave open the possibility for multiple treatments. However, I recognize the limitations of this term, because the word *compulsive* is retained even though not all the behaviors of the syndrome are driven by obsessive-compulsive mechanisms.

While I continue to use the term *compulsive sexual behavior,* I hope it is understood that this is still a description of a set of symptoms waiting for a better term to replace it.

Classification of Compulsive Sexual Behavior

Compulsive sexual behaviors can be divided into two main types: paraphilic and nonparaphilic.

Paraphilic Compulsive Sexual Behavior

Paraphilic behaviors are unconventional sexual behaviors that are obsessive and compulsive. They interfere with love relationships and intimacy.

In early editions of the American Psychiatric Association's *Diagnostic and Statistical Manual of Mental Disorders (DSM)*, these unconventional behaviors were referred to as sexual deviation.[10] However, influenced by Money's work, the term *paraphilia* was introduced into the classification of sexual disorders in the *DSM-III*.[11] This term was viewed as more precise and non-pejorative. As a consequence, the classification is generally accepted within clinical sexology, but not without criticism.[12]

In the recent *DSM-IV*, paraphilias (or unconventional sexual behaviors) are defined as "recurrent, intense sexually arousing fantasies, sexual urges, or behaviors involving (1) nonhuman objects, (2) the suffering or humiliation of oneself or one's partner, or (3) children or other non-consenting persons." The definition goes on to explain, "The behavior, sexual urges, or fantasies cause clinically significant distress in social, occupational, or other important areas of functioning."[13]

Although Money has defined nearly 50 paraphilias, there are currently eight paraphilic disorders recognized in the *DSM-IV*: *pedophilia, exhibitionism, voyeurism, sexual masochism, sexual sadism, fetishism, transvestic fetishism,* and *frotteurism*.[14]

Some behaviors, such as sado-masochism, when they are consensual and do not impair life functioning, are not considered a paraphilia because they do not meet all of the diagnostic criteria.

Nonparaphilic Compulsive Sexual Behavior

Nonparaphilic compulsive sexual behavior involves conventional behaviors which, when taken to an extreme, are recurrent, distressing, and interfere in daily functioning.

The *DSM-IV* describes one example under the heading of "Sexual Disorders Not Otherwise Specified" as "distress about a pattern of repeated sexual relationships involving a succession of lovers who are experienced by the individual only as things to be used."[15] Other examples include: compulsive fixation on an unattainable partner, compulsive masturbation, compulsive love relationships, and compulsive sexuality in a relationship.[16]

Not all sexual behaviors that cause problems necessarily reach a diagnostic threshold. Nor are there well-established clinical criteria to define such behavior.[17] In the past, we have used a slight alteration of the paraphilia diagnostic criteria. In my own thinking, I propose the following criteria to define non-paraphilic compulsive sexual behavior:

  a. involves recurrent and intense normophilic (nonparaphilic) sexually arousing fantasies, sexual urges, and behaviors that cause clinically significant distress in social, occupational, or other important areas of functioning; and
  b. is not due simply to another medical condition, substance use disorder, or a developmental disorder

It is important not to label "problems" prematurely and ignore intra-inter-sociocultural considerations that might better explain the behavior. In developing diagnostic criteria, we must take the norms of gender, sexual orientation, and sociocultural groups into consideration.

Behaviors in Context

In fact, there are those who do not believe in sexual addiction or even in the idea of compulsive sexual behavior as a disorder. Their main criticism of these concepts is the possibility of overpathologizing behavior. They fear that the pathologizing of sexual behaviors (either by professionals or individuals) may be driven by anti-sexual attitudes and a failure to recognize the wide range of normal human sexual expression.

Individuals might think they are suffering from compulsive sexual behavior when, in reality they are experiencing behaviors that are part of sexual development, that are sexual problems but not compulsive, or that are simply in conflict with their values.

In order to avoid overpathologizing, it is important for professionals to be comfortable with a wide range of normal sexual behavior—both types of behavior and frequency of behavior. And it is important to look at all sexual behaviors in context.

Sexual Development

Individuals might view some sexual behaviors as obsessive or compulsive when they do not view them within a developmental context. Adolescents, for example, can become "obsessed" with sex for long periods of time. Adults commonly go through periods when sexual behavior may take on obsessive and compulsive characteristics. Individuals might naturally become obsessed with their partner and feel compelled to seek out their company and to express affection in early stages of romance. These are healthy processes of sexual development and must be distinguished from compulsive sexual behavior.

Sexual Problems

It is common for people to have sexual problems that are not pathological. People can make mistakes. They can at times act impulsively. Their behavior can cause problems in a relationship. Some people will use sex as a coping mechanism, just as they may use alcohol, drugs, or eating. These patterns of sexual behavior are sometimes problematic. They are often remedied by learning from mistakes or learning healthier forms of sexual expression. By its nature, the clinical syndrome of compulsive sexual behavior is much more resistant to change.

Conflict with Values

Many patients identify that they have compulsive sexual behavior when it is more a matter of conflict over intrapersonal values. For example, they might view masturbation, oral sex, homosexual behavior, sado-masochistic behavior, or a love affair as compulsive because they disapprove of these behaviors.

It is, therefore, very important to distinguish between individuals who have a values conflict with their sexual behavior and those who engage in compulsive sexual behaviors. Similarly, individuals may have a conflict with their values and those of their partner, family, or culture. Sometimes the problem is a matter of interpersonal or intercultural conflict.

Treatment

While we are still in search of a consensus of terminology, cause, and diagnostic criteria, it is important to recognize that there are a number of types, patterns, and manifestations of compulsive sexual behavior. It is prudent to look at this as a syndrome that calls for a variety of treatment approaches.

12-Step Groups

For those who view compulsive sexual behavior as an addiction, 12-step groups modeled on Alcoholics Anonymous (AA) are a logical place to turn for treatment. There are a plethora of self-help groups such as Sexual Addicts Anonymous (SAA), Sex and Love Anonymous (SLA), and Sexaholics Anonymous (SA). Each is modeled after AA, and each uses the 12 steps and traditions of AA as a basic philosophy and guide.

There are reports that this approach is successful.[18] In fact, there are many people who seek help only through such groups. Certain practitioners base their treatment on this methodology or use these groups as an adjunct to their treatment.[19]

This method, however, remains controversial. Many feel that the "abstinence model" useful for alcoholics cannot be applied to sexuality since sexual expression is a basic need of life. Critics view the abstinence solution as an oversimplification of compulsive sexual behavior and potentially dangerous when proper medical and psychological treatment is not provided.

While I have argued about the dangers of the "addiction model" and 12-step groups,[20] my clinical experience has shown that some patients find these groups extremely helpful as an adjunct to treatment and that others find them neutral or problematic. In addition, many patients find the term "addiction" a useful metaphor to describe their problem.

Although I still have concerns about the "addiction model" and 12-step groups, I do not see 12-step groups under professional guidance as necessarily incompatible or harmful. Obviously, we are in need of more rigorous study of the effectiveness of these groups.

Psychotherapy

There are a number of psychotherapeutic treatment models. Again, given diagnostic considerations, it is important that we consider such treatment on an individual basis.

My colleagues and I have found that group therapy, augmented with individual and family therapy, has been very effective as a cornerstone of treatment.[21] However, we also individualize treatment plans within the group. And, certainly, not all patients should be treated in group, given diagnostic considerations.

My colleagues and I have also found a high rate of personality disorders in our patients—certainly a variety of personality disorder traits that are intertwined in their management or mismanagement of interpersonal relationships. Psychotherapy can prove very helpful in uncovering the sources of these management strategies and helping patients to learn more adaptive management mechanisms.

Treatment should also go beyond the removal or reduction of symptoms and help individuals learn new skills in psychosexual functioning. Beyond control of the affective states (especially anxiety and depression), in many cases more emphasis needs to be placed on addressing basic identity and intimacy functioning. Many of our patients with long-standing patterns of dysfunctional sexual behavior know very little about healthy sexuality and intimacy. Thus, a large part of treatment and after care should focus on developing a positive and healthy sexuality.

Pharmacology

There are a number of pharmacologic treatments that have proved effective in clinical case studies.[22] Antidepressants that selectively act on serotonin levels in the brain are effective in reducing sexual obsessions and compulsions and their associated levels of anxiety and depression. The newer medications interrupt the obsessive thinking and help patients control urges to engage in CSB. They also help patients use therapy more effectively. Medications that suppress the production of male hormones (antiandrogens) can also be used to treat a variety of paraphilic disorders.

John Bradford has developed an algorithm of pharmacologic treatment of paraphilic compulsive sexual behavior based upon his clinical experience in treating sexual offenders and support from the clinical literature.[23] It relies heavily on the use of SSRIs (Selective Serotonin Reuptake Inhibitors) in mild cases and on antiandrogen treatment in extreme cases.

We are in need of a similar algorithm for nonparaphilic compulsive sexual behavior. While the antiandrogens could be used in more severe cases, there are a variety of other medications and combinations of medications that could be used to control less severe cases. Although the behavior may be distressing, it does not involve sexual offending behavior. Therefore, I have significant concern about the use of antiandrogens to control nonparaphilic CSB because of side effects and the fact that it also suppresses normophilic functioning, which we are interested in enhancing. We need to look at the effectiveness of other regimens with less potential problems of side effects and those that will not interfere in normophilic functioning.

Fortunately, there is now an array of pharmacologic treatments proven effective in clinical case studies. However, we are still in desperate need of controlled clinical trials in order to develop a more evidenced-based clinical approach to pharmacologic treatment.

Conclusion

A challenge remains to understand nonparaphilic compulsive sexual behavior, find where this clinical syndrome fits in our classification of sexual disorders, determine clear diagnostic criteria, and find effective treatment approaches.

While the debate over the past few decades has been helpful, we are in desperate need of more research. Meanwhile, we must learn to recognize this clinical syndrome in individuals and know when to apply the appropriate methodology based upon our best available scientific understanding of the complexity of possible causes and treatments.

UNDERSTANDING SEXUAL ADDICTION

Patrick Carnes

During the past three decades, professionals have acknowledged that some people use sex to manage their internal distress. These people are similar to compulsive gamblers, compulsive overeaters, or alcoholics in that they are not able to contain their impulses—and with destructive results.

Definition

To facilitate classification and understanding of psychological disorders, mental health professionals rely on the *Diagnostic and Statistical Manual of Mental Disorders (DSM)* published by the American Psychiatric Association and now in its fourth edition.

Each edition of this book represents a consensus at the time of publication about what constitutes mental disorders. Each subsequent edition has reflected changes in understanding. The *DSM's* system is, therefore, best viewed as a "work in progress" rather than the "bible."

The term *sexual addiction* does not appear in *DSM-IV.* In fact, the word *addiction* itself does not appear. It condenses the criteria for addictive disorders—such as substance abuse and pathologic gambling—into three elements:

- *Loss of control (compulsivity).* "There is a persistent desire or unsuccessful efforts to cut down or control substance abuse." "Has persistent unsuccessful efforts to control, cut back, or stop gambling."
- *Continuation despite adverse consequences.* "The substance use is continued despite knowledge of having a persistent or recurrent physical or psychological problem

that is likely to have been caused or exacerbated by the substance use." "Has committed illegal acts such as forgery, fraud, theft, or embezzlement to finance gambling."

- *Obsession or preoccupation.* "A great deal of time is spent in activities necessary to obtain the substance, use the substance, or recover from its effects." "Is preoccupied with gambling."[24]

Complex Problem

Typically, individuals in trouble for their sexual behavior are not candid about whatever incident has come to light, nor are they likely to reveal that the specific behavior actually is a part of a consistent, self-destructive pattern. The nature of this illness causes patients to hide the severity of the problem from others, to delude themselves about their ability to control their behavior, and to minimize their impact on others.

Often some event will precipitate a visit to the primary care provider. Sexual excess of some type will create a physical problem. Sexually transmitted diseases, damage to genitals, unwanted pregnancies: all are among the reasons for such a visit. Most patients will say that the event is a unique situation.

The primary care provider will often treat the physical problem without probing for more information. If, however, there is sexual addiction, the problem will not disappear. A wide range of behaviors can be problematic, including compulsive masturbation, affairs, use of pornography, voyeurism, exhibitionism, sexual harassment, and sex offending.

Health care providers must understand that underneath what appears to be an isolated event may be a more complex pathologic problem with a host of related factors such as the following:

- A high incidence of depression and suicide
- The presence of high-risk and dangerous behaviors including self-harm designed to escalate sexual experiences
- The high probability of other addictive behaviors including alcoholism, drug abuse, and pathologic gambling
- Extreme disruption of the family, including battering, sexual abuse, and financial distress

Behaviors

Clinicians should remember that the discovery of something sexual does not make an addictive illness. A long-term affair, for example, would be a problem for a spouse but would not be a compulsive pattern. Likewise, a person with exploitive or violent behavior does not necessarily have an addictive illness.

I have been gathering data on sexual addiction since 1985. In the process, I have found that sexually addictive behavior clusters into 10 distinct types.

Patients often will be active in more than one cluster. That is one of the most important lessons of sexual addiction: patterns exist among behaviors.

The 10 distinctive types of behaviors are:

- *Fantasy sex.* Arousal depends on sexual possibility. The individual neglects responsibilities to engage in fantasy and/or prepare for the next sexual episode.
- *Seductive role sex.* Arousal is based on conquest and diminishes rapidly after the initial contact. It can be heightened by increasing risk and/or number of partners.
- *Voyeuristic sex.* Visual stimulation is used to escape into an obsessive trance. Arousal may be heightened by masturbation or risk (peeping), or violation of boundaries (voyeuristic rape).
- *Exhibitionistic sex.* The individual attracts attention to the body or its sexual parts. Arousal stems from the shock or the interest of the viewer.
- *Paying for sex.* Arousal is connected to payment for sex, and with time, it actually becomes connected to money itself. Payment creates an entitlement and a sense of power over meeting needs. The arousal starts with "having money" and the search for someone in "the business."
- *Trading sex.* Arousal is based on gaining control of others by using sex as leverage.
- *Intrusive sex.* Arousal occurs by violating boundaries with no repercussions.
- *Anonymous sex.* Arousal involves no seduction or cost and is immediate. It has no entanglements or obligations associated with it and often is accelerated by unsafe or high-risk environments such as parks and restrooms.
- *Pain-exchange sex.* Arousal is built around specific scenarios or narratives of humiliation and shame.
- *Exploitive sex.* Arousal is based on target "types" of vulnerability. Certain types of vulnerable people (such as clients/patients) become the focus.

In addition, in recent years people have begun to use cybersex in unexpected numbers, and many are finding themselves accessing sex in problematic ways.

Individuals suffering from sexual addiction have found sex on the Internet a natural extension of what they are already doing. They can act out any of the previously mentioned 10 types of sexual behavior on the Internet. They can find sex partners, be voyeuristic, start affairs, and swap partners, among other things.

There are also many individuals who never would have experienced sexual compulsive behavior had it not been for the Internet. Consider this:

- About 200 sex-related Web sites are added each day, and there are more than 100,000 existing sites.
- Sex on the Internet constitutes the third largest economic sector on the Web (software and computers rank first and second), generating one billion dollars annually.

- A total of 65 million unique visitors use free porn sites, and 19 million unique visitors use pay porn sites each month.
- Approximately one percent of Internet users have a severe problem that focuses almost exclusively on cybersex, with major neglect of the rest of their life's activities.[25]

Successful Treatment

A number of key factors are involved in successful recovery from sexual addition. They include:

- *A good addiction-oriented primary therapist.* Most successful recoveries involve a relationship with a therapist over a three- to five-year period, the first two years of which are very intense.
- *A 12-step sexual addiction group.* The probability of relapse is extremely high if the addict does not attend meetings.
- *A 12-step program for other addictions.* If the addict has other addictions, a 12-step program is necessary for those as well. A suggestion that makes things easier is to find a sponsor, or sponsors, who attends all of the same meetings your patient does. This way, there is a consolidation of relationships.
- *Program work, not just attendance.* Completing step work, finding a sponsor, and doing service are all key elements of recovery. Individuals should become actively involved in the program's activities. In a recent outcome study of an inpatient program for sexual addiction, researchers discovered that only 23 percent actually complete the first 9 of the 12 steps in 18 months. However, of those who did, recidivism was rare.[26]
- *Early family involvement.* Family participation in the patient's therapy improves the chance for success.
- *Spiritual support.* Addicts report that the spiritual work started in their 12-step communities and continued in various spiritual communities was critical to the changes they needed to make.
- *Exercise along with good nutrition and a healthy lifestyle.* Addicts who reduce their stress, start an exercise program, and eat more healthfully do better in their recovery.

In discussing what had helped them in their recovery, over 190 sex addicts indicated that these treatments were the most helpful (in order from most to least): a higher power (87 percent); couples 12-step group based on sexual addiction (85 percent); a friend's support (69 percent); individual therapy (65 percent); a celibacy period (64 percent); a sponsor (61 percent); exercise/nutrition (58 percent); a 12-step group based on subjects other than sexual addiction (55 percent); partner support (36 percent); inpatient treatment (35 percent); out-patient group (27 percent); therapy (21 percent); family therapy (11 percent); and after care (hospital) (9 percent).[27]

Healthy Sexuality

The goal of treatment is healthy sexuality. Some therapists insist on a period of celibacy, which does help to reduce chaos and make patients available for therapy. But recovery from sexual addiction does not mean sexual abstinence.

The objective of treatment is to help individuals develop a healthy, strong sexual life. One of the risks is that the patients may slip to a position of sexual aversion, in which they think all sex is bad. Sexual aversion, or "sexual anorexia," is simply another variant of sexual compulsive behavior.

Patients will sometimes bounce from one extreme to the other. True recovery involves a clear understanding about abstaining from certain sexual behaviors combined with an active plan for enhancing sexuality.

Recovery from sexual addiction is likened to recovery from eating disorders. Food is a necessary part of life, and recovery from eating disorders requires defining what is healthy eating and what is not. Similarly, the goal of recovery from sexual addiction is learning what is healthy sexuality for the individual.

Healthy sexuality for most sexually addicted individuals involves not only a change in behavior but also an avoidance of fantasizing about behaviors that are unhealthy. Sexual fantasizing can be healthy, particularly for a reasonably healthy couple that uses their increased excitement to move toward rather than away from the partner. However, sexual imagery that is not respectful of other human beings increases objectification, depersonalization, and destructive bonding based on hostility rather than affection. Asking patients about their "sobriety" definition and about the content of fantasies provides clues to help with treatment and recovery.

Keeping Up

To determine how well the patient is doing in establishing a healthy lifestyle, clinicians can ask some simple questions. Does the patient have tools for avoiding relapse during times of hunger, anger, loneliness, and tiredness? Is the patient attending 12-step self-help meetings? If not, what are the obstacles preventing the patient from doing so? What are the patient's perceptions of what goes on at a meeting? Does he or she have a sponsor (a person longer in recovery who can guide the newer member)?

Is the patient seeking a counselor or therapist who is knowledgeable in addiction recovery? Is there balance between work and recreation? Is the patient exercising or engaging in any sports? Is the patient actively working to improve his or her relationship with a spouse or significant other? Is the spouse also attending a self-help meeting? These are all indicators to determine if the individual is fully engaged in building a healthier lifestyle.

Conclusion

The treatment of sexual addiction has taken a long time to gain recognition and respect as an area of medical specialty.

As with other disorders, such as alcoholism or anorexia, clinicians face many challenges in learning about sexual addiction. Most who take time to learn find patients who are profoundly grateful.

In many ways, the field of sexual addiction lags behind both professional and lay awareness of alcoholism or anorexia. Yet, important strides are being made in both understanding and awareness.

Appreciating the issues and challenges of sexual addiction will help clinicians when their patients' behaviors cross the line from problems of judgment to symptoms of a clinical disorder.

NOTES

Both articles are reprinted with permission from the *SIECUS Report* (June/July 2003), Sexuality Information and Education Council of the United States, New York, NY.

1. Patrick Carnes, *Out of the Shadows*, Minneapolis, MN: CompCare Publications, 1983, p. 4.

2. R. J. Barth and B. N. Kinder, "The Mislabeling of Sexual Impulsivity," *Journal of Sex and Marital Therapy*, vol. 13, 1987, pp. 15–23.

3. M. A. Jenike, "Obsessive-compulsive and Related Disorders," *New England Journal of Medicine*, vol. 321, 1989, pp. 539–41; E. Coleman, "Compulsive Sexual Behavior: New Concepts and Treatments," *Journal of Psychology and Human Sexuality*, vol. 4, 1991, pp. 37–52; E. Coleman, "Is Your Patient Suffering from Compulsive Sexual Behavior?" *Psychiatric Annals*, vol. 22, no. 6, 1992, pp. 320–25; E. Coleman, "Treatment of Compulsive Sexual Behavior," In R. C. Rosen and S. R. Leiblum (Eds.). *Case Studies in Sex Therapy* (New York: Guilford Publications, 1995), pp. 333–49.

4. J. Bancroft, "Individual Difference in Sexual Risk Taking by Men—A Psycho-socio-biological Approach." In J. Bancroft (Ed.). *The Role of Theory in Sex Research* (Bloomington, IN: Indiana University Press, 2000), pp. 177–212; J. Bancroft and E. Janssen, "The Dual Control Model of Male Sexual Response: A Theoretical Approach to Centrally Mediated Erectile Dysfunction," *Neuroscience and Biobehavioral Review*, vol. 24, pp. 571–79.

5. S. B. Levine, "A Modern Perspective on Nymphomania," *Journal of Sex and Marital Therapy*, vol. 8, 1982, pp. 316–24; R. J. Stoller, *Perversion: The Erotic Form of Hatred* (New York: Pantheon, 1975).

6. H. Kohut, *The Restoration of the Self* (New York: International University Press, 1977).

7. J. Money, *Love and Love Sickness: The Science of Sex, Gender Difference and Pair-bonding* (Baltimore: The Johns Hopkins University Press, 1980); J. Money, *Lovemaps: Clinical Concepts of Sexual/Erotic Health and Pathology, Paraphilia, and Gender Transposition in Childhood, Adolescence, and Maturity* (New York: Irvington Publishers, 1986).

8. J. Money, (1986). *Lovemaps: Clinical Concepts of Sexual/Erotic Health and Pathology, Paraphilia, and Gender Transposition in Childhood, Adolescence, and Maturity* (New York: Irvington Publishers, 1986).

9. E. Coleman, "Sexual Compulsivity: Definition, Etiology, and Treatment Considerations," In E. Coleman (Ed.), *Chemical Dependency and Intimacy Dysfunction* (New York: The Haworth Press, Inc., 1987).

10. R. J. Stoller, *Perversion: The Erotic Form of Hatred.* (New York: Pantheon, 1975); *Diagnostic and Statistical Manual of Mental Disorders* (2nd Edition) (Washington, DC: American Psychiatric Association, 1968).

11. *Diagnostic and Statistical Manual of Mental Disorders* (Second Edition) (Washington, DC: American Psychiatric Association, 1968); *Diagnostic and Statistical Manual of Mental Disorders* (Third Edition) (Washington, DC: American Psychiatric Association, 1980).

12. *Diagnostic and Statistical Manual of Mental Disorders* (Fourth Edition) (Washington, DC: American Psychiatric Association, 1994).

13. Ibid., pp. 522–523.

14. Ibid.

15. Ibid., p. 538.

16. E. Coleman, "Is your patient suffering from compulsive sexual behavior?" *Psychiatrics Annals,* vol. 22 (6), 1992, pp. 320–425.

17. A. Goodman, *Sexual Addiction: An Integrated Approach* (Madison, CT: International Universities Press, 1998).

18. M. Hunter, *Hope and Recovery: A Twelve Step Guide to Overcoming Compulsive Sexual Behavior* (Minneapolis: CompCare Publishers, 1991); P. Carnes, *Don't Call It Love: Recovery from Sexual Addiction* (New York: Bantam Doubleday Publishing Group, Inc. 1992).

19. P. Carnes, *Out of the Shadows: Understanding the Sexual Addict* (Minneapolis: CompCare Publishers, 1983).

20. E. Coleman, "Sexual Compulsivity vs. Sexual Addition: The Debate Continues," *SIECUS Report,* vol. 7, no. 11, July 1986; E. Coleman, "Sexual Compulsivity: Definition, Etiology, and Treatment Considerations," In E. Coleman (Ed.), *Chemical Dependency and Intimacy Dysfunction* (Binghamton, NY: The Haworth Press, Inc., 1987); E. Coleman, "The Obsessive-compulsive Model for Describing Compulsive Sexual Behavior," *American Journal of Preventive Psychiatry and Neurology,* vol. 2, no. 3, 1990, pp. 9–14.

21. E. Coleman, S. M. Dwyer, G. Abel, W. Berner, J. Breiling, R. Eher, J. Hindman, R. Langevin, T. Langfeldt, M. Miner, F. Phafflin, and P. Weiss, "Standards of Care for the Treatment of Adult Sex Offenders," *Journal of Psychology and Human Sexuality,* vol. 11, no. 3, 2000, pp. 11–17; E. Coleman, T. Gratzer, L. Nesvacil, and N. Raymond, "Nefazodone and the Treatment of Nonparaphilic Compulsive Sexual Behavior: A Retrospective Study," *Journal of Clinical Psychiatry,* vol. 61, 2000, pp. 282–84.

22. J. M. Bradford and A. Pawlak, "Double-blind Placebo Crossover Study of Cyproterone Acetate in the Treatment of the Paraphilias," *Archives of Sexual Behavior,* vol. 22, no. 5, 1993, pp. 383–402; J. Cesnik and E. Coleman, "Use of Lithium Carbonate in the Treatment of Autoerotic Asphyxia," *American Journal of Psychotherapy,* vol. 43, no. 2, 1989, pp. 277–86; A. J. Cooper, "A Placebo-controlled Trial of the Antiandrogen Cyproterone Acetate in Deviant Hypersexuality," *Comprehensive Psychiatry,* vol. 22, no. 5, 1981, pp. 458–65; E. Coleman, J. Cesnik, A.M. Moore, and S. M. Dwyer, "Exploratory Study of the Role of Psychotropic Medications in the Psychological Treatment of Sex Offenders," *Journal of Offender Rehabilitation,* vol. 44, no. 2, 1992, pp. 204–17; J. P. Fedoroff, "Buspirone Hydrochloride in the Treatment of Transvestic Fetishism," *Journal of Clinical Psychiatry,* vol. 49, no. 10, 1988, pp. 408–9; J. P. Federoff, "Serotonergic Drug Treatment of Deviant

Sexual Interests," *Annals of Sex Research,* vol. 6, 1993, pp. 105–21; M. P. Kafka, "Successful Treatment of Paraphilic Coercive Disorder (a Rapist) with Fluoxetine Hydrochloride," *British Journal of Psychiatry,* vol. 158, 1991, pp. 844–47; M. P. Kafka, "Successful Antidepressant Treatment of Nonparaphilic Sexual Addictions and Paraphilias in Males," *Journal of Clinical Psychiatry,* vol. 52, no. 2, 1991, pp. 60–65; M. P. Kafka and R. Prentky, "Fluoxetine Treatment of Nonparaphilic Sexual Addictions and Paraphilias in Men," *Journal of Clinical Psychiatry,* vol. 53, no. 10, 1992, pp. 351–58; D. J. Stein, E. Hollander, D. T. Anthony, F. R. Schneier, B. A. Fallon, M. R. Liebowitz, and D. F. Klein, "Serotonergic Medications for Sexual Obsessions, Sexual Addictions and Paraphilias," *Journal of Clinical Psychiatry,* vol. 53, no. 8, 1992, pp. 267–71; N. C. Raymond, B. Robinson, C. Kraft, B. Rittberg, and E. Coleman, "Treatment of Pedophilia with Leuprolide Acetate: A Case Study," *Journal of Psychology and Human Sexuality,* vol. 13, nos. 3 and 4, 2001, pp. 79–88; N. C. Raymond, J. E. Grant, S. W. Kim, and E. Coleman, "Treatment of Compulsive Sexual Behavior with Naltrexone and Serotonin Reuptake Inhibitors: Two Case Studies," *International Clinical Psychopharmacology,* vol. 17, 2002, pp. 201–5; F. Thibaut, B. Cordier, and J. M. Kuhn, "Effect of a Long-lasting Gonadotrophin Hormone-releasing Hormone Agonist in Six Cases of Severe Male Paraphilia," *Acta Psychiatrica Scandinavica,* vol. 87, 1993, pp. 455–60; F. Thibaut, B. Cordier, and J. M. Kuhn, "Gonadotrophophin Hormone Releasing Hormone Agonists in Cases of Severe Paraphilia: A Lifetime Treatment?" *Psychoneuroendocrinology,* vol. 21, no. 4, 1996, pp. 411–19; P. Briken, E. Nika, and W. Berner, "Treatment of Paraphilia with Leutinizing Hormone-releasing Agonists," *Journal of Sex & Marital Therapy,* vol. 27, no. 1, 2001, pp. 45–55.

23.   J. M. Bradford, "Treatment of Sexual Deviation Using a Pharmacologic Approach," *Journal of Sex Research,* vol. 37, no. 3, 2000.

24.   *Diagnostic and Statistical Manual of Mental Disorders* (Fourth Edition) (Washington, DC: American Psychiatric Association, 1994), pp. 181, 618.

25.   P. Carnes et al, *In the Shadows of the Net* (Center City, MN: Hazelden Foundation, 2001), pp. 6–7.

26.   P. Carnes, "Sexual Addiction and Compulsion: Recognition, Treatment, and Recovery," *CNS Spectrums,* Vol. 5, No. 10, October 2000, pp. 63–68.

27.   Ibid.

Chapter Sixteen

COMPULSIVE OR OTHER PROBLEMATIC SEXUAL BEHAVIOR

Richard Leedes

Early relationships affect the nature of sexual desire and sexual behaviors through adulthood. In this chapter, I will explore how two factors—fantasies and emotional attachments—influence sexuality. In particular, I will explain how these factors contribute to hypersexuality, a condition sometimes referred to as sexual addiction or sexual compulsivity.

Fantasies can be described as *compassionate,* meaning that they involve an appreciation or cherishment of the personal qualities of one's partner, or *objectified,* meaning that they focus on body parts or distinctive sexual activities. Fantasies can also be negative and anxiety producing, causing a person to avoid intimate contact or specific sexual behaviors. Through the course of this chapter, we will explore how the nature of fantasies is related to emotional attachments and how these two factors work together to form a person's *lovemap,* a developmental template that reflects an idealized lover or an idealized erotic script (Money, 1986). It has been found that people with sexual addictions have a disposition, or bias, toward objectified fantasies, and at the same time, they are uncomfortable and anxious in close relationships.

Treatment of sexual addiction should take dispositions toward fantasies and emotional attachments into consideration. At the Counseling Center at Princeton, where we see 150 patients per week who struggle with sexual addiction, our goals are to help these people reduce the negative impact of their objectified fantasies and increase their comfort level in personal relationships.

THE TWO VARIABLES OF SEXUAL DESIRE: FANTASY AND RELATIONSHIPS

The brain is a powerful sex organ. Thoughts and feelings influence our experience of sexual encounters and can enhance or inhibit sexual behavior. In this chapter, we will explore how sexual fantasies are shaped by our past experiences and have the ability to influence our current behavior.

Objectified fantasies, described above, are normal (Leitenberg & Henning, 1995). Sex addicts, however, are likely to spend a considerable about of time obsessing about objectified fantasies, as compared to non-sex-addicts (Carnes, 1983) and they are much more likely to engage in these objectified fantasies than they are in compassionate ones. Furthermore, sex addicts are often not able to distinguish these pretend relationships from authentic relationships. "Leading a fantasy double life is a distortion of reality" (Carnes, 1983, p. 4).

A person's comfort with emotional intimacy and close human relationships also affects sexual desire. Sex addicts commonly experience a pervasive feeling of loneliness and a sense of alienation from partners, friends, and family. The result is that these individuals begin to live in their fantasies, while they continue to be uncomfortable in interpersonal relationships. "The addict substitutes a sick relationship to an event or process for a healthy relationship with others. The addict's relationship with a mood altering experience becomes central to his life" (Carnes, 1983, p. 4). It has been suggested that this loneliness and distance from others is a result of what is described by Bowlby (1973, 1980, 1988), as the person's dysfunctional "internal working model." In this chapter, the term *disposition* is used to describe internal working models of attachment relationships (i.e., significant and emotionally close relationships). Sex addicts have a disposition that makes them uncomfortable or nonresponsive in interpersonal relationships, while feeling comfortable in their pseudoreality, filled with objectifications (Leedes, 1999). Kaplan (1995) describes this as a "virtual reality" (p. 46).

WHAT IS SEX ADDICTION?

Beginning in the 1980s, the terms *sexual addiction* and *sexual compulsivity* began to appear in professional publications and the popular press (Levine and Troiden, 1988). This followed the publication of Carnes' (1983) book, *The Sexual Addiction,* which many sexologists viewed as a counterreaction to the permissive cultural landscape of the 1970s. Carnes (1996) speculates that the category "sexual compulsivity" was introduced to the American Association of Sex Educators, Counselors and Therapists (ASSECT) as a less pejorative alternative to "sexual addiction." At the time, sexologists were concerned that sexual addiction research was being conducted by those who had an unscientific approach to human sexuality. Additionally, self-help programs (and some of their literature) were viewed as contributing to sexually negative stereotypes.

Although one single clinical entity has not yet been classified by the American Psychiatric Association, the concepts of sexual addiction and sexual compulsivity do have common themes that can supply an operational definition of hypersexuality. Goodman (1993) has developed a diagnostic list of criteria for sexual addiction (Table 16.1). These criteria tend to focus on the behaviors exhibited by hypersexual people rather than the chronicity of their obsessions.

The missing element of all of these interpretations of hypersexuality is insight into how this particular behavioral pattern relates to a person's sexual desire. By deconstructing fantasy, we can determine how and why specific sexual behavior patterns affect people's lives. In other words, fantasies reflect a person's life experiences and are the key to understanding sexual desire. Goodman (1993) acknowledges the diversity of sexual desire by stating,

Table 16.1
Diagnosis of Sexual Addiction

A. Recurrent failure to resist impulses to engage in a specified sexual behavior.
B. Increasing sense of tension immediately prior to initiating the sexual behavior.
C. Pleasure or relief at the time of engaging in the sexual behavior.
D. At least five of the following:

1) Frequent preoccupation with the sexual behavior or with activity that is preparatory to the sexual behavior
2) Frequent engaging in the sexual behavior to a greater extent or over a longer period than intended
3) Repeated efforts to reduce, control, or stop the sexual behavior
4) A great deal of time spent in activities necessary for the sexual behavior, engaging in the sexual behavior, or recovering from its effects
5) Frequent engaging in the sexual behavior when expected to fulfill occupational, academic, domestic, or social obligations
6) Important social, occupational, or recreational activities given up or reduced because of the sexual behavior
7) Continuation of the sexual behavior despite knowledge of having a persistent or recurrent social, financial, psychological, or physical problem that is caused or exacerbated by the sexual behavior
8) Tolerance: need to increase the intensity or frequency of the sexual behavior in order to achieve the desired effect, or diminished effect with continued sexual behavior of the same intensity
9) Restlessness or irritability if unable to engage in the sexual behavior

E. Some symptoms of the disturbance have persisted for at least one month, or have occurred repeatedly over a longer period of time.

Source: From A. Goodman, Diagnosis and treatment of sexual addiction, *Journal of Sex and Marital Therapy, 19,* no. 3 (1993): 230.

It is not the type of behavior, its object, its frequency, or its social acceptability that determines whether a pattern of sexual behavior qualifies as a sexual addiction; it is *how* this behavior pattern relates to and affects the individual's life, as indicated in the definition and specified in the diagnostic criteria (p. 231). (See Table 16.1.)

TOWARD A COMPREHENSIVE THEORY ON SEXUAL DESIRE

With the exception of Kaplan (1979, 1995, 1996), no contemporary researchers have offered a comprehensive theory on sexual desire that is able to explain both hyposexuality and hypersexuality. This presents a serious impasse for the treatment of sexual addicts. Nathan (1995) describes the error made by therapists when they try the "teach the sex addict to have sex like a normal person" approach. Whereas non-sexual-addicts are given permission to fantasize anything they like, fantasy for sexual addicts "is not an alternative to forbidden sexual activity but rather a rehearsal for it" (Nathan, 1995, p. 360). She continues that sex therapists are uncomfortable having people deny their fantasies "because it does not acknowledge the psychodynamic imperative of a person's fantasy choice, the way in which a preferred sexual fantasy reinvokes and reworks past experience" (Nathan, 1995, p. 361).

Nathan's (1995) last statement is basic to the problem. If fantasy is an internal representation assembled by psychodynamic content, then understanding fantasies and their function is key to treating sexual desire disorders. Kaplan (1995, 1996) and Stoller (1975) describe how, through fantasy, a person becomes powerful and is able to find resolution in virtual reality, whereas in the real world, resolution is elusive.

I have proposed the theory that the disposition toward fantasy and the disposition toward comforting interpersonal relationships shape sexual desire as a heuristic, or guide, for conducting sexual desire and sexual addiction research. By demonstrating a relationship between the disposition held toward objectified fantasies by sexual addicts and the uncomfortable feelings they have toward interpersonal attachments, I will be able to suggest relevant variables that comprise sexual desire.

THE NATURE OF SEXUAL DESIRE

Many researchers have recognized the psychological nature of sexual desire. Masters, Johnson, and Kolodny (1994) suggest that sexual desire is more a reflection of psychosocial forces than biological ones. Kaplan (1995) believed that dysfunction in sexual motivation, sexual avoidance, and hypersexual desire is regulated by psychological processes. Sexual addiction and compulsion researchers also suggest that hypersexuality is primarily a result of early family experiences (Carnes, 1991; Coleman, 1991).

Fantasy can be thought of as internal, symbolic representations of early and significant relationships (Kaplan, 1995; Levine, 1988, Money, 1986; Stoller 1975). Fantasy management can represent the crucial variable for interventions when attempting to change sexual avoidance and hypersexuality. Kaplan hypothesizes that sexual fantasies are

> mental representations of a person's most ardent sexual wishes and desires. As such, fantasies and desires are identical in content, differing only that fantasy remains in the realm of virtual reality or mental simulation, while desire is fantasy that may actually be put into practice (p. 46).

Kaplan (1995) asserts that fantasies can both increase, or "up-regulate," and decrease, or "down-regulate," sexual desire. As a consequence, these virtual sexual images are powerful aphrodisiacs that can enhance and add new dimensions to pleasurable experiences. Alternatively, they can metastasize a person's ability to appreciate the human qualities of one's partner. This can evolve to the chronic objectification of others.

Virtual reality can also produce "antifantasies," which are negative, fearful, or repulsive representations of selected people or erotic activities. Antifantasies result from distorted perceptions of sexual partners or spouses or from irrational ideas such as intrusive incestuous thoughts (Kaplan, 1996). Antifantasies influence brain activity as if the mental representations were real dangers and the negative emotional state, such as fear, guilt, or disgust, suppresses or down-regulates sexual desire away from the person or object that stirs up the imagery. Antifantasies can play a role in sexual avoidance whether someone has a general form of hyposexual desire disorder (HSD) or sexual aversion disorder (SAD), "sexual anorexia" (Kaplan, 1995, p. 55), or a specific avoidance, as in the case of many sexual addicts who are only sexually avoidant in the context of their loving relationships. Kaplan (1996) suggests that sexual avoidance is not the result of a passive process related to the *noncreation* of erotic fantasies but rather a dynamic process that *creates* antifantasies that down-regulate sexual desire.

Although there is some disagreement as to the nature of fantasies and antifantasies, it is clear that these are variables that can mediate either the up-regulation or down-regulation of sexual desire and sexual avoidance. People with unproblematic sexual desire use fantasies as virtual sexual inciters in order to enrich their sex lives and antifantasies as virtual sexual suppressors to exclude inappropriate opportune encounters by imagining themselves disgraced because of their inappropriate behavior.

For those persons who have negative antifantasies toward their loving partners, the nature of the antifantasy must be analyzed. Some are given insight that these representations are thought distortions based on early experiences

Table 16.2
The Two Variables of Sexual Desire (A Partitioned Love Map)

Possibilities of Sexual Desire	
Interpersonal Relationships	*Fantasy*
a disposition of either	a disposition of either
1. comfort	1. comfort
2. anxiety/obsession	2. anxiety/obsession
3. avoidance	3. avoidance

that are unrelated to their partners. Others are given insight that their disposition toward idealized fantasies is disproportional to their disposition toward compassionate elements of their partners. In the latter case, techniques need to be deployed to refocus their disposition.

The two components of sexual desire: the disposition toward fantasy and the disposition toward interpersonal attachments, can be categorized as comfortable, anxious, or avoidant (see Table 16.2). Antifantasy (fear or repugnance toward someone) is the mechanism that makes a person uncomfortable toward relationships, individual persons, or particular sexual acts.

The two components in Table 16.2, interpersonal relationships and fantasy, each have the following characteristics:

1. Both components are "hard wired" (refractory to change).
   This derives from (1) oxytocin's role in obsessive compulsive behaviors (Leckman et al., 1994), (2) the human sexual response, and (3) attachment behaviors.
2. Both components derive from early experiences and project into adulthood.
   The degree of comfort a person has toward interpersonal relationships derives from attachment theory—attachments are invariable, "from cradle to grave" (Hazan & Shaver, 1987; Hazan & Shaver, 1994; Main, 1991).
   The degree of comfort a person has toward sexuality derives from sexual development theorists: Money (1986), Stoller (1975), Weinrich (1988), and others.

THE DEVELOPMENT OF THE LOVEMAP

Early in life, as we begin to have mental imageries, a depiction of idealized love and erotic scripts begins to develop. Money (1986) called these early representations *lovemaps*. The development of the lovemap involves a biologically driven bonding process, which may be facilitated by the release of the hormone oxytocin (Leedes, 1999). Though infants are biologically predisposed to develop a particular type of bond, the environment plays a role as well. If a child's environment is supportive and nurturing, this bonding process is more likely to take place in interpersonal relationships with primary caregivers.

If something goes wrong in this process, a person may bond to objectified fantasies, which take the place of interpersonal relationships. I have hypothesized that lovemaps can be partitioned with varying degrees of intensity toward these two components (Leedes, 1999). Interpersonal attachments are developed within the first year or so of life (Ainsworth, Blehar, Water, & Wall, 1978; Bowlby, 1988), and objectified fantasies are developed within the first few years of life (Money, 1957; Weinrich, 1988). Money believed that these lovemaps were fixed, although recent anecdotal observations indicate that these early developmental representations can change dramatically. This is particularly true for those persons who chronically use Internet pornography who develop fetishes or dispositions toward underage persons.

ATTACHMENT RELATIONSHIPS

Bowlby (1973, 1980, 1988) claims that the responsiveness of a primary caretaker determines the degree to which a child will feel safe and secure. This idea derives from the study of ethology, the biological basis of behavior: parent-infant attachment is fundamental for survival. Attachments allow a caregiver to reduce a child's stress and ensure that an infant will stay near the caregiver. A protective caregiver is also able to provide support and a secure base to return to after exploration. Attachments ensure an emotional bond and physical closeness between a responsive caretaker and an infant.

This close relationship is represented internally for the infant by an internal working model (IWM) that allows the infant to predict responsiveness of a caregiver by past availability. Bowlby (1973) asserts that "the model of the attachment figure and the model of the self are likely to develop so as to be complementary and mutually confirming" (p. 238). In other words, the beliefs that a child forms about the self, such as "I am worthy of care," are regulated by the responsiveness of the primary caregiver. IWMs are in place by the second or third year of life (Ainsworth et al., 1978) and serve as a prototype for future relationships.

The way a caregiver responds to an infant predicts, in part, the kind of attachment that will develop. Ainsworth et al., (1978) have categorized three styles of attachment that are linked to caregiver responsiveness. The first style of infant-caregiver attachment is categorized as *secure*. This is the prototype for infant-caregiver attachment and is marked by proximity maintenance and comfort seeking. When securely attached, an infant is likely to explore and be sociable. This pattern of attachment represents 60 percent of American samples (Campos, Barret, Lamb, Goldsmith, & Sternberg, 1983). This distribution as well as the others listed below was replicated by Hazan and Shaver (1987) with adult samples.

The second style of infant-caregiver attachment is categorized as *anxious/ambivalent*. This infant-caregiver relationship is marked by inconsistent patterns (i.e., at times caregivers are unavailable, at times they are available, and at other times they are intrusive). The behavior patterns of the infant are marked with anxiety and anger. Further, these infants are hypervigilant about their caregiver's availability and proximity, and this inhibits their desire to explore. These infants are preoccupied with reestablishing close contact by pleading, and once reengaged, they exhibited clinging patterns. Campos et al. (1983) found that this pattern of attachment represents 15 percent of American samples.

The third style is categorized as *anxious/avoidant*. This infant-caregiver relationship is marked by the consistent rejection of an infant's request for comfort and bodily contact by the caregiver. Infants in this kind of relationship exhibit little interest in exploration and a lack of motivation to reestablish emotional attachment. These infants appear not to be fearful of separation. Campos et al. (1983) found that this pattern accounts for 25 percent of the American sample.

Infants are predisposed, through biological programming, to develop a particular kind of attachment, though the attachment system can be substantially modified by interpersonal experiences. These attachment styles conform to varying oxytocin levels present in the limbic structures, which are involved in emotion, motivation, and memory. Ideal levels of oxytocin correspond to adaptive or secure interpersonal bonds, overexpression leads to obsessive compulsive symptomatology, and an underexpression leads to the avoidance of interpersonal bonds (Leckman et al., 1994). It is speculated that anxious and avoidant styles of interpersonal bond formation interrupt the biological programming from serving its purpose of forming close relationships.

ATTACHMENTS AND SEXUAL RELATIONSHIPS

Biological programming, with the support of ideal caregiver-infant interaction, produces a comfortable, affectionate bonding experience. In this scenario, the person develops a positive emotional disposition and derives comfort and feelings of security from interpersonal bonding (Leedes, 1999). The endpoint of attachment formation (2–3 years old) is marked by the development of a symbolic representation of the attachment figure (i.e., an internal working model that is able to internally represent the caregiver's secure presence). This endpoint coincides with an eroticization process, in which an erotic representation becomes "hardwired," explained by Weinrich's (1988) and Money, Hampson, and Hampson's (1957) concept of imprinting. If warmth, bonding, and security are not evoked by the caregiver, it is likely that the child will develop a discomforting internal representation of a human bond and a comforting internal representation of an erotic depiction.

Once these processes are underway, a person is motivated to maintain the attachment system, whether to a real attachment or an attachment-like idealization, for the purposes of homeostasis. The homeostasis, or status quo, encourages proximity maintenance toward the attachment or attachment-like figure and produces feelings of security. Disruption of the status quo is associated with protest behaviors and the deactivation of other behavioral systems until proximity maintenance is reestablished.

The development of psychological closeness with an adult partner is remarkably similar to the attachment process of infants. Initially, there is a preoccupation with the responsiveness of the prospective partner. As the attachment process advances, the need for close bodily contact is replaced by a symbolic representation of the partner as a reliable and comfortable safe haven. After an extended period of time, the relationship can mirror a secure base provided by the protective caregiver. "In adults as well as children, attachments appear to be relationships critical to continuing security and so to the maintenance of emotional stability" (Weiss, 1991, p. 75). Attachment formation in adulthood is characterized by a progression: proximity seeking is followed by the establishment of comfortable "safe haven" and concludes with a contextualized "secure base" which is able to sustain a felt sense of security (Hazan and Shaver, 1994).

Hazan and Shaver (1987) have demonstrated that differences in infant attachment styles predict adult romantic attachment styles. When asked to characterize their most important love relationships, subjects depicted as secure lovers described these relationships as particularly happy, friendly, and trusting. Anxious/ambivalent lovers experienced love with obsession, emotional highs and lows, and extreme sexual attraction and jealousy. Avoidant lovers had a fear of intimacy. Additionally, they believed that happiness was not contingent on having a romantic partner—"I can get along quite well by myself" (p. 519).

Hazan and Shaver (1994) examined categories of interpersonal attractiveness (i.e., the attachment system, the caregiving system, and the sexual attraction system) in order to explain how early attachments project into the future and are refractory to change. Individuals with an emotional disposition toward comfortable interpersonal attachments pay attention to information from partners that is consistent with their schemas. Schemas operate within a default strategy (i.e., new information is easier accommodated by integrating it with existing schemas rather than converting that which has been assimilated).

Secure individuals are more likely to evaluate partners based on caregiving and the sense of feeling worthy of care that was instilled by the primary caretaker in childhood. In addition, they are more likely to choose people who are available to give care in return rather than giving primacy to sexual attraction.

A person whose early relationships were characterized by anxiety and ambivalence will have a confused emotional predisposition toward personal relationships, as caregivers were sometimes available, sometimes unavailable, and other times intrusive (Ainsworth et al., 1978). Their symbolic representation of bonding and comfort is likely to be associated with idealized or objectified schemas in order to defend against rejection. When the reality of the relationships is contradictory to the ideal (i.e., unavailable or intrusive), anxious/ambivalent people are likely to engage in obsessive protests and yearn for the elusive idealization. If the goal of the attachment system is finding a secure base, attachment behaviors (i.e., protest and obsessive searching), become a chronic condition among anxious/ambivalent individuals. It is likely that no amount of caring will satisfy their comfort requirement as bonding has been schematized with the ideal, not reality. This is supported by Hazan and Shaver's (1994) findings that anxious/ambivalent lovers are obsessive and live in the extremes. Their behavior is parallel to their childhood, where they engaged in clinging patterns. Their extreme jealousy is viewed as a corresponding behavior to the screaming protests of anxious children who are fearful of separation.

Avoidant adults, like their childhood counterparts, will lack motivation to (re)establish interpersonal attachments. They are not anxious about separation; they prefer it. For these people, interpersonal attachments are characterized by consistent rejection (Ainsworth et al., 1978). As a result, avoidant individuals are likely to form relationships that are not intimate (Hazan and Shaver, 1987). Alternatively, avoidant individuals may be too fearful to enter relationships at all. In either case, both types of insecure individuals are more vulnerable to form primary relationships with depersonalized objectifications for a source of comfort and security. Having a primary relationship with interpersonal attachments seems an intrusion on their ability to control for comfort and security. The reality of authentic interpersonal relationships is inconsistent with their idealized objectified and comforting fantasies.

THE TWO VARIABLES OF SEXUAL DESIRE APPLIED TO SEX ADDICTS

In a study conducted at the University of Pennsylvania, I tested the hypothesis that as sex addicts were able to increase their comfort with interpersonal relationships, they would be able to reduce the negative influence of their objectified fantasies. This was accomplished by participation in guided imagery exercises in which participants were induced into a state of relaxation and asked to recall a time in their lives when they experienced comforting and safe feelings toward another human being. They were asked to amplify these feelings through customary guided imagery techniques and later completed a posttest.

As explained earlier in this chapter, the most significant negative influence of chronic fantasizing is that fantasies, not people, become reinforced as emotionally comforting to a sex addict. Sex addicts want to maintain proximity to their fantasies, rather than be close to people. Sex addicts experience a feeling of withdrawal when they are asked not to fantasize, especially during times of stress. They also protest when fantasy thought-stopping techniques are employed by therapists.

Major Findings and Conjectures

1. Some 95 percent of sex addicts have insecure attachment styles (either avoidant or anxious).
2. Objectified fantasies, for sexual addicts, are surrogates for interpersonal attachments.
3. As comfort toward interpersonal attachments increases, the negative influence of objectified fantasies is diminished. Sexual addicts were able to reduce the negative influence of their fantasies and were able to modify the discomfort they experienced toward interpersonal relationships by participating in an imagery restructuring exercise.
4. The virtual reality hypothesis: Sex addicts go to virtual reality for what they find elusive in the real world—close, attachment-like internal representations (fantasies) characterized by responsiveness, affirmation, and emotional access.

Individuals who experience discomfort toward interpersonal relationships are at risk for forming a comfortable disposition toward objectified fantasies.

TREATMENT OF SEXUAL ADDICTION

The cognitive/behavioral treatments that are used for other dependencies (e.g., chemical dependence, compulsive overeating, and compulsive gambling), are used in the initial stages of treatment for sex addicts. Some of these techniques are (1) challenging thought processes that contribute to denial and minimization; (2) abstinence techniques, which involve calling another recovery person when there is an urge to act out; (3) reframing cognitive distortions (e.g., "I'm just a sexually liberated person"); (4) relapse prevention strategies, which involve identifying and avoiding specific people, places, and things; (5) as well as attending 12-step groups.

These techniques are effective for managing many addictive behaviors. Most clinicians would agree, however, that without resolving the underlying cause of these addictive or compulsive behaviors, they are likely to return. In order to produce long-term, positive treatment outcomes, it is important to examine the underlying psychodynamic cause for a person's sex addiction. The treatment strategies outlined in this section follow from the theories and research discussed earlier in this chapter.

GOALS OF TREATMENT

The following goals of treatment address the underlying cause of sexual addiction and usually follow the successful completion of the cognitive behavioral goals outlined above:

1. Patients will be able to describe how distorted thoughts about the self and others were formed.
2. Patients will experience a reduction in shame as a result of analyzing their early childhood experiences.
3. Patients will be able to analyze how early experiences have shaped their current anxious and avoidant attitudes, thoughts processes, and behaviors.
4. Patients will have a heightened awareness about how entrenched ways of thinking contribute to maladaptive default behaviors.
5. Patients will be able to access their inherent ability to experience comfort with other persons.
6. Patients will engage in activities that reinforce an experience of comfort toward others.

TREATMENT STRATEGIES

Carnes (1997) describes a detailed information-gathering technique in which patients draw what he calls a "trauma egg." The trauma egg encompasses vignettes of childhood traumatic experiences and discomfort during the person's development. The patient then labels each anecdotal vignette with two or three negative core beliefs chosen from a universal list. Some examples are I don't fit in, I am stupid, something is wrong with me, the world is not safe, no one really cares about me, no one understands me, no one can meet my needs.

After interviewing the patient about each vignette, the therapist analyzes the entire trauma egg in order to list the primary negative core beliefs the person has developed. This serves two purposes: (1) understanding the concept of introjection helps the patient see how distorted thoughts about the self and others were formed, and (2) feelings of shame, fear, anger, and sadness are reduced as patients connect these negative feelings to outside forces or events, rather than something inherently faulty about themselves. This technique addresses the first goal and contributes to an ongoing progression to address the second "process" goal.

After the detailed history is gathered, the therapist with the help of the patient, analyzes the major introjected negative core beliefs along with the associated feelings that they produce. This is accomplished by introducing the concept of trauma reenactment. Trauma reenactment refers to the idea that people tend to reenact, throughout their lives, behaviors that reinforce their introjected negative core beliefs. This can happen in many ways: (1) the person picks a partner whose behaviors resemble his perpetrator, (2) the person induces someone to act in a way that resembles his perpetrator, and (3) the person recreates the original trauma in his minds, even though the environment is safe. The following case study is an example of this third mechanism of trauma reenactment.

CASE STUDY

A 24-year-old woman complained to me during an individual session that the men in her therapy group were phony and that they did not represent themselves accurately during their group interactions. She told me that although they appeared to be supportive during group, they were actually punishing and rejecting. Late one evening, they had ignored her in the hallway after the group was over. When she walked through my foyer, she found the men "huddled in a corner together" disallowing her to join them in an after-group discussion. She promptly left the building and cried through the night feeling the acute rejection. I suggested that she bring up this issue in group.

When she told the story to the men in the group the following week, they explained to her in a convincing way that they simply had not seen her in the hallway. My center conducts several groups simultaneously, and the foyer can be crowed. The men were not huddled keeping others out but rather were confined to a small space in a crowded hallway. The patient had interpreted their behavior as a cue that triggered her primary negative core beliefs: no one really cares about me, something is wrong with me, and the world is not a safe place. Her trauma egg revealed that during her childhood, her divorced mother had a parade of men visiting her, all of whom viewed her as a pest or distraction to their agendas with her mother.

This patient had recreated the trauma in two ways. The first was by making up a story about the men in her group being rejecting and punishing. The second was by provoking the men with her scathing comments about their phoniness when she retuned to group the following week. She induced the men—at first—to give uncaring feedback, which further convinced her that the group was "not a safe place."

(Continued)

(Continued)

It took several weeks of processing this issue for the patient to understand how she had created this reenactment. All the group members in our sobriety/trauma groups have an understanding of trauma reenactment. Through nondefensive sharing about their own experiences of similar trauma reenactments, this issue was eventually resolved. It is through experiences such as these that the third and fourth goal of treatment can be internalized. Often, several years of group therapy are necessary in order to help patients remain in the reality of life and not escape into either the virtual reality of erotic fantasy or the virtual reality of trauma reenactment.

Experiential techniques and talk therapy that induce feelings are important modalities for trauma resolution. These evocative therapies contribute to the completion of the fifth goal of treatment.

When patients enter treatment, even though they may love their partners dearly, there is a discrepancy between the desire that they have toward their objectified/idealized fantasies and the desire that they have toward their loving partner. This discrepancy can change temporarily by using the following intervention. After a brief relaxation induction, the patient is asked to recall the last time he experienced poignancy with his partner and allow this vision to be enhanced. He is then asked to amplify this vision of comfort and connectedness. Immediately following this experience, he is asked to rate the power of his erotic fantasies. Invariably, he responds that the power is greatly diminished.

After the use of these experiential exercises, which allow patients to access their inherent ability to experience comfort from other people, patients are encouraged to become involved with activities with other recovery persons to creating bonding, cohesiveness, and real connection. Examples of these interpersonal activities are going to 12-step meetings, group therapy, phone calls to other recovering persons, being sponsored by a person with successful recovery, and marital therapy after being in treatment for awhile. This is a formidable task to patients because of their anxious or avoidant attachment styles of relating to others. However, it is a necessary step to achieving goals five and six.

As part of an overall strategy, we encourage patients to go to 12-step meetings designed for sex addicts, or sexaholics. In this 12-step model, step one states that, "We were powerless over our sex addiction and that our lives have become unmanageable." Trauma therapy usually does not commence until the patient has terminated his sexually addictive behaviors. When the person is able to sustain sobriety from acting out his behaviors, he becomes acutely aware that the first step is about acceptance. Further, it becomes clear that the behavior resulting from his powerlessness goes against his core values and that these behaviors have devastated his life. This is a paradigm shift, not simply behavior modification. Powerlessness becomes internalized as the patient sees, "I just can't do this anymore." The paradox is that by accepting powerlessness, he becomes more powerful to manage his addictive thoughts and resulting behaviors

Because of the success of this 12-step model on patients' out-of-control default sexual behaviors, they are asked to apply this model to their trauma reenactments. They begin to see that the unmanageability and isolation caused by their trauma reenactment behaviors is a price that they can no longer tolerate. The strategy of escaping into virtual reality reenactment fantasies and behaviors no longer works. Once persons begin to think consciously, rather than in default ways, they are motivated to act according to their values.

Because trauma reenactment behaviors are similar to addictive behaviors, the trauma resolution mechanism works in a similar way to addiction resolution. There is (1) a trigger (someone devalues the patient or makes him feel unsafe), (2) obsession (ruminations and reoccurring resentment), (3) acting out (fighting or flight), (4) despair (an emotional hangover from the obsessions and fight or flight behaviors). The primary intervention is to reframe the obsession toward someone else as his own powerlessness over an environmental trigger. The patient begins to see more accurately the cause of his apprehension: "It's not about the trigger; it's about me and my trauma."

LIMITATION OF THIS CHAPTER

A limitation of this chapter is the lack of a description of current principles for the treatment of partners and family members that explains how marriage/family therapy works, a strategy for rehabilitation, disclosure principles, and healthy sexuality. Some of these resources can be found at the following websites: www.gentlepath.com, www.Pinegrove-treatment.com, and www.pcsearle.com.

SUMMARY AND RECOMMENDATIONS FOR CLINICIANS

This chapter contributes to the understanding of sexual addiction as it relates to (1) nosology, (2) fitting it into an overall theory of sexual desire, (3) explaining some relevant research, (4) and suggesting how treatment can flow from theory and research. I hope that some of my inferences related to sexually compulsive behavior are helpful to the reader who thinks that he or she or a person he or she cares about may be sexually compulsive.

To those of us who treat persons with sexual dysfunctions, we also have to live life on life's terms. It is clear that funding sources for sexual research will continue to be marginal. Our primary sources for the development of pragmatic information will likely depend on journal articles, conferences, and an undertaking such as this collection of writings from sexologists, researchers, and sexuality educators. An initial step to further this limited form of qualitative research would be for the members of the Society for the Advancement of Sexual Health (formerly the National Council of Sexual Addiction/Compulsivity) and the American Association of Sexuality Educators, Counselors and Therapists to develop joint programs to enhance the knowledge of their members. Our two professional organizations are frustrated at times with one another, which adds little real understanding to this apparently growing problem in our culture. Sexual addicts understand the most important slogan to their recovery is, "I am responsible for my recovery." Hopefully, the leaders of each of our organizations will echo a variation on this refrain: We are responsible to meet the needs of all persons who experience dysfunction with their sexual expressiveness. We need to continue our efforts with well thought out and formalized interactive activities.

REFERENCES

Ainsworth, M. D. S., Blehar, M. C., Water, E., & Wall, S. (1978). *Patterns of attachment: A psychological study of the Strange Situation.* Hillsdale, NJ: Erlbaum.

Bowlby, J. (1973). *Attachment and loss: Vol. 2. Separation.* New York: Basic Books.

Bowlby, J. (1980). *Attachment and loss: Vol. 3. Sadness and depression.* New York: Basic Books.

Bowlby, J. (1988). *A secure base.* New York: Basic Books.

Campos, J. J., Barrett, K., Lamb, M. E., Goldsmith, H. H., & Stenberg, C. (1983). Socioemotional development. In P. H. Mussen (Ed.), *Handbook of child psychology: Vol. 2. Infancy and developmental psychobiology* (pp. 783–915). New York: Wiley.

Carnes, P. J. (1983). *The sexual addiction.* Minneapolis: CompCare Publishers.

Carnes, P. J. (1991). *Don't call it love.* New York: Bantam Books.

Carnes, P. J. (1996). Addiction or compulsion: Politics or illness. *Sexual Addiction & Compulsivity: The Journal of Treatment and Prevention, 3*(2), 127–150.

Carnes, P. J. (1997). *The betrayal bond: Breaking free of exploitive relationships.* Deerfield Beach: Health Communications Inc.

Coleman, E. (1991). Compulsive sexual behavior: New concepts and treatments. *Journal of Psychology and Human Sexuality, 4*(2), 37–52.

Goodman, A. (1993). Diagnosis and treatment of sexual addiction. *Journal of Sex and Marital Therapy, 19*(3), 225–251.

Hazan, C., & Shaver, P. R. (1987). Romantic love conceptualized as an attachment process. *Journal of Personality and Social Psychology, 52*(3), 511–524.

Hazan, C., & Shaver, P. R. (1994). Attachment as an organizational framework for research on close relationships. *Psychological Inquiry, 5*(1), 1–22.

Kaplan, H. S. (1979). *Disorders of sexual desire.* New York: Brunner/Mazel.

Kaplan, H. S. (1995). *The sexual disorders: Dysfunctional regulation of sexual motivation.* New York: Brunner/Mazel.

Kaplan, H. S. (1996). Erotic obsession: Relationship to hypoactive sexual desire disorder and paraphilia. *American Journal of Psychiatry, 153*(7), 30–41.

Leckman, J. F., Goodman, W. K., North, W. G., Chappell, P. B., Price, L. H., Pauls, D. L., Anderson, G. M., Riddle, M. A., McDougle, C. J., Barr, L. C., & Cohen, D. J. (1994). The role of central oxytocin in obsessive compulsive disorder and related normal behavior. *Psychoneuroendocrinology, 19*(8), 723–749.

Leedes, R. A. (1999). Fantasy and the internal working models held toward "comfortable interpersonal attachments" shape sexual desire: A theory applied to persons with hypersexuality. (Doctoral dissertation, University of Pennsylvania, 1999). *Dissertation Abstracts International,* 60, 186B.

Leitenberg, H., & Henning, K. (1995). Sexual fantasy. *Psychological Bulletin, 117* (3), 469–496.

Levine, M. P. & Troiden, R. R. (1988). The myth of sexual compulsion and addiction. *Journal of Sex Research, 25,* 347–363.

Main, M. (1991) Metacognitive knowledge, monitoring, and metacognitive singular (coherent) vs. multiple (incoherent) model of attachment. In C. M. Parkes, J. Stevenson-Hinde, & P. Marris (Eds.), *Attachment across the life cycle* (pp. 127–159). London: Routledge.

Masters, W. H., Johnson, V. E., & Kolodny, R. C. (1994). *Heterosexuality.* New York: HarperCollins Publishers.

Money, J., Hampson, J. G., & Hampson, J. L. (1957) Imprinting and the establishment of gender role. *AMA Archives of Neurology & Psychiatry, 77*(3):333–336.

Money, J. (1986). *Lovemaps: Clinical concepts of sexual/erotic health and pathology, paraphilia, and gender transposition in childhood, adolescence, and maturity.* New York: Irvington Publishers.

Nathan, S. G. (1995). Sexual addiction: A sex therapist's struggles with an unfamiliar clinical entity. In R. C. Rosen & S. R. Leiblum (Eds.), *Case studies in sex therapy* (pp. 333–367). New York: The Guilford Press.

Stoller, R. J. (1975). *Perversion: The erotic form of hatred.* New York: Pantheon Books.

Weinrich, J. D. (1988). The periodic table model of the gender transpositions: Part II. Limerent and lusty sexual attractions and the nature of bisexuality. *The Journal of Sex Research, 24,* 113–129.

Weiss, R. S. (1991). The attachment bond in childhood and adulthood. In C. M. Parkes, J. Stevenson-Hinde, & P. Marris (Eds.), *Attachment across the life cycle* (pp. 66–76). London: Routledge.

APPENDIX: THE EVOLUTION OF DEFINITIONS FOR WOMEN'S SEXUAL DISORDERS

Beverly Whipple and Annette Fuglsang Owens

Definitions of men's and women's sexual disorders are reconsidered as new research findings emerge. This appendix serves to summarize the most recent efforts to develop a terminology and concepts for identifying various sexual problems concerning women.

The term *sexual disorders* is preferred for women rather than *sexual dysfunctions*. This terminology was recommended at the World Association for Sexual Health World Congress held in Montreal in 2005. In this appendix, *sexual dysfunctions* will be used in its historical context.

The current classification of sexual disorders (Table A.1) in the *Diagnostic and Statistical Manual of Mental Disorders* (American Psychiatric Association, 2000), or *DSM-IV-TR,* is based on an older, linear model of human sexual response, which describes a sequence of mainly genitally focused events (desire, arousal, orgasm) (Kaplan, 1979; Masters & Johnson, 1966; Figure A.1). The concept of the linear model was based on research conducted on males and does not fit well with female sexual responses (Basson, 2001a, 2001b, 2006; Sugrue & Whipple, 2001; Tiefer, 1988). Hence, the current *DSM-IV-TR* guidelines for classification and diagnosis of sexual disorders are not as appropriate when it comes to addressing and/or diagnosing female sexual disorders as they are with male sexual "dysfunctions."

Two international consensus development conferences were held in 1998 and in 2003 in order to revise the definitions for women's sexual dysfunction. The first consensus panel was convened prior to the 1998 meeting of

Table A.1
DSM-IV-TR **Sexual Dysfunctions**

Sexual Desire Disorders
Hypoactive Sexual Desire Disorder
Sexual Aversion Disorder

Sexual Arousal Disorders
Female Sexual Arousal Disorder
Male Erectile Disorder

Orgasmic Disorders
Female Orgasmic Disorder
Male Orgasmic Disorder
Premature Ejaculation

Sexual Pain Disorders
Dyspareunia*
Vaginismus*

Sexual Dysfunction Due to a General Medical Condition
Female Hypoactive Sexual Desire Disorder Due to**
Male Hypoactive Sexual Desire Disorder Due to**
Male Erectile Disorder Due to**
Female Dyspareunia Due to**
Male Dyspareunia Due to**
Other Female Sexual Dysfunction Due to**
Other Male Sexual Dysfunction Due to**
Substance-Induced Sexual Dysfunction
Sexual Dysfunction NOS (Not otherwise specified)

The following specifiers apply to all primary sexual dysfunctions:

Lifelong Type/Acquired Type
Generalized Type/Situational Type
Due to Psychological Factors/Due to Combined Factors

* (Not Due to a General Medical Condition)

** (Indicate the General Medical Condition)

Source: American Psychiatric Association, (2000), *Diagnostic and statistical manual of mental disorders* (4th ed., text revision) (Washington, DC: American Psychiatric Association), pp. 22–23.

the Female Sexual Function Forum (FSFF), now named the International Society for the Study of Women's Sexual Health (ISSWSH). This consensus panel consisted of 19 interdisciplinary experts in female sexual dysfunction from five countries. The goal of the consensus development conference was to evaluate and revise the existing *DSM* definitions and classifications of female sexual dysfunction as well as those from the World Health Organization's

Figure A.1
Female Sexual Response Model Developed by Masters and
Johnson (1966)

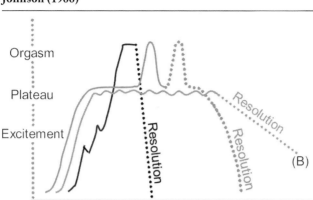

Note: This model reflects the different responses different women may
have or an individual woman may have on different occasions. For instance,
Woman A has a smooth transition from excitement to plateau to orgasm
to resolution and has multiple orgasms on this occasion. Woman B (or
Woman A on a different occasion) has a smooth transition up to plateau but
does not experience an orgasm. This is not a problem if it is an occasional
occurrence (e.g., if it is Woman A, who sometimes experiences orgasm) but
would be diagnosed as a sexual disorder if this occurs every time Woman
B has a sexual experience. Woman C has a different pattern of transition
from excitement through orgasm and resolution than either A or B—again
possibly reflecting the same woman on another occasion or three different
women.

Source: Reprinted by permission from W. H. Masters and V. E. Johnson,
Human sexual response (Boston: Little, Brown & Co., 1966).

*International Statistical Classification of Disease and Related Health Problems-10
(ICD-10)* from a psychogenic and organic perspective and to provide clinical
end points and outcomes for research and therapy. The 1998 consensus classification is summarized in Table A.2 (Basson et al., 2000).

Although, as compared to the *DSM* and *ICD-10* guidelines, "personal distress" was added as a criterion, and a new category of noncoital sexual pain
disorder was added, these guidelines were not readily accepted (Sugrue &
Whipple, 2001). One of the main problems with this classification of female
sexual dysfunction was that it is based on the triphasic functional pattern of
desire, arousal, and orgasm. This is the sexual response that was described by
Masters and Johnson and later modified by Kaplan (Figure A.1).

Although the triphasic model has widespread acceptance, it is based on
the male linear model of sexual function, which may not describe the sexual

Table A.2
First International Consensus Development Conference Definitions of Women's Sexual Dysfunction (1998)

Sexual Desire

Sexual desire disorders include:

A. Hypoactive sexual desire disorder (HHSD), defined as the persistent or recurrent deficiency (or absence) of sexual fantasies and/or desire for, or receptivity to, sexual activity, which causes personal distress.

B. Sexual aversion disorder (SAD), defined as the persistent or recurrent phobic aversion to and avoidance of sexual contact with a sexual partner, which causes personal distress.

Sexual Arousal

Female sexual arousal disorder (FSAD) is the persistent or recurrent inability to attain or maintain sufficient sexual excitement, causing personal distress. It may be expressed as a lack of subjective excitement or a lack of genital lubrication/swelling or other somatic response.

Orgasmic Disorder

Orgasmic disorder is the persistent or recurrent difficulty, delay in, or absence of attaining orgasm following sufficient sexual stimulation and arousal, which causes personal distress.

Dyspareunia

Dyspareunia is recurrent or persistent genital pain associated with sexual intercourse, which causes personal distress.

Vaginismus

Vaginismus is recurrent or persistent involuntary spasm of the musculature of the outer third of the vagina that interferes with vaginal penetration, which causes personal distress.

Noncoital Sexual Pain

Noncoital sexual pain disorder is recurrent or persistent genital pain induced by noncoital sexual stimulation, which causes personal distress.

Source: Basson et al., (2000), Report of the international consensus development conference on female sexual dysfunction: Definitions and classifications, *Journal of Urology, 163,* 888–893.

experience of women. Women can experience sexual arousal, orgasm, and satisfaction without sexual desire, and they can experience desire, arousal, and satisfaction without orgasm. If a woman has sexual satisfaction and does not go through all of the linear phases of the sexual response cycle, should she be considered as having a sexual dysfunction? In addition, this model does not take into account the documented variety of ways that women respond sexually (Whipple, 2002).

Nonlinear models of sexual response have been proposed by Whipple and Brash-McGreer (1997) based on Reed's model and Basson (2001a, 2001b; see Figure A.2). These various models are further discussed in the Association of Reproductive Health Professionals' (ARHP) Clinical Proceedings (2005).

Figure A.2
Nonlinear Model of Female Sexual Response Developed by Basson (2001b)

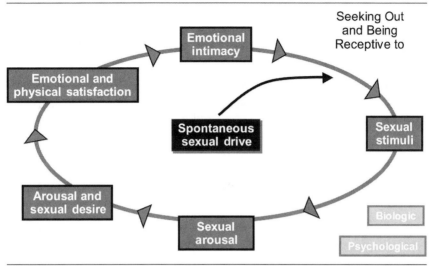

Note: Basson's nonlinear model acknowledges how emotional intimacy, sexual stimuli, and relationship satisfaction affect female sexual response.

Source: Reprinted with permission from R. Basson, Female sexual response: The role of drugs in the management of sexual dysfunction, *Obstetrics and Gynecology, 98*(2001b): 350–353. The figure appears on page 351 and is Figure 2.

Following the first consensus development meeting, Sugrue and Whipple (2001) pointed out the need to begin with identifying and defining what is normal before any pathology can be discussed:

One could argue that based on what women report to researchers, clinicians, and peers, normal sexual function for a woman, free of physical or psychological impediments, would include:

- capacity to experience pleasure and satisfaction independent of the occurrence of orgasm;
- desire or receptivity to experience sexual pleasure and satisfaction;
- physical capability of responding to stimulation (vasocongestion) without pain or discomfort;
- capability of experiencing orgasm under suitable circumstances (the desire to orgasm, lack of distraction, effective stimulation, erotic focus, and so forth).

If the above descriptors, or ones similar to them, were viewed as characteristic of normal sexual function, then the persistent absence or modification of any of the above descriptors would constitute a sexual dysfunction. (p. 224)

Table A.3
Second International Consensus Development Conference Definitions of
Women's Sexual Dysfunction (2003)

Women's Sexual Interest/Desire Disorder. There are absent or diminished feelings of sexual interest or desire, absent sexual thoughts or fantasies, and a lack of responsive desire. Motivations (here defined as reasons/incentives) for attempting to have sexual arousal are scarce or absent. The lack of interest is considered to be beyond the normative lessening with life cycle and relationship duration.

Subjective Sexual Arousal Disorder. Absence of or markedly diminished feelings of sexual arousal (sexual excitement and sexual pleasure) from any type of sexual stimulation. Vaginal lubrication or other signs of physical response still occur.

Combined Genital and Subjective Arousal Disorder. Absence of or markedly diminished feelings of sexual arousal (sexual excitement and sexual pleasure) from any type of sexual stimulation as well as complaints of absent or impaired genital sexual arousal (vulval swelling, lubrication).

Genital Sexual Arousal Disorder. Complaints of absent or impaired genital sexual arousal. Self-report may include minimal vulval swelling or vaginal lubrication from any type of sexual stimulation and reduced sexual sensations from caressing genitalia. Subjective sexual excitement still occurs from nongenital stimuli.

Persistent Sexual Arousal Disorder. Previously considered extremely rare, the complaint of intrusive spontaneous genital throbbing unrelieved with orgasm is being increasingly encountered in clinical practice. Therefore, the committee proposed the following definition.

Spontaneous intrusive and unwanted genital arousal (e.g., tingling, throbbing, pulsating) in the absence of sexual interest and desire. Any awareness of subjective arousal is typically, but not invariably, unpleasant. The arousal is unrelieved by one or more orgasms and the feelings of arousal persist for hours or days.

Women's Orgasmic Disorder. Despite the self-report of high sexual arousal/excitement, there is either lack of orgasm, markedly diminished intensity of orgasmic sensations, or marked delay of orgasm from any kind of stimulation.

Vaginismus. The persistent or recurrent difficulties of the woman to allow vaginal entry of a penis, a finger, and/or any object, despite the woman's expressed wish to do so. There is often (phobic) avoidance and anticipation/fear/experience of pain, along with variable involuntary pelvic muscle contraction. Structural or other physical abnormalities must be ruled out/addressed.

Dyspareunia. Persistent or recurrent pain with attempted or complete vaginal entry and/or penile vaginal intercourse.

Source: Basson et al. (2004), Revised definitions of women's sexual dysfunction, *Journal of Sexual Medicine, 1*(1), 45.

The Second International Consultation on Sexual Medicine was held in Paris in July of 2003. An International Definitions Committee of 13 experts from seven countries proposed a number of fundamental changes to the existing definitions of women's sexual disorders and presented their new definitions, which are summarized in Table A.3 (Basson et al., 2004). A more thorough discussion of the evolution of these models can be found in the ARHP's Clinical Proceedings (2005).

REFERENCES

American Psychiatric Association. (2000). *Diagnostic and statistical manual of mental disorders* (4th ed., text revision). Washington, DC: Author.

Association of Reproductive Health Professionals. (2005). Women's sexual health in midlife and beyond. *Association of Reproductive Health Professionals Clinical Proceedings*. Washington, DC: Association of Reproductive Health Professionals.

Basson, R., Berman, J., Burnett, A., Degrogatis, L., Ferguson, D., Foucroy, J., Goldstein, I., Graziottin, A., Heiman, J., Laan, E., Leiblum, S., Padma-Nathan, H., Rosen, R., Segraves, K., Segraves, R. T., Shabsigh, R., Sipski, M., Wagner, G., & Whipple, B. (2000). Report of the international consensus development conference on female sexual dysfunction: Definitions and classifications. *Journal of Urology, 163,* 888–893.

Basson, R. (2001a) Human sex-response cycles. *Journal of Sex & Marital Therapy, 27,* 33–43.

Basson R. (2001b). Female sexual response: The role of drugs in the management of sexual dysfunction. *Obstetrics and Gynecology, 98,* 350–353.

Basson, R., Leiblum, S., Brotto, L., Derogatis, L., Fourcroy, J., Fugl-Meyer, K., et al. (2004). Revised definitions of women's sexual dysfunction. *Journal of Sexual Medicine, 1*(1), 40–48.

Basson, R. (2006). Sexual desire and arousal disorders in women. *New England Journal of Medicine, 354,* 1497–1505.

Kaplan, H.S. (1979). *Disorders of sexual desire.* New York: Brunner/Mazel.

Masters, W.H., & Johnson, V.E. (1966). *Human sexual response.* Boston: Little, Brown & Co.

Sugrue, D.P., & Whipple, B. (2001). The consensus-based classification of female sexual dysfunction: Barriers to universal acceptance. *Journal of Sex & Marital Therapy, 27,* 221–226.

Tiefer, L. (1988). A feminist critique of the sexual dysfunction nomenclature. *Women and Therapy, 7,* 5–21

Whipple, B. (2002). Women's sexual pleasure and satisfaction: A new view of female sexual function. *The Female Patient* (Primary Care Edition), *27*(8), 39–44; and (OB/GYN Edition) *2,*(8), 44–47.

Whipple, B., & Brash-McGreer, K. (1997). Management of female sexual dysfunction. In M. L. Sipski & C. Alexander (Eds.), *Sexual function in people with disability and chronic illness: A health professional's guide* (pp. 511–536). Gaithersburg, MD: Aspen Publishers.

World Health Organization. (1992). *ICD 10: International statistical classification of disease and related health problems.* Geneva: World Health Organization.

SEXUAL HEALTH RESOURCES

Many additional resources are listed in individual chapters.

BOOKS

Bancroft, J. (1989). *Human sexuality and its problems* (2nd ed.). New York: Churchill Livingstone.

Kleinplatz, P. J. (Ed) (2001). *New directions in sex therapy. Innovations and alternatives.* Philadelphia, PA: Brunner-Routledge; Taylor & Francis Group.

Komisaruk, B. R., Beyer-Flores, C., & Whipple, B. (2006). *The science of orgasm.* Baltimore, MD: Johns Hopkins University Press.

Leiblum, S. R., & Rosen, R. C. (Eds.) (2006). *Principles and practice of sex therapy* (Fourth Edition). New York, London: The Guilford Press.

Levine, S. B., Risen, C. B., & Althof, S. E. (Eds.) (2003). *Handbook of clinical sexuality for mental health professionals.* New York: Brunner-Routledge.

Maurice, W. L. (1999). *Sexual medicine in primary care.* St. Louis, Missouri: Mosby.

Ross, M. W., Channon-Little, L. D., Rosser, B. R. S., & Ross, M. W. (2000). *Sexual health concerns: Interviewing and history taking for health practitioners* (2nd ed.). Sydney; Philadelphia: MacLennan + Petty.

ORGANIZATIONS

The American Association of Sexuality Educators, Counselors, and Therapists (AASECT); Phone (804) 752–0026, Fax (804) 752–0056, http://www.aasect.org. AASECT facilitates contact to certified sexuality educators, counselors and sex therapists in the United States and other selected countries. Provides certification and continuing education for professionals in the sexuality field.

Sexuality Information and Education Council of the United States (SIECUS); Phone: (212) 819–9770, Fax: (212) 819–9776, http://www.siecus.org. This key organization provides links to current sexuality resources and educational materials about sexuality and religion, parenting, teenagers, disability, etc.

The Society for the Scientific Study of Sexuality (SSSS), http://www.sexscience.org. This international organization is the oldest professional society dedicated to the advancement of knowledge about sexuality.

Other Organizations

The Alexander Foundation for Women's Health, http://www.afwh.org

American Association of Marital and Family Therapists, http://www.aamft.org/index_nm.asp

American Psychological Assn's page on Sexuality, http://www.apa.org/topics/topicsbehavior.html

American Social Health Association, http://www.ashastd.org

Association for Reproductive Health Professionals, https://www.arhp.org

International Society for Sexual Medicine (ISSM), http://www.issm.info

International Society for the Study of Women's Sexual Health (ISSWSH), http://www.isswsh.org

National Sexuality Resource Center, http://nsrc.sfsu.edu

Planned Parenthood, www.plannedparenthood.org

The Society for Sex Therapy and Research, http://www.sstarnet.org

The Women's Sexual Health Foundation, http://www.twshf.org

World Association for Sexual Health, http://www.worldsexology.org

WEBSITES

Alternate Sexuality

BDSM Café, http://www.bdsmcafe.com

Deviant Desires, http://www.deviantdesires.com

Fetish Exchange, http://www.fetishexchange.org

Gloria Brame.com, http://gloria-brame.com

Educational Programs

Human Sexuality Education Opportunities (SSSS), http://www.sexscience.org/publications/index.php?category_id=438.
Comprehensive list of Doctorate and Masters programs that have a strong sexual health component compiled by the Society for the Scientific Study of Sex.

Institute for Advanced Study of Human Sexuality, http://www.iashs.edu
Located in San Francisco, this independent "free-standing" graduate institute offers a range of training programs as well as a wealth of resource materials in human sexuality and erotology.

Kinsey Institute, http://www.indiana.edu/~kinsey/
Information about Indiana University's world-famous Kinsey Institute for Sex, Gender & Reproduction in Bloomington, IN.

Maimonides University, to http://www.esextherapy.com

Located in southern Florida, this graduate program trains professionals who have already achieved at least a masters degree, and who are licensed in their home state, to specialize and achieve doctoral training in sex therapy.

Widener University, http://www.widener.edu (search for "Doctor of Education in Human Sexuality Program")

Located in Philadelphia, this program offers masters and doctoral degrees in two tracks—one that is specifically focused on training sexuality educators, and one that is specifically focused on training sexuality counselors and sex therapists.

Masturbation

The Clitoris.com, http://www.the-clitoris.com
Betty Dodson Online, http://www.bettydodson.com
Jackinworld, http://www.jackinworld.com
Masturbation Techniques, http://www.masturbation-techniques.net

Pain

International Pelvic Pain Society, http://www.pelvicpain.org
National Vulvodynia Association, http://www.nva.org
Sex without Pain.com, http://www.sexwithoutpain.com

Religion

Belief Net, http://www.beliefnet.com/
Not a sexuality website, per se, but gives good information regarding a variety of religious views on sexuality-related topics.

The Center for Sexuality and Religion, http://www.ctrsr.org
Religious Institute on Sexuality, Morality, Justice, and Healing, http://www.religious institute.org
Religious Tolerance, http://www.religioustolerance.org/
Not a sexuality website, per se, but gives good information regarding variety of religious views on sexuality-related topics.

Sexual Abuse

Association for the Treatment of Sexual Abusers, http://www.atsa.com
American Professional Society on the Abuse of Children (APSAC), www.apsac.org
Child Abuse & Neglect Outreach Project, http://www.disability-abuse.com/
HealthySex.com, http://www.healthysex.com
An educational site developed by renowned therapist Wendy Maltz to promote healthy sexuality—sex based on caring, respect, and safety.

International Society on Child Abuse & Neglect (ISPCAN), http://www.ispcan.org

Sexual Health—General

Archive for Sexology, http://www2.hu-berlin.de/sexology
Love and Health, http://loveandhealth.info
Sexual Health Network, http://www.SexualHealth.com
Sexuality.org, http://www.sexuality.org

Sexual Orientation

Bentvoices.org, http://www.bentvoices.org
> A website by and for gay and bi men with disabilities

Bisexual.org, http://www.bisexual.org/

Parents, Families & Friends of Lesbians & Gays (PFLAG), http://www.pflag.org/

Sex Workers

Bay Area Sex Worker Advocacy Network (BAYSWAN), http://www.bayswan.org
> Bay Area Sex Worker Advocacy Network, is a collaborative project providing information for sex workers and about the sex industries.

Network of Sex Work Projects, http://www.nswp.org/
> The Network of Sex Work Projects is an international organization that promotes sex workers' health and human rights.

Surrogates

International Professional Surrogates Association, http://surrogatetherapy.org

Teen

Advocates for Youth, http://www.advocatesforyouth.org

I Wanna Know, http://www.iwannaknow.org/
> Teen site by the American Social Health Association

Scareleteen, http://www.scarleteen.com/
> Advice about sex for teens

Sex Etc., http://www.sxetc.org/

Teenwire, http://www.teenwire.com/

Transgender

The Renaissance Transgender Association, http://www.ren.org/

Transgender Care, http://www.transgendercare.com/

Transgender Tapestry, http://www.ifge.org/

Other

The Body, http://www.thebody.com

Human Rights Campaign, http://www.hrc.org/

Updates following the Surgeon General's Call to Action to Promote Sexual Health and Responsible Sexual Behavior (2001), http://www.Satchercalltoaction.com

INDEX

ABOUT THE CONTRIBUTORS

BARBARA ALTEROWITZ, Dipl., Volkswirt, is a certified sexuality counselor (AASECT) working primarily in sexual rehabilitation after cancer. Her focus has been on informing cancer patients and couples about dealing with relationship issues and medical aspects for resuming sexual relations in light of male erectile dysfunction and female problems after cancer. Ms. Alterowitz, a sought-after speaker, is coauthor of the acclaimed book *The Lovin' Ain't Over* and its follow-up, *Intimacy with Impotence,* and cofounder and codirector of The Center for Intimacy After Cancer Therarpy Inc (C-I-ACT). She holds a postgraduate degree from Freiburg University in Germany.

RALPH ALTEROWITZ, BA, MEA, is a certified sexuality counselor (AASECT) specializing in counseling and research in sexual rehabilitation after cancer. His private practice concentrates on counseling and conducting workshops for couples on renewing their intimacy after cancer treatment. His innovative philosophy is reflected in his counseling protocols, which embrace therapeutic advances. In his medical technology work, he applied telemedicine to craft long-distance cardiac monitoring systems. Mr. Alterowitz is coauthor of the acclaimed book *The Lovin' Ain't Over* and its follow-up, *Intimacy with Impotence,* and cofounder and codirector of The Center for Intimacy After Cancer Therarpy Inc (C-I-ACT). He holds degrees from the University of Iowa and George Washington University.

TAREK ANIS, MD, is a professor of andrology and sexology in the faculty of medicine, Cairo University. Additionally, Dr. Anis is the senior consulting andrologist to the Nasser Institute of Health and a cofounder of the IVF center of the Women's Medical Hospital. He maintains an independent practice in Cairo, specializing in men's health.

Currently, Dr. Anis is the chief editor of the "Sexual Health Update" an international literature review service. Dr. Anis is also president of the Pan-Arab Society for Sexual Medicine (PASSM), which includes members from 22 Arabic-speaking nations.

ELIZABETH A. BARON-KUHN, MD, FACOG, is a fellow of the American College of Obstetricians and Gynecologists and is board certified in obstetrics and gynecology. She has been in private practice for 20 years in the suburbs of Chicago and recently started to work at Riverside Medical Center in Waupaca, Wisconsin. She has special expertise in the treatment of PMS and menopause as well as all areas of women's midlife health.

CAREY ROTH BAYER, EdD, RN, earned a bachelor of science degree in nursing from Xavier University, and both a master's degree in adult education and a doctorate in human sexuality education from Widener University. Carey has lectured on sexual/reproductive anatomy, contraception, sexual dysfunction and its treatment at the community college and university levels. She has written sexuality curriculums for teaching parents and college students and has studied nurses' perceptions of addressing sexuality with patients in a pediatric intensive care unit.

MARIANNE BRANDON, PhD, is a clinical psychologist and a diplomat in sex therapy through AASECT. She completed her doctoral training at Ohio University and her internship at the University of Connecticut School of Medicine. Dr. Brandon is a graduate of a postdoctoral fellowship in eating and weight disorders from the Sheppard and Enoch Pratt Hospital in Baltimore. She is codirector of the Sexual Wellness Center in Annapolis, Maryland. Dr. Brandon coauthored *Reclaiming Desire: 4 Keys for Finding Your Lost Libido,* published in June of 2004. She is currently in private practice in the Baltimore-Annapolis area.

PATRICK CARNES, PhD, CAS, a nationally known speaker and author on addiction and recovery issues, is the primary architect of Gentle Path treatment programs for the treatment of sexual and addictive disorders. He is currently the executive director of the Gentle Path program at Pine Grove Behavioral Center in Hattiesburg, Mississippi. Dr. Carnes is also the chief executive officer of New Freedom Corporation and New Freedom Publications in Carefree, Arizona.

SANDRA COLE, PhD, is professor, sexologist, and gender specialist at the University of Michigan Medical School. Dr. Cole is past president of the American Association of Sexuality Educators, Counselors and Therapists; and a certified sexuality educator and sexuality counselor. Since 1983 she has been a strong advocate and ally with the transgender community, teaching—training, lecturing, and consulting. Her focus is on social justice, public policy, partner/spouse concerns, couple relationship and intimacy issues, and the necessity for adequate and reliable mental and medical health care for transgender and transsexual people and their families. In 1993, she and her team established the University of Michigan Comprehensive Gender Services Program, where she served as director until 2000.

ELI COLEMAN, PhD, is professor and director of the Program in Human Sexuality, Department of Family Medicine and Community Health, University of Minnesota Medical School in Minneapolis. He is the author of numerous articles and books on compulsive sexual behavior, sexual offenders, sexual orientation, gender dysphoria, chemical dependency and family intimacy, and on the psychological and pharmacological treatment of a variety of sexual dysfunctions and disorders. Professor Coleman is the founding and current editor of the *Journal of Psychology of Human Sexuality* and the *International Journal of Transgenderism*. He is a past president of the Society for the Scientific Study of Sexuality (SSSS), the Harry Benjamin International Gender Dysphoria Association (HBIGDA), and the World Association for Sexual Health (WAS).

DALLAS DENNY, MA, is a writer and activist who lives in Georgia. After 20 years as a licensed psychological examiner, she recently retired her license to practice psychology in Tennessee. Dallas has been editor of the journals *Chrysalis* and *Transgender Tapestry* and has been published widely on transgender issues, often with her coauthors, Sandra Cole and Jamison Green. She is board chair of the nonprofit Real Life Experiences Inc. and is a founding board member of the nonprofit Gender Education & Advocacy, Inc.

AHMED EL-SAKKA, MD, is an associate professor of urology, Suez Canal University, Ismailia, Egypt. He graduated from medical school at that university and completed a residency-training program in urology and andrology. He was trained as a fellow in male sexual function and dysfunction at the University of California, San Francisco. Dr. El-Sakka is an internationally recognized expert in the area of male sexual dysfunction. His list of publications includes over sixty original research studies and over twenty book chapters and review articles. He is also a reviewer for over fifteen scientific journals. He has received several national and international awards and prizes.

CAROL RINKLEIB ELLISON, PhD, is a psychologist in private practice in Oakland, California; an AASECT certified sex therapist; a fellow of the Society for the Scientific Study of Sexuality; and an instructor of human sexuality courses for nurses and mental health professionals. She coauthored the Ellison/Zilbergeld sexuality survey of 2,632 women and wrote *Women's Sexualities: Generations of Women Share Intimate Secrets of Sexual Self-Acceptance:* a chapter on intimacy-based sex therapy in *New Directions in Sex Therapy;* a chapter on facilitating orgasmic responsiveness in *Handbook of Clinical Sexuality for Mental Health Professionals;* and a chapter in *A New View of Women's Sexual Problems.*

HUSSEIN GHANEM, MD, is a professor of andrology, sexology, and STIs at Cairo University. Dr. Ghanem graduated from medical school at Cairo University, Egypt, in 1982 and completed the residency program in andrology. He trained as a fellow in male reproductive medicine and surgery at University of Iowa Hospitals (1987–1988) and Baylor College of Medicine in Houston, Texas (1988–1989). Dr. Ghanem obtained a doctorate (1990) in andrology, sexology, and STDs. His publications include over thirty articles in various international medical journals. He is a member of the International Society of Sexual Medicine and serves on several of its committees, including the communication and standards committees.

ANDREW T. GOLDSTEIN, MD, graduated from the University of Virginia and the University of Virginia School of Medicine. He completed his residency in obstetrics and gynecology at the Beth Israel Medical Center. He is on the faculty of the Division of Gynecologic Specialties at the Johns Hopkins School of Medicine. In 2002, he became the director of the Centers for Vulvovaginal Disorders in Washington, DC, and in New York City. Goldstein has been elected to the International Society for the Study of Vulvovaginal Disorders (ISSVD) and is a grant recipient of the National Vulvodynia Association (NVA). He is actively involved in research on vulvar and sexual pain disorders.

JAMISON GREEN is an author, educator, public speaker, and policy consultant specializing in transgender and transsexual issues. He conducts educational programs on transgender awareness for corporations, law enforcement agencies, government agencies, religious institutions, and professional groups such as physicians, psychologists, and attorneys. His book *Becoming a Visible*

Man (2004) is a primary text for transgender studies in numerous colleges and universities. He serves as a director on the boards of several organizations, including the Transgender Law and Policy Institute and the Harry Benjamin International Gender Dysphoria Association, and he is currently pursuing a PhD in law at Manchester Metropolitan University in England.

RAVEN JAMES, EdD(c), MEd, has been a sexuality educator for over twelve years. Raven is a master trainer for the Office of Alcohol and Substance Abuse Services (OASAS) in New York State and was certified as a prevention professional. She has written curricula and lectured on such topics as dying and death, STI counseling issues, HIV prevention, hepatitis C, and LGBT issues in substance abuse. Raven is currently a doctoral candidate in human sexuality education from Widener University. She is also a member of the Society for the Scientific Study of Sexuality.

RICHARD LEEDES, PhD, CSAT, is the director of the Counseling Center at Princeton. He is a certified sex addiction therapist and is on the faculty of Robert Wood Johnson Medical School, Department of Addiction Psychiatry. Leedes has been appointed by the Federal District Court of New Jersey as a director for pretrial and probation sexual offender treatment. He has spoken throughout the country on the topic of sex addiction and has contributed to the *Journal of Sexual Addiction & Compulsivity.*

GINA OGDEN, PhD, is a licensed marriage and family therapist and a board-certified sex therapist in Cambridge, Massachusetts. She is author of *The Heart and Soul of Sex: Making the ISIS Connection,* which is based on results of her nationwide survey on sexuality and spirituality. She is also author of *Women Who Love Sex: An Inquiry into the Expanding Spirit of Women's Erotic Experience.*

ANNETTE FUGLSANG OWENS, MD, PhD, is certified as a sexuality counselor by the American Association of Sexuality Educators, Counselors, and Therapists (AASECT). She hails from Denmark where she earned both of her degrees and is cofounder and chief medical officer of The Sexual Health Network (www.SexualHealth.com). Besides addressing sexuality issues with clients, she also delivers sexual health education content online—in both written and video formats—and has written articles and chapters on the subject of sexual health. Owens is editor-in-chief of *Contemporary Sexuality* (AASECT's monthly newsletter), and serves as secretary on the AASECT board of directors. She is an active member of various national and international sexuality organizations.

TALLI YEHUDA ROSENBAUM, PT, is a physical therapist specializing in urogynecological and pelvic floor rehabilitation and is an AASECT-certified sexuality counselor. She serves on the board of the Women's Health Section of the Israel Physiotherapy Society and is a delegate to the International Organization of Physiotherapists in Women's Health. She is on the professional advisory boards of the Women's Sexual Health Foundation and the Alexander Foundation for Women's Health. Ms. Rosenbaum manages a private practice with offices in Jerusalem and Tel Aviv, Israel.

DAVID SATCHER, MD, PhD, completed his four-year term as the 16th Surgeon General of the United States in February 2002. He also served as Assistant Secretary for Health from February 1998 to January 2001, making him only the second person in history to have held both positions simultaneously. In January 2002, Dr. Satcher was named the director of the new National Center for Primary Care at the Morehouse School of Medicine in Atlanta, Georgia, and in December 2004, Dr. Satcher was appointed as the interim president of the Morehouse School of Medicine.

As Surgeon General and Assistant Secretary for Health, Dr. Satcher spearheaded the development of *Healthy People 2010*, which included the elimination of racial and ethnic disparities in health as one of its two goals. He also released fourteen Surgeon General's reports on topics that included tobacco and health, mental health, suicide prevention, oral health, sexual health, youth violence prevention, and obesity. Dr. Satcher would most like to be known as the Surgeon General who listened to the American people and responded with effective programs. His mission continues to be to make medicine and public health work for all groups in this nation.

ROBERT TAYLOR SEGRAVES, MD, PhD, has spent most of his career studying and treating sexual disorders. He was on the American Psychiatric Association Taskforce on Psychosexual Disorders for DSM III R and DSM IV, is past president of the Society for Sex Therapy and Research, and is the current editor of the *Journal of Sex and Marital Therapy*. He has written over two hundred publications in the area of human sexuality, made numerous national and international presentations, and authored four texts (including *Sexual Pharmacology: Fast Facts*, published in 2003). He is currently professor of psychiatry at Case Western Reserve University and chairperson of psychiatry at MetroHealth Medical Center in Cleveland, Ohio.

RANY SHAMLOUL, MD, graduated from medical school at Cairo University in 1998 and completed a four-year residency/internship training program in andrology, sexology, and sexually transmitted diseases. He then obtained his master's degree in the same field and was appointed as an assistant lecturer in the Andrology Department at Cairo University. Dr. Shamloul has published extensively in a number of international journals, including the *International Journal of Impotence Research,* and the *Journal of Sexual Medicine and Human Reproduction.* He is also a reviewer for the *Journal of Sexual Medicine.* Currently, he is involved in a research project on new vasorelaxant drugs at the University of Saskatchewan, Canada.

JULIAN SLOWINSKI, PsyD, ABPP, has been active professionally in the field of human sexuality for more than thirty-five years as an educator, clinician, author, lecturer, editor, and clinical researcher. He is a clinical assistant professor in the Department of Psychiatry at the University of Pennsylvania School of Medicine and is senior clinical psychologist at Pennsylvania Hospital in Philadelphia, where he is in private practice. He has made many media appearances and contributions to the professional literature. Dr. Slowinski is also coauthor of two books: *The Sexual Male: Problems & Solutions* and *The Good Sex Guide.*

MITCHELL S. TEPPER, PhD, MPH, is assistant director of The Center of Excellence for Sexual Health, Morehouse School of Medicine, National Center for Primary Care, Atlanta, and is founder and president of The Sexual Health Network, Inc., a Web-based company that provides information and guidance to the public via the company's Web site (www.SexualHealth.com). Dr. Tepper has a special interest in sexual health and the intersection of chronic conditions and disability. He is a former board member of the American Association of Sexuality Educators, Counselors and Therapists, SIECUS, and the International Society for the Study of Women's Sexual Health (ISS-WSH), and he holds degrees from Yale University and the University of Pennsylvania..

BEVERLY WHIPPLE, PhD, RN, FAAN, is a certified sexuality educator, sexuality counselor, and sex researcher, and the coauthor of the international best seller, *The G Spot and Other Discoveries about Human Sexuality.* She has written five other books, has delivered over 500 talks and keynote speeches, and has published over 160 research articles and book chapters. She is the recipient of many awards and has served as president, vice president, or board member in various international sexuality organizations. She is a professor emerita at Rutgers, The State University of New Jersey.

ABOUT THE EDITORS AND ADVISORS

MITCHELL S. TEPPER, PhD, MPH, is assistant director, The Center of Excellence for Sexual Health, Morehouse School of Medicine, National Center for Primary Care, Atlanta under the direction of former Surgeon General Dr. David Satcher. Tepper is also the founder of The Sexual Health Network, an organization of health professionals and educators providing information and guidance to the public via the Web site www.Sexualhealth. com, as well as providing resources and training to health professionals. Tepper, who holds an MPH from Yale University and a PhD in human sexuality education from the University of Pennsylvania, is a leading advocate for the provision of comprehensive sexual health care to people with disabilities or chronic conditions. Tepper has served on the board of directors of the American Association of Sexuality Educators, Counselors and Therapists, SIECUS, the International Society for the Study of Women's Sexual Health (ISSWSH), and The Women's Sexual Health Foundation. He also serves on the editorial board of *Sexuality and Disability* and *American Journal of Sexuality Education*. Tepper has been a guest lecturer at the Yale University School of Medicine, and is now an adjunct assistant professor of physician assistant education at Quinnipiac University. He has been featured on television networks such as CNN, Discovery, and PBS—as well as in magazines including *Good Housekeeping, Cosmopolitan,* and *GQ.*

ANNETTE FUGLSANG OWENS, MD, PhD, is certified as a sexuality counselor by the American Association of Sexuality Educators, Counselors and

Therapists (AASECT). She hails from Denmark, where she earned both of her degrees, and is cofounder and chief medical officer of The Sexual Health Network (www.SexualHealth.com). In 1999, Owens founded the Charlottesville Sexual Health & Wellness Clinic (www.CvilleWellness.com) where she provides sexuality counseling to clients. She also delivers sexual health education content online—in both written and video formats—and has written articles and chapters on the subject of sexual health. Owens is editor-in-chief of *Contemporary Sexuality* (AASECT's monthly newsletter), and serves as secretary on the AASECT board of directors. She is an active member of various national and international sexuality organizations. She has been featured in *Glamour* magazine, *Good Housekeeping*, and *USA Today*, among other publications.

ALAN M. ALTMAN, MD, is an assistant clinical professor of obstetrics, gynecology and reproductive biology at Harvard Medical School. He is a board-certified gynecologist with a private practice specializing in peri- and postmenopausal care and midlife sexuality issues. A distinguished and sought-after speaker, Dr. Altman lectures frequently throughout the country on such topics as menopause, perimenopause, sexuality, state-of-the-art developments in hormone therapy, and treatment of complicated postmenopausal symptoms in patients. He is an outspoken advocate for providing health information to the public, and was co-founder and president of the Women's Healthcare Video Library, Inc. Dr. Altman wrote and co-produced the highly acclaimed video sets: *Transitions; Preparing for Menopause, Adolescence; A Woman's First Transition,* and *Fertility; Pathways and Obstacles to Pregnancy.*

An expert on women's sexual health issues, Dr. Altman has been quoted and interviewed over the past fifteen years by a variety of publications and television programs. His first book, *Making Love the Way We Used To . . . or Better; Secrets to Satisfying Midlife Sexuality,* was published in March, 2001, and covers the perimenopausal transition, menopause, hormones and their collective impact on sexual function, and sexual dysfunction. His second book, *The Betrayal of American Women: Don't Throw away Your Hormones so Quickly!* is due out in 2006.

ELI COLEMAN, PhD, is professor and director of the Program in Human Sexuality, Department of Family Medicine and Community Health, University of Minnesota Medical School in Minneapolis, Minnesota. He is the author of numerous articles and books on compulsive sexual behavior, sexual offenders, sexual orientation, gender dysphoria, chemical dependency, and family intimacy, as well as on the psychological and pharmacological treatment of a variety of sexual dysfunctions and disorders. Professor Coleman is the founding and current editor of the *Journal of Psychology of Human Sexuality* and the *International Journal of Transgenderism*. He is one of the past-presidents of the Society for the Scientific Study of Sexuality (SSSS), the Harry Benjamin International Gender Dysphoria Association (HBIGDA), and the World Association for Sexual Health (WAS). He has been a frequent technical consultant on sexual health issues to the World Health Organization (WHO) and the Pan American Health Organization (the regional office of the WHO). He has recieved numerous awards, including the US Surgeon General's Exemplary Service Award for his role as senior scientist on *Surgeon General's Call to Action to Promote Sexual Health and Responsible Sexual Behavior*, released in 2001. He was given the Distinguished Scientific Achievement Award from the SSSS and the Alfred E. Kinsey Award by the Midcontinent Region of the Society for the Scientific Study of Sexuality (MRSSSS) in 2001.

ANNAMARIA GIRALDI, MD, PhD, earned her degrees from the University of Copenhagen, Denmark. Trained in clinical pharmacology and sexology, she has conducted research on vascular and smooth muscle function in the male and female sexual response, on pharmacological treatment of erectile dysfunction and female sexual desire and arousal disorder, and within the field of somatic disease and sexuality. She currently works at the Sexological Clinic in Copenhagen. She is president-elect of the International Society for the Study of Women's Sexual Health, serves on the board of the European Society for Sexual Medicine, and is an associate editor of the *Journal of Sexual Medicine*.

GILBERT HERDT, PhD, is director and professor of human sexuality studies at San Francisco State University, and is director of the National Sexuality Resource Center. Herdt is an internationally recognized anthropologist and Fulbright, NIMH, and Guggenheim Fellow. He currently is conducting a study of sexual health policy in the United States.

JEAN D. KOEHLER, PhD, is a licensed marriage and family therapist and certified sex therapist in private practice. Additionally, she is an assistant clinical professor of psychiatry and behavioral sciences in the University of Louisville medical school, where she teaches clinical sexology to psychiatry, ob-gyn, and family medicine residents. She is a past president of the American Association of Sexuality Educators, Counselors, and Therapists and a founding board member of the North American Federation of Sexuality Organizations. Dr. Koehler has presented locally and nationally on the topic of sexual dysfunction for several decades. She serves on the Archdiocese of Louisville

Sexual Abuse Review Board, the International Scientific Committee of the 17th and 18th World Congress Procter of Sexology, the Procter and Gamble Regional Consultant's Board, the board of the Women's Sexual Health Foundation, the female sexual dysfunction advisory board for Ortho-McNeil Pharmaceuticals, and is a contributing expert for the Alexander Foundation for Women's Health. She was involved in the stage-three clinical trials for the Procter and Gamble testosterone patch for women.

JUDY KURIANSKY, PhD, is a clinical psychologist at Columbia University Teachers College and Columbia Medical Center; a visiting professor at Peking University Health Sciences Center; and an honorary professor in the University of Hong Kong's department of psychiatry. A diplomate of the American Board of Sexology, a follow of the American Academy of Clinical Sexology (AACS), and a winner of the AACS Medal of Sexology for Lifetime Achievement, she is a pioneer of sex diagnosis and sex therapy evaluation. Her credits include membership on the Diagnostic and Statistical Manual of Mental Disorders III (DSM-III) committee, evaluative work on early Masters and Johnson therapy, and an extensive experience with sex-related radio and TV call-in advice shows. A cofounder of the Society for Sex Therapy and Research (SSTR) and a past board member of the American Association of Sexuality Educators, Counselors, and Therapists (AASECT), Kuriansky has authored hundreds of articles in professional journals and mass market publications. She has developed and led numerous workshops about sexuality around the world, including workshops on integrating Eastern and Western safe sex and relationship enhancement techniques. Her many publishing credits include *The Complete Idiot's Guide to Tantric Sex and Generation Sex: America's Hottest Sex Therapist Answers the Hottest Questions About Sex*, as well as several books about sex and relationship in Japan and China.

JUNE MACHOVER REINISCH, PhD, was director of The Kinsey Institute for Research in Sex, Gender & Reproduction from 1982 to 1993. Since then she has served as director emerita and a senior research fellow and was a member of the Institute's board of trustees for two years. She has held professorships at Rutgers, the State University of New Jersey, and Indiana University, both in the colleges and medical school. She is the founder, director, and principal investigator of The Prenatal Development Projects, which does research in Denmark and the United States, and she is a senior researcher at the Institute of Preventive Medicine, Danish Epidemiological Science Center, Copenhagen. Dr. Reinisch serves as director of acquisitions and new exhibitions, Museum of Sex, New York City and as the vice president of scientific affairs. She is also the executive director, of the Health and Science Advisory

Board of the online adult sexuality education Web site, http://loveandhealth. info.net. She is president of R² Science Communications, Inc., a company that consults with business, media, and the legal profession. Dr. Reinisch lectures extensively to academic, scientific, and general public audiences in the United States, Europe, and Asia.

WILLIAM R. STAYTON, MDiv, ThD, PhD, is director of the graduate human sexuality program in the Center for Education, School of Human Service Professions at Widener University, Pennsylvania. He is a founding board member of the Center for Sexuality and Religion, and he serves on the National Advisory Council, an organization working to implement the former Surgeon General's *Call to Action to Promote Sexual Health and Responsible Sexual Behavior*. Dr. Stayton is board chair of Planned Parenthood of southeastern Pennsylvania and a former president of the board of directors of both AASECT and SIECUS. He is the author of numerous articles and book chapters on sexuality, theology, sexual orientation, and gender identity. He is a frequent guest on radio and television programs.

BEVERLY WHIPPLE, PhD, RN, FAAN, a certified sex educator, sex counselor, and sex researcher. She is the coauthor of the international best seller *The G Spot and Other Discoveries about Human Sexuality,* which has been translated into 19 languages and was republished as a classic 23 years later in 2005. Her other books are *Safe Encounters: How Women Can Say Yes to Pleasure and No to Unsafe Sex, Smart Women, Strong Bones, Outwitting Osteoporosis* and *The Science of Orgasm.* Dr. Whipple has delivered over 500 talks and keynote speeches and has published over 160 research articles and book chapters. She is the recipient of many awards and was the president of AASECT (1998–2000), was the vice president of the World Association for Sexology (2001–2005), was on the board of the International Society for the Study of Women's Sexual Health (2002–2004), was the president of SSSS (2002–2003), and is currently the secretary general of the World Association for Sexual Health (2005–2009). She is also a fellow of the Society for the Scientific Study of Sexuality and a fellow in the American Academy of Nursing. She is a professor emerita at Rutgers, The State University of New Jersey.